Computational Methods in Psychiatry

Gopi Battineni • Mamta Mittal
Nalini Chintalapudi
Editors

Computational Methods in Psychiatry

Springer

Editors
Gopi Battineni
Clinical Research Centre, School of Medicinal and Health Products Sciences
University of Camerino
Camerino, Macerata, Italy

Mamta Mittal
Data Analytics and Data Science
Delhi Skill and Entrepreneurship University (under Government of NCT Delhi)
New Delhi, Delhi, India

Nalini Chintalapudi
Clinical Research Centre, School of Medicinal and Health Products Sciences
University of Camerino
Camerino, Macerata, Italy

ISBN 978-981-99-6636-3 ISBN 978-981-99-6637-0 (eBook)
https://doi.org/10.1007/978-981-99-6637-0

This Springer imprint is published by the registered company Springer Nature Singapore Pte Ltd.
The registered company address is: 152 Beach Road, #21-01/04 Gateway East, Singapore 189721, Singapore

Paper in this product is recyclable.

Contents

About the Editors

Gopi Battineni is a research associate at the Clinical Research Centre, School of Medicinal and Health Products Sciences, University of Camerino, Italy since 2022. A master's degree (with honours) in Computer Science and Engineering from Sheffield Hallam University, UK in 2016; a master's degree (with honours) in Enterprise Engineering from the University of Bordeaux, France in 2018; and a PhD in One health at the University of Camerino in 2021. His research area includes telemedicine, predictive analystics, process mining, natural language processing, data mining, big data, and machine learning. Dr. Battineni is a member of the European Research Committee and has published more than 90 research papers in SCI, SCIE, and Scopus-indexed journals and attending conferences, seminars, and guest talks on an international platform. He is a reviewer of many reputed international journals from different popular publishing houses such as Elsevier, MDPI, Wiley, Dove, plus one, and BMJ. He managed and chaired different international conferences. He is an Associate Editor with reputed SCIE-indexed journals: Journal of Personalized Medicine and Algorithms (MDPI, Switzerland).

Mamta Mittal is working as Head and Associate Professor (Data Analytics and Data Science) at Delhi Skill and Entrepreneurship University (under the Government of NCT Delhi), New Delhi. She received PhD in Computer Science and Engineering from Thapar University, Patiala. She has been teaching for the last 18+ years with an emphasis on Data Mining, Machine Learning, DBMS, and Data Structure. Dr. Mittal is a Lifetime member of CSI and published and communicated more than 90 research papers in SCI, SCIE, and Scopus-indexed Journals. She holds five patents and two copyrights in Artificial Intelligence, IoT, and Deep Learning. Dr. Mittal has edited/authored many books with reputed publishers like Springer, IOS Press, Elsevier, and CRC Press and working on DST approved Project "Development of IoT-based hybrid navigation module for mid-sized autonomous vehicles" with a research grant of 25 Lakhs. Currently, she is guiding PhD scholars in Machine Learning, Computer Vision, and Deep Learning. She is the book Series editor of *Health Informatics & Healthcare: using AI & Smart Computing & another Series Edge AI in Future Computing with CRC Press*, Taylor & Francis, USA.Dr. Mittal is an Editorial Board member with InterScience, Bentham Science, Springer, and Elsevier and has Chaired several Conferences. She is Associate Editor with reputed SCIE-indexed journals: Earth Information Science (Springer) and Dyna (Spain).

Nalini Chintalapudi is a postdoctoral researcher at the Clinical Research Centre, School of Medicinal and Health Products Sciences, University of Camerino in Italy. She earned a degree (with first-class distinction) in Computer Science from Jawaharlal Nehru Technological University, India; A master's degree (with honours) in Computer Science and Engineering from the same university in 2015. She completed PhD in Computer Science and Mathematics at the University of Camerino in 2023. Her research area includes text mining, natural language processing, data mining, big data, and machine learning. Dr. Nalini Chintalapudi is a member of the European Research Committee and has published more than 45 research papers in SCI, SCIE, and Scopus-indexed journals.

Mental Health in Italy During the Pandemic: A Shift from Self-determination to Solidarity?

Roberto Garetto and Maurizio Di Masi

Abstract The State of Exception caused by the pandemic constitutes an indispensable starting point of a redefinition of the relationship between public and private spheres in the perspective of protection of right to mental health. The authors trace the evolution of the right to health, in the international, European and domestic context and deepen the theme of the protection of the right to health of persons with mental illness. The Italian constitutional framework represents a peculiarity since it is characterised by a strong solidarity-based character and a specific attention on the right to health. Its constitutional formulation outlines a twofold role: fundamental right of the human person and interest of the community. The Italian legal system has given primary importance to mental illness, starting with the so-called Basaglia Law. The pandemic emergency has prompted the Italian government to adopt a series of welfare measures that do not always fully protect mental health. For this reason, the authors call for a reorganisation of the national health care system that can enhance the solidaristic principle.

Keywords Mental health · Right to health · Self-determination · COVID-19 · Solidarity

R. Garetto (✉)
Istituto Giuridico Internazionale Torino, Torino, TO, Italy
e-mail: roberto.garetto@igito.it

M. Di Masi
Dipartimento di Giurisprudenza, Università degli Studi di Perugia, Perugia, PG, Italy
e-mail: maurizio.dimasi@unipg.it

G. Battineni et al. (eds.), *Computational Methods in Psychiatry*,
https://doi.org/10.1007/978-981-99-6637-0_1

1 Coronavirus and State of Necessity

The lockdown imposed by the pandemic emergency has had significant repercussions on mental health and on the legal relationships that concern them [1]. It therefore appears central to analyse the impact that the emergency legislation imposed by the spread of the COVID-19 syndrome has had on mental health.

It has been acutely observed that the coronavirus has led to a measurement of the quality of the possible or impossible relationship. If the physicality of the encounter contains within itself the 'germ' of a potential infection—if, therefore, the contact now holds in the form of a substantial contamination—, the reason for the detachment must prevail. Indeed, in this period, social and family relations also had to compare the reasons for social distancing, a new form of solidarity capable of stemming the spread of the pandemic and thus protecting individual and collective health [2]. Nevertheless, the social distancing itself has over time led to heavy repercussions in terms of mental health. Such mental health repercussions have ended up calling into question the public/private dichotomy, both with respect to the role of the State and the exercise of personal freedoms.

The theme of the relationship between pandemic, democracy and State of Emergency has been the subject of an animated Italian cultural debate. In particular, the discussion was opened by an article by the philosopher Giorgio Agamben, where he started from the observation that the institutional reaction to the pandemic shows itself—once again—the growing tendency to use the State of Exception (SoE) as a normal paradigm of government [3], p. 11. The effect of the decree-law immediately approved by the Italian government 'for reasons of hygiene and public safety' in fact was a real militarisation of the municipalities and areas in which at least one person is positive. In such cases, the source of transmission was unknown or the case was not attributable to a person coming from an area already affected by the virus infection.

Although Agamben has probably underestimated the risks and the real extent of the disease, he starts from a correct perspective of analysis: that which sees the need for security of the population as an instrument of government [4].

From a technical-legal point of view, the SoE constitutes a limit situation of suspension of the constitutional order in force, or of a segment of it [5]. In this circumstance, the figure of a supreme decision-maker emerges, whose role is to arbitrarily declare the SoE, defining its content and the methods of exercising power itself. The entire legal system therefore ends up falling back on the will of the decision-maker, who unlimitedly centralises every power and prerogative within himself. This definition, typical of Western legal thought, has its roots in the reflections of two thinkers, Carl Schmitt and Santi Romano.

In particular, Carl Schmitt defines the SoE as the dictatorship itself [6], associating this institution to the concept of sovereignty: the sovereign is the one who decides on the SoE [7]. In this way, sovereign power compensates for the absence of law. According to Schmitt, within the SoE, there would be an eclipse of the rule in favour of the decision alone, while maintaining a correlation with the law [6]

Santi Romano, on the other hand, makes an attempt to reconcile law and a SoE, through the paradigm of the State of Necessity. In fact, it would not be an eclipse of the legal system, but a constitutional condition of *ordinary* emergency, internal to the system itself and necessary to overcome a crisis situation [8].

On the contrary, this position is rejected by Giorgio Agamben, who affirms that necessity does not fall within the category of sources of law [3], p. 23. There would therefore be no relationship between the production of law and the State of Necessity. The latter remains relegated to the space of the non-juridical, which sees citizens at the mercy of the sovereign's will. In reiterating its incompatibility with the law, Agamben also observes how the paradigms of the SoE have become more and more normalised, turning into ordinary instruments of governance. This would also happen on the occasion of the recent pandemic. In fact, we would be faced with a substantial suspension of constitutional guarantees, in which the production of law is entrusted primarily (if not exclusively) to decrees of the President of the Council of Ministers (rules that formally are not law) [9]. From Agamben's point of view, the pandemic emergency situation could therefore be easily brought back within the framework of the SoE, having the executive power assumed the role of supreme decision-maker. In this space of non-juridicality, the individual would be perceived as a potential infected, allowing an arbitrary compression of his freedoms and rights [2, 3].

Moreover, the coronavirus pandemic has brought to light the importance of investigating the public/private dichotomy, analysing how the relationship between the two has changed and what role the public sphere tends to assume. The neoliberal myth that the best regulation would be that left to private self-regulation now emerges in all its fragile ideology. What happened seems to have brought out a generalised 'need for the State'. This perception has been exacerbated by a growing sense of insecurity, due to the severe economic crisis engendered by the lockdown and the prolonged paralysis of several productive sectors. This has led to a rethinking of the role of the State, calling for its more incisive intervention in income support and supplementation policies.

To better understand this scenario, however, it is necessary to analyse the particular evolution of the fundamental right to health.

2 The Right to Health as a Fundamental Human Right

The right to health is an essential part of internationally recognised fundamental human rights. The right of every person to enjoy the best conditions of physical and mental health that he or she is capable of attaining was first mentioned in 1946 in the Constitution of the World Health Organization (WHO), whose Preamble defines the concept of health as 'a state of complete physical, mental and social well-being and not merely the absence of disease or infirmity'. The Preamble further states that 'the enjoyment of the highest attainable standard of health is one of the fundamental rights of every human being without distinction of race, religion, political belief, economic or social condition'. The Preamble thus defines the right to health and explicitly connotes it as a fundamental right [10].

The right to health will find explicit recognition, 2 years later, in the Universal Declaration of Human Rights (UDHR). Everyone has the right to living standards that are appropriate for his or her own health and the welfare of his or her family, including nutrition, accommodation, and medical treatment, according to Article 25 of the Universal Declaration of Human Rights (UDHR), which was approved by the General Assembly of the United Nations (UN) on 10 December 1948.

In addition to these two documents, the provisions of the International Covenant on Economic, Social and Cultural Rights (ICESCR) must also be taken into account. This document was written according to the directions of the United Nations and was opened for signature by General Assembly resolution 2200 A (XXI) of 16 December 1966. It became effective only on 3 January 1976.

The 1966 Covenant, instead adopting the WHO definition of right to health, provided its own definition mentioning that everyone has the right to the enjoyment of the highest attainable 'standard' of physical and mental health (Article 12(1)). Further, it specifies how this right must be guaranteed including reducing stillbirth rates and infant mortality for child health development; better environmental and industrial hygiene; epidemics, endemics, occupational diseases and other problems should be prevented, treated and controlled; and make sure you get all the medical care that individuals need (Article 12(2)).

Although the three mentioned documents identify health as a fundamental human right, they do not provide the jurist with precise parameters to connote the right in question. It is unclear what is concretely meant by 'standard' of health, and as a result, the specific content of international obligations still remains a debated issue. Albeit having to respect, protect and realise the right to health are the basis for understanding the obligations of State parties, the actions to be taken in practice are less clear. This gives rise to a second issue: the lack of clarity on obligations risks leaving State Parties with a dangerous margin of discretion. If there is no obligation to allocate a specific number of resources in the health system, the State, especially if it is a developing country, can claim an absence of resources and thus justify not allocating money in the health sphere. This problem is often highlighted, but still unsolved: people in poor countries tend to have less access to health services than those in better-off countries [11]. However, investing in health for a developing country represents a great opportunity for economic growth and State health budgets should be as sizable as possible, as that makes investing in wealth returns. It has also been shown that in reality, measures to improve the health *status* of individuals are not a costly operation for States, quite the opposite. In 1993, the World Bank stated that 'spending on health can also be justified on purely economic grounds. Improved health contributes to economic growth in four ways: it reduces production losses caused by worker illness; it permits the use of natural resources that had been totally or nearly inaccessible because of disease; it increases the enrollment of children in school and makes them better able to learn; and it frees for alternative uses resources that would otherwise have to be spent on treating illness' [12].

Despite the difficulties highlighted above in identifying an objective standard in health, it is remarkable to note that the Court of Justice of the European Union (CJEU) explicitly resorted to the above-mentioned WHO's definition issuing the judgement in the case *United Kingdom of Great Britain and Northern Ireland v Council of the European Union* (Case C-84/94, judgement of 12 November 1996), which concerned occupational health and safety matters [13].

While it is unquestionably assumed that the right to health is a fundamental right, it should nevertheless be kept in mind that the concrete needs for health protection, although they may be *latu* sensu common, are profoundly different depending on the geographical areas taken that, despite being broadly ubiquitous, the actual demands for health protection vary greatly depending on the regions that are being considered.

On the other hand, however, the right to health, like the majority of human rights commitments, everyone is entitled to the right to health, regardless of their *status* as a person in the eyes of the law. Stateless people, detainees, and unauthorised migrants are all covered. The realisation of the right to health shall be gradual and progressive, similar to other social and economic rights. Under Article 2(1) of the ICESCR Covenant, states that ratify the covenant must take all necessary steps to gradually realise every facet of this right, including enacting legislative measures.

The provision of a gradual realisation of this right (*verbatim* 'progressively') implicitly entails that the implementation of any cultural, social or economic right must be fully realised through time; it is not achievable in the short term. Each State Party is only required to realise the right to health in as gradual a manner as possible rather than instantly implementing it in its entirety. This right indeed cannot be realised at once, unlike other rights such as the right to life. In other words, the complete realisation of a right that falls under the area of economic, social and cultural rights, like the right to health, requires a longer term strategy across time.

This does not mean, however, that State Parties do not have obligations to individuals. States, in ratifying any human rights convention, must meet three requirements: respect, protect and realise the fundamental rights and freedoms enshrined in the agreement. The right to health is no exception, as specified by General Comment No. 14 of the Committee on Economic Social and Cultural Rights. Indeed, it makes it clear that: 'health is a fundamental human right indispensable for the exercise of other human rights. Every human being is entitled to the enjoyment of the highest attainable standard of health conducive to living a life in dignity'. Recognising health human rights implies that the State Party must not interfere, directly or indirectly, with the enjoyment of the right. For example, the State may not discriminate (implicitly or explicitly) against individuals or grant access to the right to health only to certain categories, as it would constitute interference with the right. Protecting health as a human right also requires affirmative action by the State: it must take steps to prevent third parties from undermining the exercise of this right. Operating on the human rights level requires a more dynamic approach, demanding the State Parties to take concrete action through the adoption of legislative, administrative and financial measures to realise progressively the right to health to the fullest. This means that the State must commit to allocating a certain number of resources for health and must create laws that lead to the highest enjoyment of the right to health.

More broadly, the right to health also presupposes an additional obligation: cooperation. States must cooperate as much with international organisations, such as WHO or the UN, as with non-governmental organisations and other States. As a progressive right, the right to health needs joint actions, for without them there could be no question of success in respecting, protecting and realising rights. If a State has the means to influence other countries about the enjoyment of the right to health, it should attempt to cooperate as much as possible.

2.1 Implementation of the Right to Health at International Level

It was outlined above how health should be regarded as a human right. As a result, it stands as an underpinning for all other fundamental rights. Due to the pivotality of the right to health, States and their bodies are held responsible for far more than just managing health systems. They ought to take it upon themselves to detect and identify the elements that have a detrimental effect on everyone's well-being through proper cooperation. Nevertheless, they should implement those that have a favourable effect. The fulfilment of ad hoc initiatives by the WHO is crucial for the progressive implementation of the right to health. Two approaches, in particular, have been adopted since the 1980s.

They are, respectively, known under the name of 'Health for All' strategy and 'Health Promotion', or Ottawa Charter. These measures are intended to achieve two strategic goals: illness prevention and health promotion.

In 1981, the WHO Assembly unanimously adopted the 'Global Strategy for Health for All by the Year 2000'. This document states that: 'as a minimum *all* people in *all* countries should have at least such a level of health that they are capable of working productively and of participating actively in the social life of the community in which they live'. To achieve these goals, it is stated that: 'every individual should have access to primary health care and through it to all levels of a comprehensive health system' [14].

A few years later, in 1986, the First International Conference on Health Promotion conference was held in Ottawa. The Conference outlined strategies for a global, coordinated effort focused on the person's physical and psychological welfare. As a prominent outcome of this Conference, the Ottawa Charter was subsequently signed by the WHO Member States. The human being is at the centre of the Ottawa Charter. The Charter is based on a comprehensive understanding of the human being as a whole, rather than as a combination of its own parts. In line with this, social organisation is seen as a cohesive totality.

In this light, in order for everyone to reach their full health potential, they must be placed in the most favourable situation. Any stakeholder (governments, private and public health organisations, as well as whatever non-governmental organisations) can actively participate in the implementation of this new approach to the right to health, ordered to equity. According to the Ottawa Charter, health promotion is the process of empowering people to exert more control over and enhance their well-being. As a result, health develops into an essential asset for daily living and an outcome that improves the world itself. Everyone needs to develop his or her capacity to take care of both himself or herself and the others. In this manner, the Ottawa Charter supports a social health accomplishment aimed at establishing the optimal conditions for a healthy human development at all stages of life and under all circumstances.

3 The Right to Health in the European Context

In the European context, it should be borne in mind that in 1998 the WHO Regional Office for Europe (WHO/Europe) adopted the 'Health for All in the 21st Century'. The document is also known as 'Health 21' not only because it deals with health in the twenty-first century, but also because it lays out 21 'targets' for improving the health of Europeans. Keeping the findings of the 'Health for All' strategy of two decades earlier, this document aims to achieve a successful translation of policy to action, taking the European framework as a reference. With the awareness that the range of strategies available to improve health is wide and the availability of resources is constrained, the WTO/Europe requires States to carry out a priority-setting [15].

In addition to WHO/Europe, reference must be made to the Council of Europe and the European Union (EU) when it comes to health in Europe. With respect to the former, as noted by Harris et al. [16], the right to health, similar to the other 'social rights', is not explicitly stated in the 'European Convention on Human Rights' (the ECHR), in force since 3 September 1953. This is precisely why it was necessary for the European Court of Human Rights (the ECtHR) to intervene.

By way of an evolving and thorough interpretation of other sections of the Convention, especially Article 3 (the prohibition of torture) and Article 8 (respect for private and family life), the ECtHR has gradually increased the protection of the right to health.

The limits of this indirect means of defence are, however, evident. Purely on its own, the right to health is not safeguarded. It is only when its violation takes the form of the infringement of another right expressly recognised by the Convention that a broad protection can include the right to health. The ECtHR jurisprudence clearly shows this pattern. See the following cases in particular: ECtHR, *Kudla v Poland*, application no. 30210/96, Judgement of 26 October 2000; ECtHR, *Poltoratskiy v Ukraine*, application number 38812/97, Judgement of 29 April 2003; ECtHR, *Bensaid v UK*, application no. 44599/98, Judgement of 6 February 2001; ECtHR, *Vo v France*, application no. 53924/00, Judgement of 8 July 2004; ECtHR, *Pretty v UK*, application no. 2346/02, Judgement of 29 April 2002; ECtHR, *Tysiac v Poland*, application no. 5410/03, Judgement of 20 March 2007; ECtHR, *Ashot*

Harutyunyan v Armenia, application number 34334/04, Judgement of 15 June 2010; ECtHR, *K. H. v Slovakia*, application no. 32881/04, Judgement of 28 April 2009; ECtHR, *Evans v UK*, application no. 6339/05, Judgement of 7 March 2006; ECtHR, *Dybeku v Albania*, application no. 41153/06, Judgement of 18 December 2007.

Instead, the 'European Social Charter' (ESCr), a Council of Europe instrument that was adopted in 1961 and later amended by additional protocols, establishes everyone's entitlement to the right to health [17]. The text of the treaty was also completely revised in 1996. The ESCr, Part I (11), provides that: 'everyone has the right to benefit from any measures enabling him to enjoy the highest possible standard of health attainable'. Additionally, the ESCr has a clause in Article 11 that specifically mentions the 'right to protection of health'. The 'appropriate measures' of the States Parties, who vowed to uphold the right to health, are outlined in the wording of the conclusive part of Article 11, that (without any claim to completeness) enumerates the following:

- To eliminate the root causes of ill-health as much as feasible
- To offer resources for guidance and education aimed at promoting health
- To encourage personal responsibility for the individual's health
- To eradicate endemic, epidemic, and other diseases as much as possible

In particular, the States Parties undertake the above-mentioned measures either directly or in conjunction with public or private organisations.

It should be borne in mind that this treaty is characterised by a so-called *a la carte* system, whereby single States can decide which specific articles to bind themselves to. This obviously diminishes its impact. With reference to Article 11, only one of the 43 States Parties decided not to bind. Namely, Armenia [17].

By adopting 'appropriate measures', the States Parties are obligated to guarantee 'the effective exercise' of the right to health under Article 11 of the ESCr. The 'Statement of Interpretation of Article 11 - Conclusions 2005' (Council of Europe, 2018) by the European Committee of Social Rights made it clear that in order to fulfil the duty to ensure the right to health protection, positive measures (i.e. legislative, administrative, technical measures) must be taken that are appropriate for achieving the goals specified by the provision.

Along these lines, the Social Rights Committee stated that States Parties ought to consider taking measures to eliminate the causes of poor health as a positive obligation. Therefore, they must ensure that everyone who needs healthcare can get it and afford it. Such access cannot be limited by a lack of financial means. As a result, States Parties that have ratified the ESCr are required to ensure that all people with no income have free access to healthcare.

Concerning the actual implementation of the right to health by the Council of Europe, one more significant document must also be mentioned: the 'Convention for the Protection of Human Rights and Dignity of the Human Being with regard to the Application of Biology and Medicine', opened for signature on 4 April 1997 in Oviedo (the Oviedo Convention).

Ratification of the Convention is not limited to States Parties to the Council of Europe, but is extended to all States that participated in the preparatory work. The provisions of the Oviedo Convention effectively respond to the challenges of a constantly changing medical field and the risk of indiscriminate use of bio-medical technologies. The Oviedo Convention reaffirms the centrality of the right to health: at Article 2 it states that '[t]he interests and welfare of the human being shall prevail over the sole interest of society or science'.

At the European level, the protection of the right to health guaranteed by EU regulations must also be kept in mind. The highest level of protection is provided by the Treaty on the Functioning of the European Union (the TFEU), which implements cross-cutting actions. Also worthy of particular attention regarding the right to health in the EU context is the 'Charter of Fundamental Rights of the European Union' (CFR), ratified 7 December 2000 and entered into force on 1 December 2009. Moreover, more recently, precisely in 2017, the EU Commission adopted the 'European Pillar of Social Rights' (EPSR).

In the TFEU, Article 6 assigns to the EU competence to carry out actions aimed at supporting, coordinating or supplementing the Member States' measures. The preservation and enhancement of human health is one of the areas covered by such initiatives. Article 9 states that the EU is required to define and implement its policies and activities, taking its actions and protocols, taking into consideration standards related to the development of a high level of human health protection.

Furthermore, Title XIV of the TFEU in its heading explicitly refers to public health and, in its provisions, assures that all EU actions and protocols will provide a high level of health protection for people. According to Article 168(1), EU action must complement national protocols and be focused on enhancing public health, mitigating both mental and physical diseases, and eliminating sources of risk to one's physical and mental well-being. It follows from this provision that, instead of establishing health policies, the EU operates as a coordination body.

Furthermore, according to Article 168(2), the EU will foster collaboration among Member States in the area of health protection and, when deemed necessary, shall lend support to their action. The CFR, at Article 35, establishes within the EU the right of everyone to have 'access to preventive health care and the right to benefit from medical treatment under the conditions established by national laws and practices', and provides that a 'high level of human health protection' will be ensured through implementation of health policies and activities.

The EPSR, dating back to 2017, upholds the right to health in relation to the workplace. The EPSR outlines 20 principles on the related factors affecting health, such as social protection and equitable workplace conditions. With this regard, Chap. 2 (10) states that workers have the right to a high level of protection of their health.

4 Protection of the Right to Health of Persons with Mental Illness in the International Law

Within the general context of the right to health, special attention should be paid to mental health. The debate leading to a pronouncement on the international level has been extensive and time-consuming [18]. In 1991, the UN General Assembly adopted the 'Principles for the protection of persons with mental illness' (MI principles) [19]. This is a detailed international statement that provides agreed (but non-legally-binding) basic standards of care for mental illness. The MI principles ensure the best medical and psychiatric care available, including respect for people's dignity, non-discrimination, protection from exploitation, abuse, and any other kind of degrading treatment are fundamental freedoms and rights [20].

The MI principles recognise the difficulties associated with protecting human rights in mental health facilities and emphasise that assistance should, whenever possible, be carried out within the community. This bias is motivated by the duty to treat patients in the least restrictive environment possible. The aim is to allow the patients' personal autonomy to be preserved as much as possible. The MI principles define a set of legal standards and procedural safeguards for involuntary patients. In this way, the MI principles clearly establish under what circumstances a person may be subjected to involuntary admission [21]. To ensure that involuntary admission or retention meet the requirements set out in the MI principles, a patient must be put in a position to conduct a procedure as provided by domestic law before an impartial and independent court or review body. This corresponds to a fundamental option: the MI principles offer strong protection in the case of involuntary admission or retention, as they are aimed at achieving a balance between autonomy and coercion [22].

In any case, the MI principles guarantee persons with a mental illness a range of civil and political rights, including rights of confidentiality, full respect, privacy, information access of individual health, freedom of communication and of religion or belief. Besides, these principles ensure specific social, economic and cultural rights like the right to social services appropriate to health needs, an individualised treatment plan, recreational and educational services. In this respect, it can be easily inferred that psychiatric facilities must be allocated resources comparable to those provided for other health facilities [23]. As pointed out by some scholars [24], civil and political rights are provided for the benefit of all persons with mental illness. Every person with a mental illness shall have the right to exercise all civil, political, economic, social and cultural rights.

In addition to the MI principles, the United Nations has promulgated numerous other sources of soft law whose application is intended to improve the condition of the mentally ill. Among these sources, it is worth mentioning declaration on the rights of mental retarded, and the standard rules on the rights and equal opportunities for disabled persons [25–27]. The 'Declaration on the Rights of Disabled Persons', in particular, broadly defines a person with a disability as 'any person unable to ensure by himself or herself, wholly or partly, the necessities of a normal individual and/or social life, as a result of deficiency, either congenital or not, in his or her physical or mental capabilities'. It contains, as well, an extensive list of civil, political, economic, social and cultural rights, including 'the right to medical, psychological and functional treatment' and 'the right to economic and social security and to a decent level of living'.

Lastly, the World Conference on Human Rights, which was held in Vienna in 1993, adopted the 'Declaration and Program of Action' [28]. This Declaration recognised that disabled persons are entitled, 'without distinction of any kind', to all human rights and fundamental freedoms, in line with the UDHR 'common standard' for everyone [29]. Furthermore, this Declaration provides an action program aimed at raising awareness of human rights in the context of disability.

5 The Right to Health in the Italian Constitution

The right to health is established in the Italian Constitution at Article 32(1) mentioning that the State safeguards health as a fundamental right of the individual and as a collective interest, and guarantees free medical care to the indigent. Article 32(2) states that nobody can be forced to receive medical care unless it is mandated by law and that, in any event, the law cannot go beyond the bounds set by the dignity of the human person.

Article 32 intends to configure a balance between the individual and the collectively; the former's rights correspond to the latter's interest. Precisely, it emphasised the centrality of the individual's right to health, while putting it in necessary relation to the interest of the collectivity. From this it follows that within the Italian legal system, there cannot be a right to health that concerns only the individual by his or her own. This right on the contrary requires establishing a relationship between the individual and the collectivity.

Whilst the Italian Constitution directly regulates health at the constitutional level in Article 32, the text's underlying concept of health appears to imply that it ought to be regarded as an integral part of the human person. We are therefore faced, in the words of Pietro Perlingieri [30], with a unitarian value. The Italian Constitution's Articles 2 and 3 must be considered in combination with Article 32. Therefore, in the framework of the principle of solidarity, it is necessary to recognise the right to health as a fundamental human right for everyone, and any discrimination will not be admitted [30]. Four subjective legal dispositions are thus established in such a brief text: an individual right to freedom, a communal interest, and two distinct social rights, as correctly noted by Papa [31]. The right to obtain essential treatments is included in the first type of provisions referred to as the individual right to freedom, as does the right not to necessarily receive treatments if one chooses not to be treated.

In correspondence with this right, can be inferred the requirement to refrain from any positive conduct, which burdens, as pointed out by D'Aloia [32], everybody so as to permit the self-determination of the individual. The second type of regulations relating to the collective interest guarantees that the right to make personal health decisions independently will not compromise the common interest in health.

As remarked by Papa [31] in order to care for the human person, the State must consequently develop a reasonable balance of interests when deciding whether or not require compulsory medical treatments [31]. When prescribed to avert the transmission of an infectious disease, such as when it is in the prodromal phase of wide diffusion, the requirement to undergo this kind of mandatory treatments must be regarded as legal. Instead, the argument over preventative therapies, including vaccinations, is still controversial, despite their function is not limited to preventing citizens from getting sick while simultaneously avoiding them from harming the entire community [33]. The issue arises with particular complexity with regard to mental illness, since in this case the patient may express consent or dissent with respect to the vaccine that may be compromised by his or her contingent mental health condition. Not only does this affect the patient's future prospects for good health, but in general terms it has a reverberation on the community's interest in health.

This tangled issue imposes the implementation of the principle of precaution. Article 191 TFEU states this principle. It directs the selection of the proper safety measures to provide security in the healthcare sector. However, it is not enough to respond to a potential health danger. It is instead recommended to act in advance to prevent future risks [30], p.101. The application of the precautionary principle raises complex hermeneutical issues, as one cannot disregard a balancing of principles of constitutional significance. Furthermore, this balancing operation among constitutional principles needs to be accomplished with consideration of the principle of proportionality, that is crucial in an uncertain situation like the health one. It is important to consider the above-mentioned issues in regard to the CoVID-19 epidemic, which the WHO classified to be a pandemic on 11 March 2020 [34]. The pandemic had a peerless impact on collective health, as it has not happened. It had an adverse global impact on individuals' psychological health [35] and also involved working environments [36].

Beginning in 2021, the vaccine campaign received widespread and unexpected backing from citizens. However, it simultaneously led to broad responses from many individuals who refused to receive the vaccine. Such unfavourable responses call for a compromise between two constitutional principles in the framework of the Italian Constitution: individual freedom and self-determination and a common interest in health [33]. Anyways, this requires special attention when persons with mental distress are involved [1], p.16.

To conclude the analysis of Article 32 of the Italian Constitution, it should be noted that two social rights are established such as the right to receive health care treatments, and medical care with no costs. This is deemed applicable to both Italian and foreign citizens [37]. Finally, it should be kept in mind that the notion of the right to health that can be deduced from Article 32 of the Italian Constitution cannot be limited to the physical aspect and medical implications. In other words, this notion must not be restricted to treating illnesses, but it comes to involve the well-being of the human person in a broad perspective, as a single, indissoluble psycho-physical entity [30], p.131.

6 From Medical Paternalism to *Homo Dignus*: The Central Role of the Basaglia Law in the Italian Legal System

Together with personal freedom, and self-determination, the right to health will play a pivotal role. While recognising health as a fundamental right of the individual and as an interest of the community provides that no one can be obliged to a specific health treatment except by law. Furthermore, neither can the law violate the limits imposed from respect for the human person. This way the primacy of the individual over his own body is restored, avoiding functionalization of health, which risks appearing paternalistic. The right to health, on the other hand, shows its subversive potential from the outset, entailing on the one hand the guarantee of the habeas corpus by the State and local authorities, as clearly emerges from the Law No. 833/1978 establishing the National Health Services (NHS) [38]. This clarifies not only that the Republic protects health as a fundamental right of the individual and collective interest through the NHS, but also the protection of physical and mental health according to dignity and freedom. Accordingly, the Basaglia law imposed the closure of all mental hospitals in Italy and regulated compulsory health treatment, establishing public mental health services [39], p.26.

Provisions on voluntary and compulsory medical examinations and treatments have not only determined a new consideration of the mentally ill, but also affirmed the cardinal rule regarding compulsory health treatments. This is based on to which they must be disposed of in compliance with the dignity of the person and the civil and political rights guaranteed by the constitution, including as far as possible the right to free choice of doctor and place of treatment. The Italian NHS is implemented and broadened in scope in the sense that even compulsory health treatment must always be accompanied by initiatives aimed at ensuring consent and participation. Persons who are obliged to do so and in the course of compulsory medical treatment, the patient has the right to communicate with anyone he deems appropriate. These norms have forced us to reconsider the relationship between the mentally ill and society, since it has introduced the mentally ill person into civil society as had never happened for centuries, forcing the person to social relations with all other subjects of the community [38, 40].

The attention that developed in Italy in the 1970s for mental illness and the protection of the dignity of persons who are unable to understand and express their will will lead to a reconfiguration of the same relationship between physician and patient. Shifting the gaze of the law on mental illness has allowed Italy to personalise the dialogue between the physician and the patient with mental illness (and not only), calibrating it according to the level of understanding of the person and above all adapting the semantics of communication to the patient's level of understanding [41]. This however explains because also law scholars were the first to tackle the relevance of the right to health above all from an individualistic point of view, focusing on the specialty of the relationship of care between physician and patient, to guarantee health self-determination of the latter. Lastly, freeing it from traditional medical paternalism. In this sense, the bio-juridical debate has moved, from issues concerning procreative self-determination (medically assisted procreation and gestation for others) to the end of life (advance directives for treatment and assistance in suicide).

It follows that the debate in recent years has mostly marginalised the aspect of health protection as an interest of the community, improving instead the role of the patient in the therapeutic relationship [42]. Starting from the nineteenth-century codifications, which subjected patients to the physician's authority, until the emergence of the personalist principle and the resulting revolution of 'informed consent', which shifted the focus on patients and was finally recognised [43]. Indeed, in the eighteenth century, people's lives became an object of study and government for medical science, which ended up 'medicalizing' life itself, that is to say, translating into medical terms those issues that could have been dealt with by social measures [44]. That means exploiting dependence on the doctor's help for domain purposes, and ultimately, using knowledge in terms of power over the patient [45]. In fact, the therapeutic relationship entails functional subjection to treatment, which has historically implied the non-recognition of patients' authority over their bodies; indeed, the etymology of the term 'patient' refers to those who passively accept other people's actions [42]. Throughout almost the whole twentieth century, the healthcare professional was considered to have technical and scientific knowledge, which placed him or her in a dominant position, compared to the patient, who needs care and assistance. Thus, the physician–patient relationship is seen by the jurist as very similar to a family law relationship, characterised by the physician's authority as opposed to the patient's subjection [45].

The growing attention to people's bodies and human life, in the modern State, also led to the progressive widening, beyond the State of Exception, of the decision on 'bare life', to the point of reaching an area of indistinction between fact and law, where sovereignty enters in a more intimate symbiosis not only with the jurist but also with the physician, the scientist, the expert, the priest [5, pg. 135]. Therefore, who rules the ill citizen's body? [46] Following the atrocities that emerged during the Nuremberg Trial [47], as well as the principles outlined in post-conflict Constitutions, it can be argued that, in the Italian legal system, each citizen rules his own body [48]. Apparently, sovereignty over the citizen's body passes from the State, and thus from a public law discipline to the citizen, hence to a private law discipline. However, this is the legacy of what Michel Foucault called the 'microphysics of power', referring to the power that branches into all social relationships, becoming widespread [49]. And not without reason, concerning the different power devices, which tend to curb and define human subjectivity, the philosopher stressed that the 'right' to life, to the body, to health, to happiness, to satisfy basic needs, the 'right' to regain, beyond all the oppressions or 'alienation', what we are and what we might be, this 'right' that is so incomprehensible to the traditional legal system, is the political reply to all these new political procedures [50]. Although in a changing rules and principles scenario, the patient's self-determination in his relationship with the physician, will be a further hypothesis of 'juridification' of the human person [46, 51].

The growing importance of the personalistic principle, following the 1947 Constitution's enactment, led to a noteworthy modification of the physician–patient relationship [52]. This change will then strengthen what we may call the 'bioethical' paradigm [53], which tends to distance medical knowledge from exclusive science and insiders' competence, to recognise a specific competence of the patient [54]. The peculiarity of this new paradigm is that morality is intended as a social, not a natural institution, consisting of a set of rules and shared values in a given society, aimed at promoting coexistence, as well as a dignified level of well-being and self-fulfilment; namely 'quality of life' [55, 56].

This moral approach involves not only the decay of the sanctity of life and the irrelevance of finalism but also the distinction between biological and biographical life, as well as the loss of the almost sacredness of medical acts. Nevertheless, the most interesting scenarios of the change in the power relation between physician and patient seem related to the recent developments of informed consent. The Italian Constitutional Court gave it a prominent role, being the synthesis of two fundamental rights of the patient: the right to health and to personal self-determination [57].

As Stefano Rodotà has masterfully pointed out, we may believe that self-determination is the foundation of free governance of the self, and sovereignty over our bodies [55, pg. 267]. Naturally, self-determination has its limits since it can restrict the freedom of others and can be contradictory. The subject of imposing limitations is a particularly delicate point because it immediately produces hostility towards 'paternalistic' Legislators, who have no right to invade the sphere of personal freedom [56], p. 250. Furthermore, only since the 1990s, the privileged system of medical malpractice has been facing a deep crisis, caused by both criminal [58] and civil case-law, after the affirmation of the patient's right to individual self-determination, within the therapeutic relationship [59]. Thus, in the context of the 'constitutionalization' of the person [51, 56], informed consent ends up entailing a substantial legal paradigm shift, by reshaping the private law relationship between the healthcare professional and the person assisted, restoring the patient's control power over himself/herself and his/her health. In this way, the physician–patient relationship switches from a paternalistic perspective [60] to a potentially equal approach, based on cooperation. While the first one sees the physician as the only one competent to determine whether the damage exists and how much it amounts to, the second view is summarised by the expression 'therapeutic alliance' between patients and physicians.

Furthermore, the developments in case-law regarding informed consent are deeply affected by the ambiguous nature of such consent, which assumes different functions, of using different narrative stratifications, depending on the case. It may be considered as a condition and foundation of the legitimacy of the medical act, and thus an essential requirement of the relationship concerned; it can be taken as a criterion for transferring the risk of treatment from physician to patient, through consent [61]; finally, it may be seen as the expression and exercise of people's fundamental rights, such as health and self-determination [62–64]. Therefore, in recent studies, the information obligation represents an integral part of the therapeutic performance, as well as a sort of independent (and not accessory) healthcare, just like the diagnostic intervention [65]. The emergence of the patient's self-determination in the care relationship has increased the number of subjective legal situations that physicians can harm in their work. The right to self-determination represents a form of respect for the freedom of the individual and, at the same time, a means to pursue his or her best interests. It consists not only of the right to choose between different possibilities of medical treatment but also to possibly refuse therapy and to consciously decide to interrupt it, considering the personalistic principle, which animates the Italian Constitution. This sees a human being as an ethical value in itself, which must be respected at any time of his life and in his entirety, in the light of the set of ethical, religious, cultural and philosophical convictions that guide his volitional determinations [46, 66]. Furthermore, the violation of the right to self-determination has become fully independent from the infringement of the right to health. This means that the lack of informed consent to medical treatment can take on significance for compensation purposes, although there is no damage to health, or if such damage is not causally connected to the violation of that right, in all cases involving negative consequences (which must be quite serious, in case of non-material damage) resulting from the violation of the fundamental right to self-determination, considered by itself [67]. Thus, in this perspective, the right to informed consent represents one aspect of the inviolable right to personal freedom, since the *homo juridicus* has acquired the *homo dignus* legal identity, according to an axiological interpretation not only of constitutional rights but also of those mentioned in European sources.

By accepting the authoritative doctrine, the judges of the Italian Court of Cassation recalled the legislative sources underlying the right to informed consent, a genuine right of the person. Thereby, following Stefano Rodotà's reconstructive proposal, the Court of Cassation identified human dignity as an inevitable common denominator, a legacy of the constitutionalism of the second post-war period, drafting both a new *status* of the person and a new framework of constitutional duties [56, pg. 179]. First of all, *homo dignus* is a self-determined man, who is enabled to define his life project. Hence, in a legal system based on the anthropological model of *homo dignus*, no external will can replace that of the person concerned, especially in the physician–patient relationship. Then, under living law as laid down by the constitutional statements and by the Italian Court of Cassation, as well as by the osmosis between interpretation, on the one hand, and internal and international rules, on the other, concerning healthcare interventions on patients, the State and its institutions, including the judge, have a duty to ensure a *focus* on the dimension of the human person in its concrete existentiality, due to its dignity, that governs fundamental rights, and without which these rights may be subject to limits capable of downgrading their impact. It also represents an axiological value, which underpins the legal system as a whole and thus, *a fortiori*, each ordinary rule. Therefore, if *homo juridicus* is now *homo dignus*, as held by Italian Court of Cassation in judgement No. 7237/2011, by accepting the authoritative doctrine and by starting from various provisions on human rights, case-law is further improved in these hypotheses. In any case, the jurisprudence crystallised the principle according to which the omitted or insufficient information with a healthy intervention represents a violation of the right to personal self-determination which, however, becomes compensable only if the patient attaches that, due to this, he or she has suffered a truly harmful consequence in terms of subjective suffering and contraction of the freedom to self-determination.

After many years of bioethical, deontological and bio-juridical reflection, on 14 December 2017, the Senate of the Italian Republic finally approved the legal text 'Rules on informed consent and advance treatment provisions', carefully legislating on ethically sensitive issues, such as the care relationship and the end of life [68]. Although medically assisted death and assisted suicide are still not recognised, the law approved by the Senate appears to be consistent with regulations aimed at protecting *homo dingus*. Indeed, it is keen to ensure the patient's self-determination and dignity, which have primacy over 'other' choices of the healthcare professional or the interested party's family, under Articles 2, 13 and 32 of the Italian Constitution, and Articles 1 ('Human dignity'), 2 ('Right to life') and 3 ('Right to the integrity of the person') of the CFR of the EU. Overall, by incorporating the main supranational directions and the best national court decisions, the law introduces significant innovations in the Italian legal system.

7 Solidarity as a Principle for Reinterpreting Health and Other Fundamental Rights

Regarding the theory of the State of Exception, essentially centred on the restriction of individual freedom, there is a need for a more aware reconstruction of the concreteness of the pandemic situation [69]. In particular, these measures, by the very nature of the epidemic phenomenon, must operate a prudent balance, which takes into account the protection of individual freedoms and ensures the effectiveness of the rights of the community within which these freedoms are exercised [70]. A reasonable and proportional compression of some individual rights could therefore be justified, in the specific case, by the solidarity need for the protection of public health. This is true, in particular, for the subjects most vulnerable to the risk of possible contagion. Beyond any theoretical reconstruction, there is a need for a concrete solidarity perspective, [71] which adequately considers the general constellation of interests that gravitate around the pandemic.

Health, in a collective sense, has instead been brought to the centre of attention with respect to the case of compulsory vaccinations. A question regarding the issues of constitutional legitimacy raised by the Veneto Region, ten compulsory vaccinations were provided for minors up to 16 years of age, including unaccompanied foreign minors, with simultaneous provision, for cases of non-compliance, administrative pecuniary sanctions, and the prohibition of access to services educational for children. In this regard, the Italian Constitutional Court found the question unfounded, since the laws that provide for vaccination obligations if they coordinate the protection of collective health with the individual right to health, as well as, in the specific case of compulsory vaccinations, with the interest of the child, which also requires protection against parents who do not fulfil their care duties. The coordination of these multiple fundamental rights and principles, therefore, leaves room for the discretion of the Legislator in choosing how effective prevention of infectious diseases is ensured.

The issue of vaccines has also been questioned by Italian scholars with special reference to persons with mental frailty and the mentally ill. Here too, therefore, the criterion to be affirmed is that the person concerned, even when mentally different from others, will need only himself or herself, even in the case of coronavirus, to express valid consent to vaccination [1, 33]. It is clear, on the other hand, that the pandemic has put on the balancing plate not only the right to health, in its individual and collective dimension but a whole series of constitutional freedoms, whose compression seems to be justified in conformity with the principle of social solidarity under Article 2 of the Italian Constitution.

Among the 'new generation' fundamental rights that risk being compressed due to the lockdown, for example, there is the protection of personal data. In this regard, it is interesting to underline the issue of the processing of personal data: in the case of data tracing, a treatment that seems necessary to monitor and contain the spread of the pandemic can be highly problematic, due to the need for a balance with the rights and freedoms of all and of each. On the other hand, health data, unlike other sensitive data, see the fundamental right of the person concerned not to disclose his medical and health situation to be more clearly contrasted with the interest of the community or of third information parties [1, 70].

The need to balance these opposing legal situations at stake, however, confirms that no information is valid for itself, but for the context in which it is inserted, for the purposes for which it is used, and for the other information to which it is connected [70]. Even the coronavirus, then, places us in front of the need to balance interests that lean in favour of collective health already by the provision of Article 9 of the General Data Protection Regulation (i.e. EU Regulation No. 2016/979), which allows the use of personal data even without the consent of the interested party just when the processing is necessary for reasons of public interest in the public health sector [1], p.101.

That no fundamental right is incompressible, on the other hand, is confirmed by Article 52 of the CFR of the European Union, where it is envisaged that, in compliance with proportionality, fundamental rights and freedoms may be limited where necessary and for purposes of general interest. 'General interest', 'public interest' and 'community interest' are all notions that, in an emergency and uncertain situation such as that caused by COVID-19, require broadening the scope of the duty of solidarity [71, 72].

8 The National Health System to the Test of the Pandemic

The health emergency due to the pandemic has left its mark on the emotional and psychological spheres of many persons. A considerable number of persons found themselves dealing with disorders such as anxiety, depression, stress and psychological fragility, more or less directly related to the situation and a suddenly uncertain and changing context. Although in all countries, the knowledge on the impact of the pandemic on mental health is still limited and mostly derived from experiences only partially comparable to the current epidemic, the demand for psychosocial interventions will likely increase significantly in the coming months and years. Investing in nationwide mental health services and programs, which have suffered from limited funding for years, is therefore now more important than ever. The past few months have brought many challenges, particularly for healthcare professionals, students, family members of COVID-19 patients, people with mental disorders, and more generally people in disadvantaged socioeconomic conditions, and workers whose livelihoods have been threatened.

At the EU level is of interest the report 'The impact of the CoVID-19 pandemic on the mental health of young people', published by the EU Commission on the occasion of the European Year of Young People (2022) [73]. This research analyses how European countries have addressed the challenges posed by the pandemic to the mental and emotional well-being of young people.

According to the report, member States took a proactive approach to address the mental health of young people during the pandemic emergency. One of the most common measures taken was to strengthen psychological support in schools, both by increasing the number of psychologists and counsellors available to students and by training school staff to recognise and address signs of mental distress. Six sectors were mainly involved: mental health protection, education, information on the impact of the pandemic on psychological well-being, youth work, leisure, and sports. To concretely help citizens in combating these issues, the Italian Legislature, by decree-law of 30 December 2021, converted by Law No. 15/2022, introduced as an additional form of economic support the 'psychologist *bonus*'. The measure is designed to provide help in supporting expenses related to psychological and psychotherapeutic care pathways. It should be noted that there is no age distinction for obtaining the psychologist *bonus*, and this is a particularly important aspect of the facility, given that it is precisely minors and children who have often suffered from psychological distress due to the major changes that the pandemic has brought to their daily lives. One need only think of distance education, which while it has allowed school teaching programs to continue, it has also taken young and very young people away from direct contact with their peers [74]. The psychological *bonus* measure appears important, but it is an intervention with an occasional and temporary character. The advantage of the *bonus* is that it opens up the possibility of those who have no resources to meet with a professional figure. But the sessions allowed by the *bonus* sums allow 4 to 12 sessions, realistically few for those facing a serious psychic problem.

As regards services, an intervention program to manage the impact of the epidemic was promoted as part of the Working Group 'Mental health and CoVID-19 emergency', established by decree of the President of the 'Istituto Superiore della Sanità' in April 2020 of COVID-19 on mental health and an Intervention Program for the management of anxiety and perinatal depression in emergency and post-emergency COVID-19. Both programs were aimed at ensuring the care of persons with psychiatric disorders or at high risk of anxiety disorders and depression. In particular, as regards the perinatal mental health program (which includes screening and early intervention of proven efficacy), it was proposed to adapt it to facilitate its integration—in the current emergency—within the different program's interventions at the regional level. The Working Group also provided indications for the management of the needs of family members of patients admitted to COVID-19 hospital wards [74].

About taking charge of citizenship in general and the management of anxiety and stress deriving from isolation and the fear of the consequences of the pandemic, the Working Group assessed the state of first- and second-level telephone services, drawing up two reports that collect recommendations and critical issues on the matter that are important for the management of subsequent pandemic waves or other emergencies. The Working Group is currently engaged with the Ministry of Health and the main scientific societies in the field of psychiatry in a fact-finding investigation on the functioning of mental health services since the beginning of the epidemic, to verify whether patients have been offered continuity of care and in what way. The survey, which will be addressed to all Mental Health Departments throughout the country, will be important to reorganise care and assistance in light of the persistence of emergency conditions.

Also, to facilitate access to mental health services, the Working Group has also started collaboration with the Ministry of Health for the preparation of the Italian Health Equity Status Report with the coordination of the WHO/Europe. Factors such as lower education, low-quality employment, poverty and the resulting income inequalities can have an impact on mental health because they affect access to services both for prevention and treatment of acute episodes [75]. However, putting the principle of solidarity at the centre of the problems caused by the pandemic implies reconsidering the relationship between the NHS and the right to health, a fundamental right which—as already noted—in the Italian Constitution is protected in the dual capacity of individual law and collective interest. This double dimension, which therefore also implies the social dimension, is also found in the law establishing the NHS, a law reformed starting in the 1990s and which, also due to the allocative choices imposed—more or less directly—from the EU, it requires a reflection on the effectiveness of the right to health [39, 69].

The allocative choices of the NHS, as highlighted by the pandemic, are shown in all their tragedy. The problem is that of now structural tension between supply and demand concerning treatment since the demand has made the need for treatments increasingly complex, and more and more expensive, either due to the ageing of the population or because the treatments are technologically more sophisticated. Given the relevance of the human person and his fundamental rights, among which health is the main one, it is necessary to ask oneself if financially there are the resources to make the right to health emotional. The Italian Constitutional Court also intervened, recognising the legitimacy of the balance between available resources and the protection of the right to health [76].

From a constitutional point of view, however, there is a problem of balancing. Here the crucial problem arises, which we will discuss in the coming years: the renewed role of the State. If before the pandemic, the hegemonic role of the market seemed prominent in the dichotomy State/market, today it is questioned. Furthermore, the market tends to be considered as responsible for the deterioration of the NHS. In this sense, some scholars invite us to reconsider the origins of the NHS and the idea of participation that characterised its conception [77]. In this regard, the idea of the NHS as a 'commons' (i.e. the idea according to which a different articulation of the territorial fabric that involves the enhancement of participation can and should also work on the level of the NHS and the protection of collective health) is of renewed interest [78].

The problem is that we have faced emergency management of the pandemic, which pushes us to make tragic choices, due to a lack of planning accompanied by effective action in the definition of the health service. Today we are facing the need to rethink a health service in which health is rewarded and where therefore produces healthy effects in all social policies. The debate appears polarised: on the one hand, there are power groups who are asking to resume production in all ways, on the other hand, those who ask for more caution and mapping of the circulation of the virus. Added to this is the clash between those who would like to continue privatising health care and the forces that oppose it, who are aware that health is the product of social struggles—as Chiara Giorgi well underlines [79].

If the NHS was born from social and political struggles, today it is necessary to implement the model, to guarantee primary prevention activities through a defence of the environmental matrices in which we live, and to rethink, through advanced common management, a health system that promotes the health and not the disease. The idea of participation and social control of the population was present in the NHS at its origins. Moreover, the implementation law found a problem in its implementation precisely about political participation in health management, a principle affirmed by Giulio Maccacaro (one of the greatest interpreters of the 'Medicina Democratica' movement) [80]. This participation was immediately declassified as a representative of political parties, hence all the criticisms made since the 1980s on the 'patronage' management of local health companies (so-called USL). This was one of the causes that later led to the progressive corporatization of the USL, to their transformation into companies with the 1992 counter-reform of the NHS [39], p.86.

Today, in the pandemic and post-pandemic phase, we should then rediscover the importance of collective participation to find the authentic roots of the NHS. This is the only way to give effect to the principle of solidarity [69, 72]. Hospital-centricity, whose criticism is now 20 years old, has more marked its presence in some Italian Regions, while in other contexts, it has been slowed down [81]. The capillary network model of services and institutions, built in the 1980s, has undergone continuous variations and repercussions since the 1990s, as in the rest of the Italian territory where the neoliberal model of ethics of individual responsibility, but has fortunately withstood the challenge imposed by the COVID-19 disease [82].

9 Conclusions

In conclusion, we can note that psychological well-being and mental health are deeply sensitive issues. During the pandemic, psychiatric well-being became and still is of particular importance with strong repercussions, not only in the short term. In Europe and in Italy, the issue of prevention and treatment of these disorders seems to be pivotal in achieving an inclusive and sensitive citizenship. It was precisely the spread of the CoVID-19 that demonstrated how a public health service is the only organisation that can effectively deal with an exceptional event [81]. Effective mental health protection would require structural measures, specific mental health services on the territories and opportunities for constant psychological visits.

Furthermore, it has been observed that public responsibility in health protection cannot be separated from a related responsibility in guaranteeing the other human rights [83]. This evidently should place a number of obligations on the health care organisation that go beyond the mere arrangement and provision of services and benefits instrumental to the treatment of illness. Therefore, it is desirable that in investing in an Italian health system that takes care of the persons in a proactive manner and is capable of contemplating the socioeconomic determinants of mental health, we will move rapidly towards participative and solidaristic goals.

Conflicts of Interest No author has any conflicts during preparation and publication of the manuscript.

Author Contributions RG authored paragraphs 2, 2.1, 3, 4 and 5; MDM authored paragraphs 1, 6, 7, 8 and 9.

References

1. Cendon P, editor. Pandemia e danni risarcibili. Reggio Emilia: Corsiero Editore; 2022.
2. Costantini C. Estetica della distanza e trasformazione del comune. https://cristinacostantinicc.wixsite.com/mysite. Accessed 24 Oct 2023. Ead. Ontologia dell'emergenza e politica della giurisdizione. Crisi estetiche dell'ordine globale e fenomenologia nostalgica del corpo politico. In: Giannone Codiglione G, Pierdominici L, editors. Comparative law in times of emergencies. Rome: RomaTre Press; 2022. p. 3.
3. Agamben G. A che punto siamo? Macerata: Quodlibet; 2021.
4. Di Cesare D. Anche per lo stato d'eccezione la paura è un boomerang. Il manifesto, 2020. https://ilmanifesto.it/anche-per-lo-stato-deccezione-la-paura-e-un-boomerang/. Accessed 24 Oct 2023.
5. Agamben G. Homo sacer. Il potere sovrano e la nuda vita. Torino: Einaudi; 1995.
6. Schmitt C. La dittatura. Dalle origini dell'idea moderna di sovranità alla lotta di classe proletaria. Roma-Bari: Laterza; 1975.
7. Schmitt C. Teologia politica. Quattro capitoli sulla dottrina della sovranità. Bologna: il Mulino; 1972.
8. Romano S. Sui decreti-legge e lo stato di assedio in occasione del terremoto di Messina e di Reggio-Calabria. Rivista di diritto pubblico e della pubblica amministrazione in Italia. 1909;I:251–72.

9. Azzariti G. I limiti costituzionali della situazione d'emergenza provocata dal Covid-19. Questione giustizia on-line, 2020, https://www.questionegiustizia.it/articolo/i-limiti-costituzionali-della-situazione-d-emergenza-provocata-dal-covid-19_27-03-2020.php. Accessed 24 Oct 2023.
10. Pallotta G, Battineni G, Nittari G, Amenta F. Psychological stress and mental health among seafarers. In: Gupta D, Polkowski Z, Khanna A, Bhattacharyya S, Castillo O, editors. Proceedings of Data Analytics and Management. Lecture Notes on Data Engineering and Communications Technologies, vol. 90. Singapore: Springer; 2022. https://doi.org/10.1007/978-981-16-6289-8_1.
11. Peters DH, Garg A, Bloom G, Walker DG, Brieger WR, Hafizur Rahman M. Poverty and access to health Care in Developing Countries. Ann N Y Acad Sci. 2008;1136:161–71.
12. World Bank. World Development Report. Investing in health. Oxford: Oxford University Press; 1993. p. 17.
13. Ellis E. Case C-84/94 United Kingdom of Great Britain and Northern Ireland v. council, judgment of 12 November 1996, not yet reported. Common Market Law Rev. 1997;34(4):1049–60.
14. World Health Organization. Global strategy for health for all by the year 2000. Geneva: World Health Organization; 1981. p. 15.
15. World Health Organization. Health for all in the 21st century. Copenhagen: World Health Organization; 1998. p. 30.
16. Harris D, O'Boyle M, Bates E, Buckley C. Harris, O'Boyle, and Warbrick law of the European convention on human rights. 4th ed. Oxford: Oxford University Press; 2018.
17. Council of Europe, European social charter. Collected texts (7th edition). Updated: 1st 2015. Tables of accepted provisions, p. 72.
18. Rossi S. La salute mentale attraverso lo spettro dei diritti umani. Forum di Quaderni Costituzionali/Rassegna. 2015;3:1–72.
19. United Nations General Assembly. Resolution 46/119 of 25 1993: 'Principles for the protection of persons with mental illness and the improvement of mental health care'. https://www.ohchr.org/en/instruments-mechanisms/instruments/principles-protection-persons-mental-illness-and-improvement. Accessed 24 Oct 2023.
20. Rosenthal E, Rubenstein LS. International human rights advocacy under the 'principles for the protection of persons with mental illness'. Int J Law Psychiatry. 1993;16(3–4): 257–300.
21. Fischer J. Comparative look at the right to refuse treatment for involuntary hospitalized persons with a mental illness. Hastings Int'l & Comp L Rev. 2005;29:153.
22. Perlin L. International human rights and mental disability law: when the silenced are heard. Oxford: Oxford University Press; 2011. p. 15.
23. McSherry B. International trends in mental health Laws: introduction. Law in Context. 2008;26(2):1–9.
24. Rosenthal E, Sundram CJ. International human rights in mental health legislation. NYL Sch Journal Int'l & Comp Law. 2002;21:489.
25. United Nations General Assembly. Resolution 2856 (XXVI) of 20 December 1971: Declaration on the rights of mentally retarded persons. https://www.ohchr.org/en/instruments-mechanisms/instruments/declaration-rights-mentally-retarded-persons. Accessed 24 Oct 2023.
26. United Nations General Assembly. Resolution 3447 (XXX). Declaration on the rights of disabled persons. https://www.ohchr.org/en/instruments-mechanisms/instruments/declaration-rights-disabled-persons. Accessed 24 Oct 2023.
27. United Nations General Assembly. Standard rules on the equalization of opportunities for persons with disabilities. https://www.un.org/development/desa/disabilities/standard-rules-on-the-equalization-of-opportunities-for-persons-with-disabilities.html. Accessed 24 Oct 2023.
28. United Nations, World Conference on Human Rights, Vienna, 25 June 1993. https://www.ohchr.org/en/instruments-mechanisms/instruments/vienna-declaration-and-programme-action. Accessed 24 Oct 2023.
29. Alston P. The UN's human rights record: from San Francisco to Vienna and beyond. Hum Rights Q. 1994;16(2):375–90.

30. Perlingieri P. La persona e i suoi diritti. Problemi del diritto civile. Naples: Edizioni Scientifiche Italiane; 2005.
31. Papa A. La tutela multilivello della salute nello spazio europeo: opportunità o illusione? Federalismiit. 2018;16(4):80–99.
32. D'Aloia A. Diritto di morire? La problematica dimensione costituzionale della 'fine della vita'. Politica del diritto. 1998;29(4):601–36.
33. Garetto R, Allegranti I, Cancellieri S, Coscarelli S, Ferretti F, Nico MP. Ethical and legal challenges of telemedicine implementation in rural areas. In: Mittal M, Battineni G, editors. Information and communication technology (ICT) frameworks in telehealth. TELe-health. Cham: Springer; 2022. https://doi.org/10.1007/978-3-031-05049-7_3.
34. Nicola M, Alsafi Z, Sohrabi C, Kerwan A, Al-Jabir A, Iosifidis C, et al. The socio-economic implications of the coronavirus pandemic (COVID-19): a review. Int J Surg. 2020;78(15):185–93. https://doi.org/10.1016/j.ijsu.2020.04.018.
35. Mittal M, Battineni G, Goyal LM, Chhetri B, Oberoi SV, Chintalapudi N, et al. Cloud-based framework to mitigate the impact of COVID-19 on seafarers' mental health. Int Marit Health. 2020;71(3):213–4.
36. Garetto R, Pascucci F. Salute della persona e organizzazione dell'attività alberghiera ai tempi del COVID-19–Person's Health and Hotel Business in Covid-19 Times. Actualidad Jurídica. Iberoamericana. 2020;12bis(55):602–13.
37. Caravita di Toritto B. La disciplina costituzionale della salute. Diritto e società. 1984;11(3):21–60.
38. Marella MR. La protezione giuridica dell'infermo di mente. Rivista critica del diritto privato. 1991:229.
39. Pioggia A. Diritto sanitario e dei servizi sociali. Turin: G. Giappichelli Editore; 2020.
40. Perlingieri P. Gli istituti di protezione e di promozione dell'‹‹infermo di mente››. A proposito dell'handicappato psichico permanente. Rassegna di diritto civile. 1985:54.
41. Mazzoni CM. Libertà e salvaguardia nella disciplina dell'infermità mentale. In: Cendon P, editor. Un altro diritto per il malato di mente. Esperienze e soggetti della trasformazione. Naples: Edizioni Scientifiche Italiane; 1988. p. 489.
42. Zatti P. «Parole tra noi così diverse». Per una ecologia del rapporto terapeutico. La Nuova giurisprudenza civile commentata. 2012;3(2):143–50.
43. Foglia M. Consenso e cura. La solidarietà nel rapporto terapeutico. Turin: Giappichelli; 2018.
44. Ongaro Basaglia F, Bignami G. Medicina/medicalizzazione. In: Ongaro Basaglia F, editor. Salute/Malattia. Le parole della medicina, Turin: Einaudi; 1982.
45. Princigalli A. La responsabilità del medico. Napoli: Jovene; 1983.
46. Di Masi M. Il fine vita. Rome: Ediesse; 2015.
47. Santosuosso A. Corpo e libertà. Una storia tra diritto e scienza. Milan: Raffaello Cortina editore; 2001.
48. Zatti P. Principi e forme del «governo del corpo». In: Rodotà S, Zatti P, editors. Trattato di Biodiritto, Il governo del corpo, vol. 1. Milan: Giuffrè; 2011.
49. Foucault M. Sorvegliare e punire. Nascita della prigione. Turin: Einaudi; 1993.
50. Foucault M. La volontà di sapere. Milan: Feltrinelli; 1984.
51. Marini G. La giuridificazione della persona. Ideologie e tecniche nei diritti della personalità. Rivista di diritto civile. 2006;3(1):359–94.
52. Cendon P. I malati terminale e i loro diritti. Milan: Giuffrè; 2003.
53. Mori M. Il caso Eluana Englaro: la Porta Pia del vitalismo ippocratico, ovvero perchè è moralmente giusto sospendere ogni intervento. Bologna: Pendragon; 2008.
54. Zatti P. Maschere del diritto volti della vita. Milan: Giuffrè; 2009.
55. Rodotà S. La vita e le regole. Tra diritto e non diritto. Milan: Feltrinelli; 2009.
56. Rodotà S. Il diritto di avere diritti. Roma-Bari: Laterza; 2013.
57. Corte costituzionale. Sentence No. 438/2008. In: Foro italiano, 2009, I, c. 1328.
58. Cassazione Penale, Section V. Sentence No. 5639/1992. In: Rivista italiana di medicina legale, 1993, p. 460.

59. Barni M, Santosuosso A, editors. Medicina e diritto. Milan: Giuffrè; 1995.
60. Caterina R. Paternalismo e antipaternalismo nel diritto privato. Rivista di diritto civile. 2005;6(2):771–96.
61. Castronovo C. Profili della responsabilità medica. Studi in onore di Pietro Rescigno, V, Responsabilità civile e tutela dei diritti. Milan: Giuffrè; 1998.
62. Cattaneo G. Il consenso del paziente al trattamento chirurgico. Riv Trimest Dirit Proced Civ. 1957;959
63. Ferrando G. Consenso informato del paziente e responsabilità del medico; principi, problemi e linee di tendenza. Rivista critica del diritto privato. 1998;1:37.
64. Carusi D. Tutela della salute, consenso alle cure, direttive anticipate: l'evoluzione del pensiero privatistico. Rivista critica del diritto privato. 2009;1:7–20.
65. Pucella R. Autodeterminazione e responsabilità nella relazione di cura. Milan: Giuffrè; 2010. p. 153.
66. Cassazione civile, Section III, 09.02.2010, No. 2847. In: Giurisprudenza italiana. 2011;4: 816.
67. Gorgoni A. Il diritto alla salute e il diritto all'autodeterminazione nella responsabilità medica. Obbligazioni e contratti. 2011;3:191–201.
68. Gristina GR, Busatta L, Piccinni M. The Italian law on informed consent and advance directives: its impact on intensive care units and the European legal framework. Minerva Anestesiol. 2019;85:401–11.
69. Marella MR, Marini G, Nivarra L. Editoriale. Rivista critica del diritto privato. 2020;1(2):3–8.
70. Rodotà S. Tecnologie e diritti. Bologna: il Mulino; 1995. p. 83.
71. Rodotà S. Solidarietà. Roma-Bari: Laterza; 2014.
72. Alpa G. Solidarietà. Un principio normativo. Bologna: il Mulino; 2022.
73. https://op.europa.eu/en/publication-detail/-/publication/be9b29b1-4ae1-11ed-92ed-01aa75ed71a1/language-en. Accessed 24 Oct 2023.
74. https://www.salute.gov.it/portale/nuovocoronavirus/dettaglioNotizieNuovoCoronavirus.jsp?lingua=italiano&menu=notizie&p=dalministero&id=5957. Accessed 23 Oct 2023.
75. https://www.iss.it/rapporti-covid-19/-/asset_publisher/btw1J82wtYzH/content/rapporto-iss-covid-19-n.-23-2020-indicazioni-di-un-programma-di-intervento-dei-dipartimenti-di-salute-mentale-per-la-gestione-dell-impatto-dell-epidemia-covid-19-sulla-salute-mentale.-versione-del-6-maggio-2020. Accessed 24 Oct 2023.
76. Di Costanzo C, Zagrebelsky V. L'accesso alle cure intensive fra emergenza virale e legittimità delle decisioni allocative. BioLaw. 2020;1S:441–6. https://teseo.unitn.it/biolaw/article/view/1472. Accessed 24 Oct 2023.
77. Cauduro A, Liberati P. Sull'emergenza (annunciata) del Servizio sanitario nazionale. GiustiziaInsieme.it, 28 March 2020, https://www.giustiziainsieme.it/it/diritto-dell-emergenza-covid-19/954-sull-emergenza-annunciata-del-servizio-sanitario-nazionale. Accessed 24 Oct 2023.
78. Marella MR. The commons as a legal concept. Law Critique. 2017;28:61–86. https://doi.org/10.1007/s10978-016-9193-0.
79. Giorgi C. La sanità da riscoprire. Le radici politiche del Servizio Sanitario Nazionale. Centro per la Riforma dello Stato. 15 March 2020, https://centroriformastato.it/la-sanita-da-riscoprire-le-radici-politiche-del-servizio-sanitario-nazionale-1/. Accessed 24 Oct 2023.
80. Maccacaro GA. Medicina democratica, movimento di lotta per la salute, relazione introduttiva al convegno costitutivo di Medicina democratica, Bologna, 15–16 May 1976. In: Maccacaro GA. Per una medicina da rinnovare. Scritti 1966–1976, Milan: Feltrinelli, 1979.
81. Giorgi C. Presente e futuro delle politiche sanitarie. In: Menabò di Etica e Economia, 2021. https://archivio.eticaeconomia.it/presente-e-futuro-delle-politiche-sanitarie/#. Accessed 24 Oct 2023.
82. Pompili R. Le infrastrutture della salute. Euronomade.info. 2020. http://www.euronomade.info/?p=13328. Accessed 24 Oct 2023.
83. Pioggia A. Diritti umani e organizzazione sanitaria. Rivista del Diritto della Sicurezza Sociale. 2011;1:21–42.

Analysis of Depression Disorder with Motor Activity Time-Series Data Using Machine Learning and Deep Learning

G. Kalyani, M. Suneetha, B. Janakiramaiah, and Gopi Battineni

Abstract The future of the healthcare system is being altered by new technology developments. Depression is a neurological condition that can cause significant emotional suffering. The way of brain working can change how much of an impact it has on the body. A person with depression typically has a low mood and may feel depressed or hopeless all the time. In response to loss or tragedy, depressive symptoms may appear briefly. However, if the symptoms persist for more than 2 weeks, it may indicate a significant depressive condition. The incidence of major depressive disorder is 350 million people worldwide (MDD). Historically, conventional techniques have been used to identify depression symptoms. Recently, research has started investigating the relationship among psychosocial characteristics, like quality-of-life scale, and mental health, that helps to identify and predict MDD earlier for better treatment. Finding the elements that contribute to depression may inspire new research and therapeutic approaches because depression is an illness that is increasingly posing a significant community health threat. In this work, we have provided comprehensive approaches to handle and examine the time series data and better understand the association between depressed aspects connected to physical activity in daily life using machine learning and deep learning techniques. There seem to be more direct links between various physical conditions and depression. These could end up being particularly interesting in terms of etiology. The two

G. Kalyani · M. Suneetha
Velagapudi Ramakrishna Siddhartha Engineering College, Vijayawada, Andhra Pradesh, India

B. Janakiramaiah
Prasad V Potluri Siddhartha Institute of Technology, Vijayawada, Andhra Pradesh, India

G. Battineni (✉)
Clinical Research Centre, School of Medicinal and Health Products Sciences, University of Camcrino, Camerino, Italy
e-mail: gopi.battineni@unicam.it

G. Battineni et al. (eds.), *Computational Methods in Psychiatry*,
https://doi.org/10.1007/978-981-99-6637-0_2

best examples are probably heart disease and stroke. The experimental results support the hypothesis that the change in the physical activity of daily life for a sequence of days is an indication of unipolar depression.

Keywords Motor activity · Unipolar · Bipolar · Depression · Physical activity · Random forest · XGBoost · LSTM

1 Introduction

According to the World Health Organization (WHO), health is a condition of total physical, mental, and social well-being and not merely the absence of disease or disability. More than 350 million individuals worldwide experience depression, which has the potential to worsen into a significant health issue, especially when it lasts for a long time and is moderate to severe in intensity. Depression may be extremely painful, interrupting daily activities like job, school, family, and relationships, as well as economic and emotional ones. In the worst instance, it may result in suicide, which accounts for about one million fatalities each year [1]. The child and young adult populations in Latin America have a high incidence of psychological problems; about 20% of these populations have disorders that call for the assistance of health services. However, this number is understated because adolescents try to conceal and hide their difficulties from adults and lack the confidence to obtain medicinal frameworks [2].

Depression is a psychological condition that is inherently characterized by a depressed mood, a lack of interest and pleasure in the good things in life, and exhaustion. These symptoms degrade their quality of life and cause problems for those who experience them in their families, places of employment, and social settings [3]. Depression can begin with key symptoms which do not involve mood changes or even cognitive performance, making it simple for anybody to experience depression [4]. Depression can also occur without regard to age, sex, or socioeconomic status. Once depression has been diagnosed, the patient must receive medication that reduces the difficulties that this illness brings on. The fact that depression might be resistant to some medications, though, is one of the difficulties that have emerged. In treatment-resistant depression, the effects of recurrent transcranial magnetic stimulation (rTMS) on cognitive ability findings suggest that this noninvasive brain stimulation can be utilized as a method for treating depression that has not responded to medication [5].

Patients' reports are used in traditional approaches to track depression in unipolar and bipolar patients. However, bias is frequently seen in this kind of monitoring. According to Sedano et al. [6], changes in behavior and perception of the outside world are also evident. Ecological momentary assessment (EMA) is an alternative to these reports as they capture behavior, emotions, and other types of activities that occur in real-life circumstances. As the number of wearable devices such as smartwatches and smartphones with motion sensors, such as gyroscopes and accelerometers, increases, EMA measurements can be performed almost instantly, allowing for the expansion of the public's availability of mental health services without the use of new, specialized devices. As an example, various strategies to combat mental illness have used cell phones and similar technology. By using two main strategies—implementing human–computer interfaces for therapeutic support and gathering pertinent data from individuals' regular lifestyles to track the current situation and progression of their mental problems.

In the discussion of how mobiles can aid in the treatment of psychological disorders, researchers concentrated on two key strategies including incorporating human–computer interfaces for therapy support and gathering pertinent data from participants' regular lifestyles [7]. Using a smartphone as a clinical medium showed that psychological therapies can lower anxiety [8]. Data on psychiatric patients' use of and interest in using mobile applications to track their mental health symptoms proved that 50% of patients across all age-groups expressed interest in using mobile apps to track the condition of their mental health [9]. Mobile phone sensors for the identification of human behavior traits, activity detection at various levels of activity abstraction, and characterized health-related behaviors including sleeping and exercising [10].

Applications in numerous sectors, including activity recognition, are developed using devices with sensors that can obtain contextual information [11]. Finding mental diseases can be aided by activity recognition. Motor activity data is used to model the patterns of schizophrenia and depression disorders [12]. Many apps have been suggested to provide sad persons with self-help. Although these apps enhance some areas of cognitive behavioral therapy (CBT) or behavioral activation (BA) evaluation, still they are debatable that highlighting the need for superior scientific, technological, and legal expertise [13]. Two intriguing reviews on mental health disorders used many sensing layers and sensor data to model behaviors and provide associated mental health states [14, 15]. Data from social media, such as social networks (such as Twitter), online forums, and public surveys are additional ways to physical sensors. Through the monitoring of these passive data about the subject's activity, these approaches attempt to detect depressive moods. All of these methods necessitate direct patient engagement, which may result in inaccurate final diagnoses. Therefore, a technique that reduces the requirement for subject contact is necessary to prevent outliers, who purposefully overfeed data.

Daily life patterns and time series of repeating biological rhythms should be regarded as complex dynamical systems. Simple linear models are rarely able to classify complex dynamical systems. Therefore, the typical approach for assessing and rating motor activity recordings has been to use mathematical techniques from the study of nonlinear complex and chaotic systems [16]. In the analysis of data from intricate dynamical systems, machine learning (ML) methods have shown encouraging results and in a long-term investigation of bipolar patients' heart rate unevenness, ML's capacity to uncover non-obvious patterns has reasonably reliably identified mood states. Similar changes in cardiovascular and autonomic systems have been discovered in manic individuals by nonlinear heart rate variability analysis. Heart rate measurements are significantly less noisy than accelerometer recordings. However, the time series of motor activity has enormous potential for a variety of ML techniques. Random forest and neural networks [17] techniques have demonstrated potential capabilities for temporal series data of activation. Millions of parameters in a mathematical model called a neural network constantly adjust themselves to maximize performance. As a result, it is challenging to understand the lines of reasoning. Some techniques do, however, provide some interpretation of neural network internals. There is doubt about a black-box system that generates calculations without explaining the field of medicine [18]. However, results from high-quality analyses of critical variables should be regarded as reliable, at least when overfitting prevention strategies have been used [19]. The Random Forest algorithm's ensemble learning method resists overfitting and can be thought of as a woodland of decision trees, where different trees focus on stochastic portions of the data. Predictions made by decision trees are transparent and comprehensible.

2 Literature Review

Subjective observations along with clinical rating measures that are semi-structured are the current methods used to evaluate mood episodes in affective disorders. The assessment of emotional symptoms should be done using objective approaches. A change in activation is a key indicator of both bipolar and unipolar depression, according to research on motor activity, which is a neutral remark of the internal physiological state represented in behavioral patterns. In comparison to healthy controls, the depressive state is frequently linked to decreased daily motor activity, greater activity level variability, and less complex activity patterns. Contradictory motor activity patterns, resembling those seen in manic patients, have been seen in a few depressed bipolar and unipolar individuals. A thermodynamic model of depressive disorder has been developed, and it is claimed that depressive issues are diseases of energy instabilities. According to a simplified version of the paradigm, two energies emerge from a shared zero point of motor-retarded depression that has been down-regulated [20]. The first excited energy is the awakening of overexcited symptoms, such as overstated self-esteem and amplified goal-directed behavior. The second agitated energy is related to heightened internal tension, anxiety, and restlessness. A manic state appears to have enhanced levels of euphoric and agitated energy [21], while one out of every five depressions, regardless of polarity, appears to have agitated energy. These findings provide evidence in support of the thermodynamic concept. Unquestionably, motor activity is an expression of daily social rhythms that are repeated in connection with a biological pace that cycle every 24 h and are interlocked with multiple ultradian pace sequence that last from 2 to 6 h [22]. Biological pace patterns that are out of sync are proposed as key signs of mood episodes [23].

In various research on the prenatal detection of depression, ML techniques have been employed. N-gram language modeling and vector amalgamation with topic analysis were recommended to classify the anxiety levels of created emotional features [24]. The bag-of-words embedding procedure is a way to identify depression using the Twitter dataset [25]. A supervised ML algorithm's effects on measuring predictors for identifying post-traumatic stress chaos were explored in [26]. A deep neural network approach to examine depression in social media like Twitter was put up [27]. Convolutional neural networks were utilized to contrast several models and they depend on linguistic metadata for the prediction of emotions [28].

Major research studies on revealing of depression rely on textual data or person-descriptive techniques that select elements from social media posts. Textual-based featuring is used to highlight the linguistic components of social media content, including words, parts of speech, N-grams, and other linguistic traits [29]. The descriptive-based featured technique places a focus on subject descriptors, which may include age, gender, employment status, income, drug or alcohol use, smoking, and other details specific to the subject or patient [30]. In [31], authors performed research that uses supervised machine learning classifiers' prediction capabilities to study how emotions interact. They used categorization techniques to group messages on social media that dealt with depression. For the bag-of-words features, Trifan Alina et al. in [32] proposed a rule-based model utilizing a Tf-IDf technique to identify sadness from the Reddit social media platform. Early depression diagnosis using historical tweets from Twitter users using bidirectional LSTM and attention model was presented in [33].

A system for tracking emotional wellness has been created called KBRS, and it employs a deep learning model and sentiment metric algorithms are used by this system to determine which sentences have negative content [34]. A few studies examine patient behavior on social media sites using data from Facebook, Instagram, and Reddit posts by combining the discriminative power of popular ML classifiers [35]. A method for classifying depressed people on social media platforms was presented that uses the hierarchical post-representation model known as the MGL-CNN [36]. For recognizing depression, another study employs DCNN and ANN for the examination of depressed symptoms, two models—the deep model and the shallow model—are put forth. This study blends deep and shallow models with text and video elements [37]. It comprises of the RF algorithm for scoring based depression categorization and is suggested to use text that is extracted from patient responses based on language in addition to speech signals to detect depression [38]. Study that analyses text data from college students to identify depression in college students by the DISVM algorithm is used to categorize data acquired from input and, in the end, identify depression as a mental disorder [39]. Some research uses multi-modal data from text, audio, and video to analyze the patient's mental condition and subsequently forecast an outcome [40]. To account for the intensity of the patient's depression, the output is classified into various depression levels [36]. These are some of the techniques used to classify text, video, and audio elements associated with depression. Some models successfully predict the symptoms of and severity of depression, others do not produce adequate findings. Based on the aforementioned literature review, researchers concluded that there are numerous scientific answers to the problem of depression detection. Since there are more depression instances, there are more treatments that have been presented, but these solutions have not yet been highly accurate, and there have been significant losses.

Few researchers utilize the data from social media platforms, which might or might not be reliable [41]. There is a risk that using online tools for depression prediction, such Twitter and Reddit, will lead to inaccurate predictions of depressive symptoms. A mistake will result if symptoms picked up from social media sites online are incorrectly predicted [42]. It is impossible to assess a specific risk of depression if the data are inaccurate. Social media users occasionally publish depressing or sad stories, either knowingly or unknowingly, which can have an impact on the system's overall ability to detect melancholy [43]. As a result, social media networks are not a reliable source for scholars. They frequently make advantage of an accurate database created when creating a system for detecting sadness. Researchers require a method for automatically detecting depression that is highly accurate and produces little system losses. The characteristics of audio samples, video samples, and text responses from a depressed patient can be combined to get precise results [44]. The deep neural network method makes it simple to forecast depression [45]. A depression detection system will only be created if the model has been trained and has learned all the aspects of audio, video, and text. These are literature reviews that address the issue of depression detection.

The work in this article is a reexamination of motor activity recordings from a group study that was previously reported in the article [46]. The wrist-worn actigraphy utilized in the dataset, to trace the integration of intensity, amount, and duration of movement in all directions, was used to record motor activity. At a sampling frequency of 32 Hz, movements higher than 0.05 g were captured. The result was expressed in units of gravitational acceleration per minute. Throughout the recording, the actigraph device was continuously worn.

3 Methods

3.1 Dataset

The data collection includes 23 patients with depression termed as the condition group. Figure 1 depicts an instance of data related to a single person over a day. 18 people were outpatients while data were being gathered, whereas 5 people were hospitalized. The Montgomery-Asberg depression rating scale (MADRS) [47] was used by a doctor to gauge the severity of continuous depression at the beginning and end of the motor activity recordings. The dataset also includes actigraphy data from 32 non-depressed volunteers termed as the control group, comprising 5 students, 4 former patients, and 23 hospital employees who are not now exhibiting any psychiatric symptoms. Figure 1 presents the activity of condition and control concerning the time.

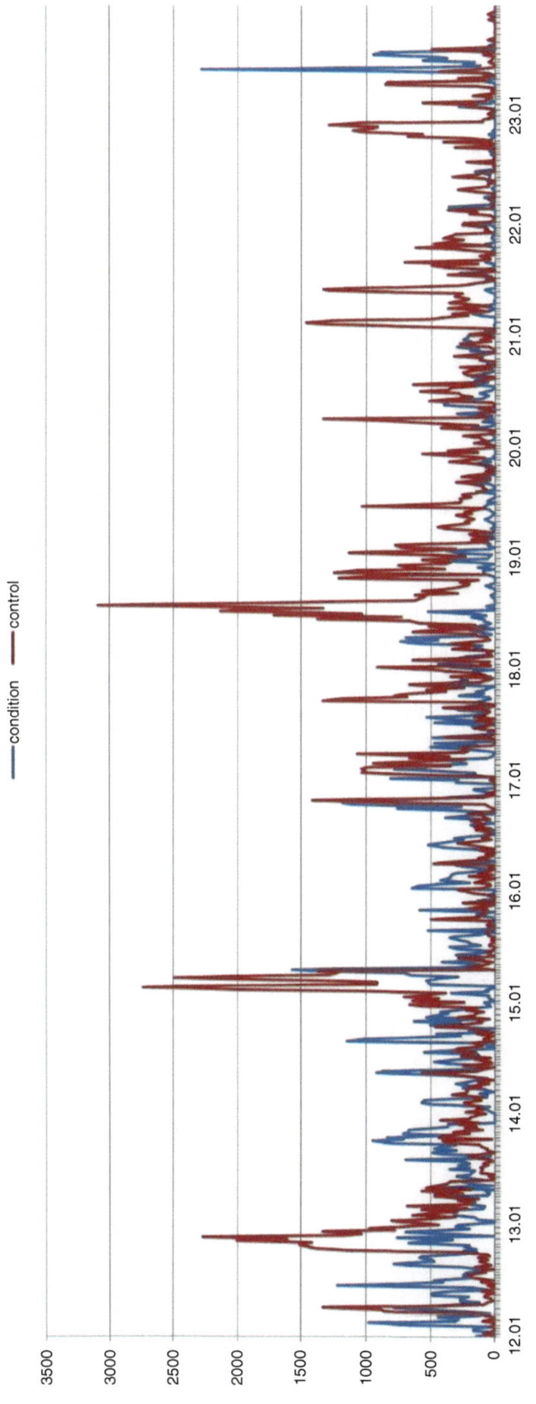

Fig. 1 Sample actigraph of 12 h for both condition and control group instance

The dataset contains the data for the condition group, and for the controls. Each patient receives a csv file containing the actigraph data that has been accumulated over time. The columns are activity, dates (the measurement day), and timestamps (1-min intervals) (activity measurement from the actigraph watch). The scores.csv file contains the MADRS results as well. The columns are number as patient id, number of measurement days, gender as 1 or 2 for female or male, age (age in age-groups), afftype as 1,2,3 for bipolar II, unipolar depressive, and bipolar I respectively, melanch as 1 and 2 for melancholia and no melancholia, respectively, inpatient as 1 and 2 for inpatient and outpatient, respectively, education grouped in years, marriage as 1 and 2 for married or cohabiting, and single, respectively, and MADRS scores at the beginning and end of the study. Figure 2 demonstrates the total number of days that each control and condition group person are tracked for motor activity data.

3.2 ML Models

3.2.1 Logistic Regression

Similar to linear regression, logistic regression employs an equation as its exemplification. To estimate an output value (y), weights or coefficient values (Beta) are linearly coupled with input values (x). The process of making the data suitable for logistic regression includes the following:

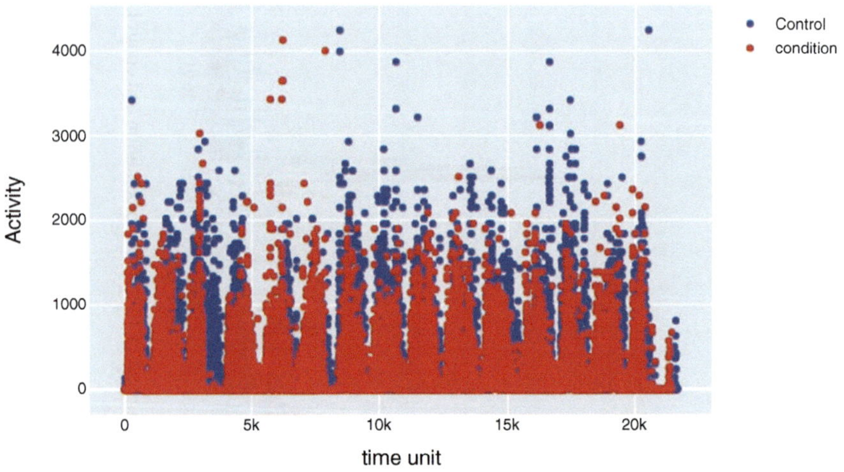

Fig. 2 Activity distribution of condition and control over time

- Reduce noise: Since the output variable (y) in a logistic regression model is assumed to be error-free, you should remove outliers and any potential misclassified cases from the training instances.
- Gaussian distribution: The input and output variables are assumed to have a linear relationship. A more accurate model may be produced by applying data transformations to your input variables that more clearly reveal this linear relationship. To better reveal this link, you may, for instance, apply log, root, Box-Cox, and other univariate transforms.
- Eliminate associated inputs: Similar to linear regression, the model can overfit if it receives several extremely correlated inputs. Study the pairwise correlations among each input and eliminate those that are extremely associated.

After preparing the data, there are "n" observations and "p" feature variables in the dataset. The feature matrix looks like this:

$$X = \begin{pmatrix} 1 & x_{11} & \cdots & x_{1p} \\ 1 & x_{21} & \cdots & x_{2p} \\ \vdots & \vdots & \ddots & \vdots \\ 1 & x_{n1} & \cdots & x_{np} \end{pmatrix}$$

where it represents the values of the jth observation's ith characteristic. The ith observation, xi, can be illustrated as follows:

$$x_i = \begin{bmatrix} 1 \\ x_{i1} \\ x_{i2} \\ . \\ . \\ . \\ x_{ip} \end{bmatrix}$$

The predicted response, denoted by h(xi), is for the ith observation, or xi. The hypothesis is the name of the formula we employ to determine h(xi).

In the case of linear regression, the prediction method we employed was

$$h(x_i) = \beta_0 + \beta_1 x_{i1} + \beta_2 x_{i2} + \ldots + \beta_p x_{ip}$$

where β_0, β_1, …, β_p are the regression coefficients

Let the vector or matrix of the regression coefficient be:

$$\beta = \begin{bmatrix} \beta_0 \\ \beta_1 \\ \beta_2 \\ \cdot \\ \cdot \\ \beta_p \end{bmatrix}$$

Afterward, in a shorter format,

$$h(x_i) = \beta^T x_i$$

The statement of the hypothesis $h(x_i)$ for logistic regression is

$$h(x_i) = g(\beta^T x_i) = \frac{1}{1 + e^{-\beta^T * x_i}}$$

The logistic regression uses the following cost function:

$$J(\theta) = -\frac{1}{m}\Sigma\left[y^{(i)}\log\left(h\theta\left(x(i)\right)\right) + \left(1 - y^{(i)}\right)\log\left(1 - h\theta\left(x(i)\right)\right)\right]$$

3.2.2 Support Vector Machine

An approach for supervised learning called the support vector machine (SVM) is employed for both classification and regression. Even if we also refer to regression issues, classification is the best fit. The technique's main goal is to locate a hyperplane in an N-dimensional space that categorizes the data points. The hyperplane's size is depending on the number of available dimensions. When there are only two input characteristics, the hyperplane is essentially a line. The hyperplane turns into a 2-D plane if the number of input characteristics is three. When there are more than three features, it gets harder to imagine. The hyperplane that best portrays the greatest gap or margin between the two classes is one logical option. Therefore, the hyperplane that maximizes the distance from it to the closest data point on each side is selected. A maximum-margin hyperplane or hard margin is said to exist if one does.

We want to optimize the distance between the data points and the hyperplane in the SVM method. The loss function known as hinge loss aids in maximizing the margin. When the expected and actual values have the same sign, then determine the loss value if they are not.

$$c(x, y, f(x)) = \begin{cases} 0, & f\ y * f(x) \geq 1 \\ 1 - y * f(x), & \text{else} \end{cases}$$

The following are crucial variables in the SVM algorithm: C: Maintaining high values of C will tell the SVM model to select a narrower margin hyperplane. The SVM model will select a larger margin hyperplane if C is not a significant value. To generate an SVM model, a kernel type must be employed. Linear, rbf, poly, or sigmoid are all possible. "rbf" is the kernel's default value and degree. It is only taken into account while using the polynomial kernel. It is the kernel function's degree for the polynomial. A degree's default value is 3.

3.2.3 XGBoost Algorithm

The XGBoost decision tree-based ensemble machine learning approach makes use of the gradient boosting methodology. In many cases, artificial neural networks perform better than all other algorithms or frameworks when it comes to unstructured data prediction problems (pictures, text, etc.). To handle small to moderate volumes of structured/tabular data, decision tree-based algorithms are now regarded as best-in-class. The following are the main algorithmic enhancements of the XGBoost algorithm: Regularization combines both L1 and L2 regularization to penalize more complex models to prevent overfitting. Sparsity awareness, which more skillfully controls various types of sparsity patterns in the data, accepts sparse features for inputs by automatically "learning" the best missing value depending on training loss. Weighted quantile sketch easily determines the best split points between weighted datasets and cross-validation at each iteration by eliminating the need to manually construct this search and to denote the specific number of boosting iterations mandatory in a single run.

The combined prediction scores of each decision tree lead to the final prediction score of the classifier. A key aspect of the example is that the two trees attempt to complement one another. We can formulate our model mathematically as follows:

$$\hat{y}_i = \sum_{k=1}^{K} f_k(x_i), f_k \in F$$

f is the functional space of F, K is the number of trees, and F is the set of potential CARTs. The following statements provide the model's objective function:

$$\text{obj}(\theta) = \sum_{i}^{n} l\left(y_i, \hat{y}_i\right) + \sum_{k=1}^{K} \Omega(f_k)$$

where the regularization parameter is the second term and the first term is the loss function. Now we apply the additive strategy, minimize the loss of what we have learned, and add a new tree, which can be summarized as follows:

$$\hat{y}_i^{(0)} = 0\,\hat{y}_i^{(1)} = f_1(x_i) = \hat{y}_i^{(0)} + f_1(x_i)\,\hat{y}_i^{(2)}$$
$$= f_1(x_i) + f_2(x_i) = \hat{y}_i^{(1)} + f_2(x_i)\,\hat{y}_i^{(t)}$$
$$= \sum_{k=1}^{t} f_k(x_i) = \hat{y}_i^{(t-1)} + f_t(x_i)$$

The following is a definition of the model's objective function:

$$\text{obj}^{(t)} = \sum_{i=1}^{n} l\left(y_i, \hat{y}_i^{(t)}\right) + \sum_{i=1}^{t} \Omega(f_i) = \sum_{i=1}^{n} l\left(y_i, \hat{y}_i^{(t-1)} + f_t(x_i)\right) + \Omega(f_t) + \text{constant obj}^{(t)}$$
$$= \sum_{i=1}^{n}\left(y_i - \left(\hat{y}_i^{(t-1)} + f_t(x_i)\right)\right)^2 + \sum_{i=1}^{t} \Omega(f_i) + \text{constant obj}^{(t)} =$$
$$= \sum_{i=1}^{n}\left[2\left(\hat{y}_i^{(t-1)} - y_i\right) f_t(x_i) + f_t(x_i)^2\right] + \Omega(f_t) + \text{constant obj}^{(t)}$$

3.2.4 Random Forest Method

As an alternative to depending solely on a single decision tree, a random forest considers the prediction from every tree and decides its prediction of the concluding output based on the majority votes of predictions. It comprises several decision trees on several subsets of the dataset and considers the average to increase the predictive accuracy of that dataset. Higher accuracy is obtained, and overfitting is avoided because of the more number of trees in the forest.

To produce the random forest, N decision trees are combined, and then, in the second step, predictions are made for every tree from the initial phase. The steps in the working process of random forest are choosing K data points at random from the training set, generating the decision trees connected to the taken data points, selecting the decision tree N that you wish to construct, Re-do 1 and 2 steps, and for any new data points, locate each decision tree's predictions for the new data point and group the new data points into the category with the maximum support.

3.2.5 Deep Neural Network

The input data is processed by the nodes in the first layer, who then output it to the neurons in the second layer, and so on, producing the output (Refer to Fig. 3). The result could be a forecast like "Yes" or "No" which is represented in probability. Each neuron in a layer, whether it be one or many, will compute a little function called an activation function. The activation process imitates the signal that should be sent to the subsequently linked neurons. The output is passed or ignored depending on whether the value produced by the input neurons exceeds a threshold. An associated weight would be present for any connection between two neurons in successive

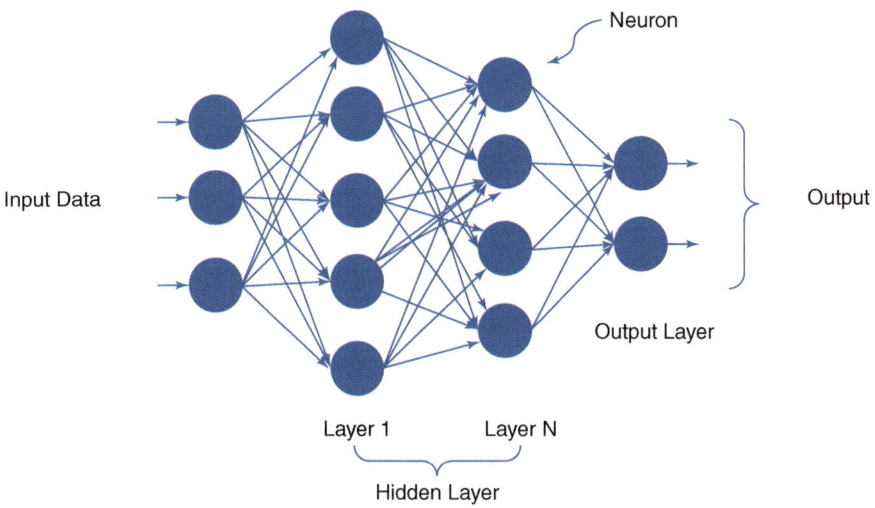

Fig. 3 The architecture of Deep Neural Network

levels. The weight identifies how the input will affect the subsequent neuron's output and, ultimately, the total result. The preliminary weights in a neural network would be completely random, however, the weights would be attuned iteratively during the model training to predict the accurate output. After breaking down the network into its parts, a few logical building blocks can be identified, such as a neuron, layer, weight, input, output, activation function, and finally a learning mechanism (optimizer), which will enable the network to gradually update its initialized weights (which were chosen at random) to weights that are better suited for accurate outcome prediction.

3.2.6 Long Short-Term Memory (LSTM) Network

LSTM is a special form of RNN that can recognize long-term dependencies. They are currently in extensive use and work amazingly well when applied to a variety of problems. LSTMs are designed specifically to avoid the long-term dependence problem. They don't have a hard time picking up new material; in fact, it's almost like it comes naturally to them to retain it for a long time. All recurrent neural networks take the form of a succession of repeating neural network modules. Typical RNNs will only have one Tanh layer in this recurring module, for example. LSTMs have a structure that resembles a chain, but the repeating module is built differently. There are four neural network layers instead of just one, and they interact in a very unique way. The memory cell and gates, which include the forget gate as well as the input gate, are the two most important parts of the LSTM. The input and forget gates regulate the inner contents of the memory cell. The contents of the memory cell would not change between the one-time step and the next gradients, assuming both segues are closed. Information may be retained over a large number of time steps thanks to gating structures, which also enable groups of information to flow across a large number of time steps. This enables the LSTM model to effectively deal with the vanishing gradient

```
Layer (type)                 Output Shape              Param #
=================================================================
lstm_35 (LSTM)               (None, 1, 256)            1737728
_________________________________________________________________
lstm_36 (LSTM)               (None, 1, 256)            525312
_________________________________________________________________
lstm_37 (LSTM)               (None, 1, 256)            525312
_________________________________________________________________
lstm_38 (LSTM)               (None, 1, 256)            525312
_________________________________________________________________
lstm_39 (LSTM)               (None, 128)               197120
_________________________________________________________________
dense_7 (Dense)              (None, 1)                 129
=================================================================
Total params: 3,510,913
Trainable params: 3,510,913
Non-trainable params: 0
```

Fig. 4 Summary of the LSTM model used in the implementation

issue that most recurrent neural network models experience. Figure 4 demonstrates the summary of the LSTM model used in the implementation.

3.3 *Experimental Setup*

With an average actigraph recording period of 12.7 days (SD = 2.8, range 5–18 days) and an average age of 42.8 years, the condition group of the experiment consists of 10 girls and 13 males. The mean MADRS score ranged from 22.7 (SD = 4.8) at the start of recordings to 20.0 (SD = 4.7) by the conclusion. Eight people were found to have bipolar disorder, while fifteen people had unipolar depression. The control group, with an average actigraph wear time of 12.6 days (SD = 3.3) and with a mean age of 38.2 (SD = 13), with involvement of 20 females and 12 males. Table 1 presents the characteristics of the experiment's data. For ML algorithms to effectively capture the important information in the original dataset, statistical features must be extracted from raw data files and reduced to a manageable amount of variables. The statistical features that were recovered for this experiment were the mean of the activity, the associated standard deviation (SD), and the fraction of minutes with the activity level as zero. Each participant's pre-normalized features from each day were utilized to get the mean values.

It is believed that the dataset accurately represents clinical data from real-world situations despite its imbalance, which includes 291 depressed and 402 non-depressed instances. Because ML algorithms tend to work better for the class that is better represented, we investigated two different class balance solutions. Oversampling is one of the two techniques used, and under-sampling is the other. Oversampling, which generates new synthetic samples at random from relevant

Table 1 Characteristics of the data considered for the experimentation

Parameter		Condition group (Depressed patients)	Control group (Healthy people)
No. of people		23	32
Gender	Male	13	12
	Female	10	20
Age	Mean	42.8	38.2
	SD	11.0	13
Total no of days tracked		291	402
Days in actigraph tracking	Mean	12.7	12.6
	SD	2.8	2.3
Label	Unipolar	15	–
	Bipolar	8	–
MADRS at start	Mean	22.7	–
	SD	4.8	–
MADRS at end	Mean	20.0	–
	SD	4.7	–
Mean activity	Mean	190.05	286.59
	SD	81.44	81.10
Proportion of zeros	Mean	0.385	0.299
	SD	0.154	0.086

neighboring areas, uses the SMOTE technique. SMOTE mixes minority instances that currently exist to produce new minority instances. It applies linear interpolation to produce additional instances for the minority class. These synthetic training records are picked at random from the k-nearest neighbors for every instance in the minority class. The NearMiss strategy is one of several under-sampling techniques that aim to balance the class distribution by arbitrarily deleting instances of the majority class. If the instances of two distinct classes are reasonably similar to one another, remove the instances of the majority class to increase the separation between the two classes. Additionally, we evaluated the effectiveness of four different machine learning classifiers: Logistic Regression, SVM, XGBoost, and Random Forest. Among the chosen techniques, XGBoost and random forest are ensemble methods, whereas logistic regression and SVM are conventional algorithms.

3.4 ML Model Hyperparameter Tuning

The hyperparameters to be tuned for the LR algorithm are four parameters for achieving the valid reasons which are the regularization parameter, regularization type, an algorithm to use in the optimization problem, and the maximum number of iterations taken for the solvers to converge. Regularization is an adjustment to a learning algorithm that aims to lower its generalization error without affecting the training error. As part of experimentation, in logistic regression, L2 regularization with a regularization parameter value of one is used. The parameter solver gives the option to select the solver algorithm for optimization. The solver algorithm used in the experimentation is LBFGS which represents BFGS with restricted RAM. This solver is more computationally efficient because it just computes an approximate value of the Hessian based on the gradient. However, because it consumes less memory than a standard BFG, it discards older gradients and only accumulates newer gradients to the extent permitted by the memory restriction. The number of iterations taken by the solver for convergence is 100.

The performance of the SVM algorithm depends on only three hyperparameters which are the regularization parameter, Kernel type, and coefficient. In the experimentation, the scale kernel coefficient which is used to scale the input data to a feature before applying it to the kernel function is used. The linear kernel function is used to transform the data with a regularization parameter value of one.

XGBoost algorithm performance is subject to the parameters no.of trees, step size shrinkage used to prevent overfitting, loss function to be optimized, function to estimate the quality of a split, and Maximum limit for depth of each tree. The number of trees constructed in the experimentation is 75. To prevent the overfitting of the constructed trees, the learning rate is tuned as 0.01 with log_loss function as the loss function for optimization, friedman_mse is used for finding the best split in the process of tree construction, and the max limit for depth of the tree is set as 3.

The hyperparameters to be adjusted for the RF algorithm are a count of trees in the forest, a metric used to estimate the quality of a split, the number of samples required at least to split an internal node, samples required at the place a leaf node, and features to be considered for the best split. 75 trees are constructed in the random forest algorithm. The number of samples plays a major role to expand a tree at any particular node. The minimum number of samples is taken as two in the experimentation, and to check the quality of splitting, Gini index measure is used. At most one sample is only required to place a leaf node by stopping the tree expansion process. The square root function is used for the total features to decide the max limit for the features to be considered at every node of the tree while selecting the best feature for splitting.

A rectified linear unit (ReLU) served as the activation function for the 10 completely connected hidden layers that made up the DNN architecture. Dropout is used with p as 0.5 after each layer, and the final layer has two units with a softmax activation function. Adam solver is used to optimize the weights with a batch size of 32 and a learning rate of 0.001. The hyperparameters of LSTM are loss, optimizer, epochs, learning rate, and batch size. The batch size is taken as 128 with a learning rate of 0.001. The binary cross-entropy loss function is used for error calculation, and the Adam optimizer is used for optimizing the weights. LSTM is implemented with 50 epochs.

3.5 Evaluation Metrics

Since the objective of the machine learning algorithms is to categorize instances as depressed mood cases or controls, the results were provided in measures of accuracy. Accuracy is the percentage of cases in the dataset with the right classification. Specificity is the proportion of controls properly classified as controls, whereas sensitivity is the percentage of appropriately classified conditions among all conditions. The harmonic mean of sensitivity and specificity is known as the F1-score. The weighted recall is a calculation that equalizes sensitivity and specificity based on sample sizes. The Predicted Positive Rate (PPR) and Predicted Negative Rate (PNR) show how many conditions (positive) or controls have been correctly classified in comparison to how many have been incorrectly classified (negative). An estimation known as weighted precision combines the predicted values based on sample sizes. Since accuracy does not take the dataset's imbalance into account when presenting results, it may offer results that are not accurate. When datasets are unbalanced, the Matthews Correlation Coefficient (MCC) is used to assess the classifiers' overall performance. In MCC, the coefficient value ranges from minus one to one, with zero denoting a random approximation.

If we consider TD: True depressed (depressed cases labeled correctly as depressive) FC: False control (depressed cases labeled as healthy cases) TC: True control (healthy cases labeled correctly as healthy FD: False depressed (healthy cases mislabeled as depressed cases), the performance metrics are defined as
Accuracy: (TD + TC) / (TD + TC + FD + FC)
Sensitivity: TD / (TD + FC)
Specificity: TC / (TC + FD)
F1-score: (2*Weighted_Precision*Weighted_Recall)/(Weighted_Precision + Weighted_Recall)
Weighted recall: (sensitivity x (TD + FC)) + (specificity x (TC + FD)) / (TD + FC + TC + FD)
Weighted precision: (PPV x (TD + FC)) + (NPV x (TC + FD)) / (TD + FC + TC + FD)
PNR: TC / (TC + FC)
PPR: TD / (TD + FD)

4 Results and Discussion

The demonstrations in Table 2 are the results of the ML algorithms experimentation. For every algorithm, three runs were done. Baseline is the algorithm implementation with the original dataset, SMOTE is the algorithm implementation with oversampling techniques to balance the dataset, and NearMiss is the algorithm implementation with the under-sampling technique for getting the balanced dataset.

As part of the conventional techniques of machine learning, SVM gives good results for identifying the depressed condition, SVM got 89.93% accuracy, 90.56% sensitivity, 88.64% specificity, and 92.32% F1-Score. SVM implementation with

SMOTE oversampling technique gives better for all the parameters except weighted precision and PPR. SVM with NearMiss under the sampling technique achieves 96.85% and 93.79% for weighted precision and PPR, respectively. SVM attains good results compared to logistic regression for Matthews Correlation Coefficient also which are 77.82%, 85.64%, and 82.03% for original, SMOTE, and NearMiss implementations, respectively.

The best performance algorithm as part of ensemble machine learning algorithms experimentation is RF with an accuracy of 94.17% on the original dataset, 95.99% with SMOTE oversampling technique, and 93.57% with the NearMiss under-sampling technique. The parameter sensitivity is highest for the XGBoost algorithm which is 92.84%, 95.44%, and 94.43% for original, SMOTE, and NearMiss implementations, respectively. Specificity is highest for random forest algorithm with 97.67%, 97.49%, and 91.6% for original, SMOTE, and NearMiss implementations, respectively. F1-score and predicted negative rate are high for the XGBoost algorithm while the remaining measures are high for the RF algorithm. In the case of Matthews Correlation Coefficient, XGBoost performance is high with 86.48%, 92.55%, and 87.83% correlation coefficient values for the original dataset, SMOTE, and NearMiss techniques, respectively.

Among the deep learning models implemented, DNN got 94.66%, 96.74%, and 94.26% of accuracy for baseline, SMOTE, and NearMiss implementations, respectively. The weighted precision is calculated as 99.46%, 88.44%, and 99.13% for

Table 2 Experimental results of ML algorithms

ML model	Class balancing	Classification results								
		Acc	Sen	Spe	F1-score	W_ recall	W_ precision	PNR	PPR	MCC
LR	Baseline	0.885	0.897	0.862	0.918	0.885	0.953	0.809	0.928	0.748
	SMOTE	0.926	0.938	0.914	0.942	0.926	0.958	0.940	0.912	0.853
	NearMiss	0.881	0.870	0.894	0.914	0.881	0.949	0.863	0.900	0.763
SVM	Baseline	0.899	0.905	0.886	0.929	0.899	0.961	0.823	0.941	0.778
	SMOTE	0.928	0.922	0.933	0.947	0.928	0.967	0.921	0.934	0.856
	NearMiss	0.909	0.888	0.933	0.938	0.909	0.968	0.880	0.937	0.820
XGBoost	Baseline	0.938	0.928	0.958	0.961	0.938	0.987	0.863	0.979	0.864
	SMOTE	0.962	0.954	0.971	0.974	0.962	0.986	0.953	0.972	0.925
	NearMiss	0.939	0.944	0.934	0.953	0.939	0.968	0.943	0.934	0.878
RF	Baseline	0.941	0.925	0.976	0.966	0.941	0.993	0.857	0.988	0.873
	SMOTE	0.959	0.945	0.974	0.973	0.959	0.988	0.943	0.975	0.920
	NearMiss	0.935	0.956	0.916	0.947	0.935	0.960	0.957	0.913	0.872
DNN	Baseline	0.946	0.930	0.980	0.970	0.946	0.990	0.867	0.994	0.884
	SMOTE	0.967	0.954	0.980	0.979	0.967	0.981	0.953	0.991	0.935
	NearMiss	0.942	0.963	0.922	0.952	0.942	0.920	0.964	0.963	0.886
LSTM	Baseline	0.953	0.937	0.988	0.975	0.953	0.994	0.881	0.997	0.900
	SMOTE	0.975	0.963	0.988	0.985	0.975	0.988	0.962	0.995	0.951
	NearMiss	0.956	0.981	0.933	0.962	0.956	0.931	0.982	0.968	0.914

baseline, SMOTE, and NearMiss implementations, respectively. The Matthews Correlation Coefficient is calculated as 93.51% for baseline, 96.35% for SMOTE, and 88.62% for NearMiss sampling techniques. LSTM got 95.39%, 97.57%, and 95.65% accuracy, respectively, for baseline, SMOTE, and NearMiss implementations. PPR is attained highest in the calculated parameters which are 99.43%, 98.88%, and 93.10%, respectively, for the three implementations. The specificity is exhibited as 98.85%, 98.85%, and 93.33%, respectively, and Matthews Correlation Coefficient is exhibited as 90.04%, 95.18%, and 91.43%, respectively, for the three experiments of baseline, SMOTE, and NearMiss techniques.

Some employ more subtle techniques, such as the one presented by Amanant et al. [48], who suggested using LSTM to forecast depression from language, semantics, and textual data. 99.0% accuracy is attained by the suggested framework. While Kour [49] projected an integrated model for depression detection utilizing CNN and biLSTM and achieved a 99.28% accuracy on standard tweets including depressive symptoms. According to the findings, there is a significant difference in the language representation of depressive and non-depressive data. Nearly everyone uses portable gadgets daily these days. Undoubtedly, the bodily motions we perform during the day are one trait that distinguishes humans. It is possible to think of this as motor activity, which is not more than recurrent social rhythms interacting with biological tempos and being controlled by the 24-h circadian clock interlaced with countless 2–6 h cycles [22]. Significant signs of mood disruption may be present if these biological rhythmic rhythms are out of balance [50]. Actigraphs, which typically record gravity acceleration units using a bracelet, are noninvasive devices that can track human activity and rest cycles. The actigraph is the tool that has been employed for the data gathering of motor activity.

In a review of studies employing EEG data to identify the two types of depression, major depressive disorder (MDD) and bipolar disorder (BD), Yasin et al. [51] used neural network and deep learning algorithms. It searched for publications that have been published over the past 10 years using a variety of source engines and a blend of different keywords, then retrieved some helpful information from those. This review's inclusion of many categories for exploited datasets, techniques for extracting features, and algorithms in publications was one of its strong qualities. The main issue in this research, especially for MMD diagnosis, was that there weren't enough articles to review; as a result, it only used about five, as claimed. Additionally, the articles that were used to support them did not adequately explain how to understand the gist of their operation.

The reviewed studies by [52] were focused on used deep learning techniques to investigate mental disorders, with depression as one of the topics, to better understand them. The four primary categories of this study were using social media data to predict the likelihood of psychological illness, using clinical data to detect mental illness, using genetic data to diagnose disease, and assessing other datasets. The electroencephalogram dataset type was only used in three papers that were specifically concerned with the identification or prognosis of depression among the selected papers that were published up through April 2019 that made use of various types of datasets. In this study, all of the analyzed datasets were fully represented. Additionally, it went into great detail on the potential and difficulties that using each dataset is likely to present. However, because it was a thorough review that focused on embracing a variety of mental disease situations, it briefly discussed a few studies on utilizing deep learning for EEG signal analysis to diagnose and forecast depression.

Khosla et al. [53] conducted a study of studies that were centered on EEG signals and other models to diagnose neurological conditions, like depression, and monitor other issues of emotion recognition. Only four papers were from an earlier period, and the majority of the papers were published between 1999 and 2019. They were obtained from a variety of sources, including journals, conferences, books, and theses. Only a few ten publications were taken into consideration in terms of the diagnosis of depression. It also included knowledge of functional neuroimaging methods. But because it covered a wide range of topics, it was unable to give each topic the attention it deserved.

5 Conclusion

The work in this article is an analysis of motor activity data for unipolar and bipolar depression classification using motor activity recordings of 23 unipolar & bipolar depression patients with 32 controls. The classification is performed using traditional machine learning, ensemble machine learning, and deep learning algorithms as well. Compared to the traditional machine learning algorithms, ensemble learning algorithms XGBoost and random forest are efficient in classifying depression disorders with actigraph data. In deep learning, LSTM and DNN are used for detecting depressive disorder. LSTM achieves good results compared to the deep neural network as it is having memory storage which is the main component while analyzing the time series data. The used machine learning and deep learning algorithms in this article are not considering non-depressive causes of reduced activity, such as injury, illness, old age, etc. These parameters also play a major role in the reduction of the activity data. Social media analysis also has been successfully investigated separately to predict depression in users based on their conversations and sharing of posts, in the future more technologically sophisticated models based on motor activity counts mixed with the subject's physical illness and social media postings can be created to accurately predict depression.

Conflicts of Interest No author has any conflicts of interest

References

1. Fisher J, de Mello MC, Patel V, Rahman A, Tran T, Holton S, Holmes W. Prevalence and determinants of common perinatal mental disorders in women in low-and lower-middle-income countries: a systematic review. Bull World Health Organ. 2012;90:139–49.

2. Navarro-Loli JS, Moscoso M. La investigación de la depresiónenadolescentesen el Perú: unarevisiónsistemática. Liberabit. 2017;23(1):57–74.
3. Cooper J, Nusslock R, Craske M, Zinbarg R, Chat IKY, Barch D, Reddy F, Green M, Horan W, Treadway M. 47. Computational models of effort-based choice in patients with major depression and schizophrenia. Biol Psychiatry. 2018;83:S19.
4. Foo JC, Redler S, Forstner AJ, Basmanav FB, Pethukova L, Guo J, Streit F, et al. Exploring the overlap between alopecia Areata and major depressive disorder: epidemiological and genetic perspectives. J Eur Acad Dermatol Venereol. 2023;37:1547.
5. Mehta S, GerasimosKonstantinou CR, Weissman ZJ, Daskalakis DV, Downar J, Mulsant BH, Blumberger DM. The effect of repetitive transcranial magnetic stimulation on suicidal ideation in treatment-resistant depression: a meta-analysis. J Clin Psychiatry. 2022;83(2):39202.
6. Sedano-Capdevila A, Porras-Segovia A, Bello HJ, Baca-Garcia E, Barrigon ML. Use of ecological momentary assessment to study suicidal thoughts and behavior: a systematic review. Curr Psychiatry Rep. 2021;23(7):41.
7. Seppälä J, De Vita I, TimoJämsä JM, MattiIsohanni KR, Feldman Y, et al. Mobile phone and wearable sensor-based mHealth approaches for psychiatric disorders and symptoms: systematic review. JMIR mental health. 2019;6(2):e9819.
8. Firth J, Torous J, Nicholas J, Carney R, Rosenbaum S, Sarris J. Can smartphone mental health interventions reduce symptoms of anxiety? A meta-analysis of randomized controlled trials. J Affect Disord. 2017;218:15–22.
9. Huckvale K, Nicholas J, Torous J, Larsen ME. Smartphone apps for the treatment of mental health conditions: status and considerations. Curr Opin Psychol. 2020;36:65–70.
10. Bayındır L. A survey of people-centric sensing studies utilizing mobile phone sensors. J Ambient Intell Smart Environ. 2017;9:421–48.
11. Nilsson MY, Andersson S, Magnusson L, Hanson E. Ambient assisted living technology-mediated interventions for older people and their informal carers in the context of healthy ageing: a scoping review. Health science reports. 2021;4(1):e225.
12. Berle JO, Hauge ER, Oedegaard KJ, Holsten F, Fasmer OB. Actigraphic registration of motor activity reveals a more structured behavioural pattern in schizophrenia than in major depression. BMC Res Notes. 2010;3:149.
13. Huguet A, Rao S, McGrath PJ, Wozney L, Wheaton M, Conrod J, Rozario S. A systematic review of cognitive behavioral therapy and behavioral activation apps for depression. PLoS One. 2016;11:e0154248.
14. Mohr DC, Zhang M, Schueller SM. Personal sensing: understanding mental health using ubiquitous sensors and machine learning. Annu Rev Clin Psychol. 2017;13:23–47.
15. Guntuku SC, Yaden DB, Kern ML, Ungar LH, Eichstaedt JC. Detecting depression and mental illness on social media: an integrative review. Curr OpinBehav Sci. 2017;18:43–9.
16. Kolosnjaji B, Eckert C. Neural network-based user-independent physical activity recognition for mobile devices. International Conference on Intelligent Data Engineering and Automated Learning. Springer; 2015.
17. Inoue M, Inoue S, Nishida T. Deep recurrent neural network for mobile human activity recognition with high throughput. Artificial Life and Robotics. 2018;23(2):173–85.
18. Bzdok D, Ioannidis JPA. Exploration, inference, and prediction in neuroscience and biomedicine. Trends Neurosci. 2019;42:251.
19. Huys QJM, Maia TV, Frank MJ. Computational psychiatry as a bridge from neuroscience to clinical applications. Nat Neurosci. 2016;19(3):404–13.
20. Sabelli HC, Carlson-Sabelli L, Javaid JI. The thermodynamics of bipolarity: a bifurcation model of bipolar illness and bipolar character and its psychotherapeutic applications. Psychiatry. 1990;53(4):346–68.
21. Adhikari SP. Factor analysis study of phenomenological subtypes of mania. Ann Psychiatr Clin Neurosci. 2019;2(1):1009.
22. Bourguignon C, Storch K-F. Control of Rest: Activity by a Dopaminergic Ultradian Oscillator and the Circadian Clock. Front Neurol. 2017;8:614.

23. Pathak J, Wikner A, Fussell R, Chandra S, Hunt BR, Girvan M, et al. Hybrid forecasting of chaotic processes: Using machine learning in conjunction with a knowledge-based model. Chaos: An Interdisciplinary. J Nonlinear Sci. 2018;28(4):041101.
24. Smys S, Raj JS. Analysis of deep learning techniques for early detection of depression on social media network—a comparative study. J Trends Comput Sci Smart Technol (TCSST). 2021;3:24–39.
25. Orabi AH, Buddhitha P, Orabi MH, Inkpen D. Deep learning for depression detection of twitter users. In: Proceedings of the Fifth Workshop on Computational Linguistics and Clinical Psychology: From Keyboard to Clinic, vol. 5. New Orleans, LA; 2018. p. 88–97.
26. Kim J, Lee D, Park E. Machine learning for mental health in social media: bibliometric study. J Med Internet Res. 2021;23:e24870.
27. Wongkoblap A, Vadillo M, Curcin V. Depression detection of twitter posters using deep learning with anaphora resolution: algorithm development and validation. JMIR Ment Health. 2021; https://kclpure.kcl.ac.uk/portal/en/publications/depression-detection-of-twitter-posters-using-deep-learning-with-anaphora-resolution-algorithm-development-and-validation(1b1ef794-5c96-4890-a0a2-04bf74323540).html
28. Un Nisa Q, Muhammad R. Towards transfer learning using BERT for early detection of self-harm of social media users. In: Proceedings of the Working Notes of CLEF 2021—Conference and Labs of the Evaluation Forum. Bucharest, Romania; 2021. p. 21–4.
29. Chiong R, Budhi GS, Dhakal S. Combining sentiment lexicons and content-based features for depression detection. IEEE Intell Syst. 2021;36:99–105.
30. Fujita, H.; Selamat, A.; Lin, J.C.W.; Ali, M. Advances and trends in artificial intelligence: from theory to practice: 34th international conference on industrial, engineering and other applications of applied intelligent systems, IEA/AIE 2021, Kuala Lumpur, Malaysia, 26–29, 2021.: Proceedings, Part II.
31. Ibitoye AO, Famutimi RF, Olanloye DO, Akioyamen E. User centric social opinion and clinical Behavioural model for depression detection. Int J Intell Inf Syst. 2021;10:69.
32. Trifan A, Antunes R, Matos S, Oliveira JL. Understanding depression from psycholinguistic patterns in social media texts. Adv Inf Retr. 2020;12036:402–9.
33. Mathur P, Sawhney R, Chopra S, Leekha M, Shah RR. Utilizing temporal psycholinguistic cues for suicidal intent estimation. Adv Inf Retr. 2020;12036:265–71.
34. Lin L, Chen X, Shen Y, Zhang L. Towards automatic depression detection: a BiLSTM/1d CNN-based model. Appl Sci. 2020;10(23):1–20. https://doi.org/10.3390/app10238701.
35. Wang Z, Chen L, Wang L, Diao G. Recognition of audio depression based on convolutional neural network and generative antagonism network model. IEEE Access. 2020;8:101181–91. https://doi.org/10.1109/ACCESS.2020.2998532.
36. Ma X, Yang H, Chen Q, Huang D, Wang Y. DepAudioNet: an efficient deep model for audio based depression classification. In: AVEC 2016 - Proc. 6th Int. Work. Audio/Visual Emot. Challenge. ACM Multimed; 2016. p. 35–42. https://doi.org/10.1145/2988257.2988267.
37. Le H-N, Boyd RC. Prevention of major depression: early detection and early intervention in the general. Population. 2022;2006:23.
38. Alghamdi NS, Hosni Mahmoud HA, Abraham A, Alanazi SA, García-Hern'andez L. Predicting depression symptoms in an Arabic psychological forum. IEEE Access. 2020;8:57317–34. https://doi.org/10.1109/ACCESS.2020.2981834.
39. Babu NV, Kanaga EGM. Sentiment analysis in social media data for depression detection using artificial intelligence: a review. SN Comput Sci. 2022;3(1):1–20. https://doi.org/10.1007/s42979-021-00958-1.
40. Alhanai T, Ghassemi M, Glass J. Detecting depression with audio/text sequence modeling of interviews. In: Proc. Annu. Conf. Int. Speech Commun.Assoc. INTERSPEECH; 2018. p. 1716–20. https://doi.org/10.21437/Interspeech.2018-2522.
41. Yang L, Pei E, Jiang D, Oveneke MC, Xia X, Sahli H. Multimodal measurement of depression using deep learning models. In: AVEC 2017—proc. 7th Annu. Work.Audio/visual Emot.

Challenge. 2017. pp. 53–54. https://doi.org/10.1145/3133944.3133948. Co-located with MM 2017, no. January 2018.
42. Lam G, Dongyan H, Lin W, City S. Context-aware deep learning for multi-modal depression detection. In: ICASSP 2019-2019 IEEE international conference on acoustics, speech and signal processing (ICASSP). IEEE; 2019. p. 3946–50.
43. Yang L, Jiang D, Sahli H. Integrating deep and shallow models for multi-modal depression analysis-hybrid architectures. IEEE Trans Affect Comput. 2021;12(1):239–53. https://doi.org/10.1109/TAFFC.2018.2870398.
44. Yang L, Jiang D, He L, Pei E, Oveneke MC, Sahli H. Decision tree based depression classification from audio video and language information. In: AVEC 2016 - Proc. 6th Int. Work. Audio/Visual Emot.Challenge. ACM Multimed; 2016. p. 89–96. https://doi.org/10.1145/2988257.2988269.
45. Yokoya S, Maeno T, Sakamoto N, Goto R, Maeno T. A brief survey of public knowledge and stigma towards depression. J Clin Med Res. 2018;10(3):202–9. https://doi.org/10.14740/jocmr3282w.
46. Garcia-Ceja E, Riegler M, PetterJakobsen JT, Nordgreen T, Oedegaard KJ, BerntFasmer O. Depresjon: a motor activity database of depression episodes in unipolar and bipolar patients. In: Proceedings of the 9th ACM multimedia systems conference; 2018. p. 472–7.
47. Montgomery SA, Asberg MARIE. A new depression scale designed to be sensitive to change. Br J Psychiatry. 1979;134(4):382–9.
48. Amanat A, Rizwan M, Javed AR, Abdelhaq M, Alsaqour R, Pandya S, Uddin M. Deep learning for depression Detection from textual data. Electronics. 2022;11:676.
49. Kour H, Gupta MK. An hybrid deep learning approach for depression prediction from user tweets using feature-rich CNN and bi-directional LSTM. Multimed Tools Appl. 2022;81:23649–23685.
50. Alloy LB, Ng TH, Titone MK, Boland EM. Circadian rhythm dysregulation in bipolar Spectrum disorders. Curr Psychiatry Rep. 2017;19:1–10.
51. Yasin S, Hussain SA, Aslan S, Raza I, Muzammel M, Othmani A. EEG based major depressive disorder and bipolar disorder detection using neural networks: a review. Comput Methods Prog Biomed. 2021;106007:106007. https://doi.org/10.1016/j.cmpb.2021.106007.
52. Su C, Xu Z, Pathak J, Wang F. Deep learning in mental health outcome research: a scoping review. Transl Psychiatry. 2020;10(1):1–26. https://doi.org/10.1038/s41398-020-0780-3.
53. Khosla A, Khandnor P, Chand T. A comparative analysis of signal processing and classification methods for different applications based on EEG signals.Biocybernet. Biomed Eng. 2020;40(2):649–90.

Intelligent Monitoring System Based on ATmega Microcontrollers in Healthcare with Stress Reduce Effect

Z. Abdiakhmetova, Zh. Temirbekova, and G. Turken

Abstract Ensuring the well-being of individuals is a crucial responsibility in today's society. The Medical Internet of Things (MIoT) plays a significant role in the field of medicine and healthcare. This research aimed to create a patient monitoring system using sensors and Arduino boards, combining both hardware and software components. The system utilized three primary sensors to collect and promptly transmit the patient's health data to a central server via the network. Whenever any abnormal data was detected, the system promptly notified the doctor with an alarm message. To check the convenience and importance of the developed system for patients, tests have currently been carried out on 150 patients. Patient data was collected in the form of a dataset with various characteristics, such as age, gender, place of residence (region), hemoglobin concentration, red blood cell count, and other data obtained during the last visit to the doctor, as well as data received daily from Arduino sensors. The effectiveness of this system was evaluated, 85% of the patients surveyed were satisfied with such a system, 7% of the test subjects were not completely satisfied, and the rest ignored the survey. The adequacy and accuracy of predicting CVD were also assessed. The convenience and simplicity of the developed system have won the hearts of patients. Respondents believe that the system is less stress resistant and more reliable. Using data in the intelligence part of the system can predict the development of cardiovascular disease and fully illustrate the progress of the disease, but more detailed research is still needed.

Keywords Intelligent system · Stress reduce · ATmega · Microcontrollers · Monitoring

---

Z. Abdiakhmetova (✉) · Zh. Temirbekova · G. Turken
Faculty of Information Technology, al-Farabi Kazakh National University, Almaty, Kazakhstan

G. Battineni et al. (eds.), *Computational Methods in Psychiatry*, https://doi.org/10.1007/978-981-99-6637-0_3

1 Introduction

Currently, in our country, there is a negative trend in the state of health of the population. The growth of life expectancy has almost negative trends, the birth rate does not justify the expected forecasts of scientists, and high mortality rates do not change from year to year. Recently, it is important to note the increase in the incidence of the population both as a result of quarantine and as a lack of a healthy lifestyle, not to mention medical examinations and monitoring the health of patients. This and other factors such as smoking, air pollution, and untimely access to doctors, are threatening factors for human health, that is, the entire future of the country and even the whole nation remain at risk.

Health issues are the foundation of global development. Healthy communities make society more stable and the economy more prosperous, but for healthy communities to be fully functional, we must ensure that everyone has the ability to afford and have fair access to high-quality health services with the help of advanced technologies, the issue of monitoring the condition of patients, which is the main one in the world health program, will always be relevant. For this reason, the improvement of patient monitoring devices is a very important topic in both healthcare and information technology [1–3].

The concept of the Medical and Health Internet of Things emerged during a time of escalating global medical expenses, leading to its swift adoption within the medical and health industry. In 2017, the world's healthcare expenditure reached approximately US $77.8 trillion, making up around 10% of the global GDP for that year. Between 2000 and 2017, the average growth rate of global medical and health expenses was 3.9%, surpassing the 3% average growth rate of the global GDP during the same period. In 2015, a study conducted by Goldman Sachs revealed that the Internet of Things for Medical and Health had the potential to significantly boost revenue and lower costs, with the potential to save the United States over 300 billion U.S. dollars annually in medical expenses. However, achieving this benefit depends on effectively transforming the vast data generated by millions of medical and health IoT devices into practical insights [4–6].

As computing power continues to advance and wireless technology becomes more compact, the Internet of Things (IoT) has evolved from a mere concept to a tangible reality, opening up diverse application scenarios. The development of innovative IoT medical equipment has greatly emphasized the crucial role of IoT technology in the medical and health industry. The increased connectivity of IoT has allowed for its implementation across various medical device categories, resulting in a substantial rise in the number of medical devices incorporating IoT capabilities. Consequently, this surge in IoT medical devices has driven advancements in sensors, IoT networks, service systems, and software to facilitate the collection and transmission of medical-grade data. As a result, a seamless integration between IoT medical devices and medical and health IT systems has been established through the Internet of Things, enabling continuous and automated transmission of medical data. This amalgamation of IoT and healthcare IT systems is known as the MIoT or smart medical care.

The IoT in the medical and health sector refers to the incorporation of various IoT-related technologies like sensors, short-range communications, the Internet, cloud computing, big data, artificial intelligence [7, 8], etc., with medical and health technologies. The goal is to create a comprehensive network that to connects doctors, health managers, residents, patients, medical devices, medicines, the environment, and other factors to facilitate automatic identification, positioning, data collection, tracking, management, and sharing of medical information. This integration aims to enhance the medical and health industry by providing comprehensive information, improving service efficiency, and enabling intelligent medical and health services centered around patients. Advancements in technology have led to the concept of gathering a patient's vital sign without requiring them to physically visit a hospital [9]. Health care monitoring systems play a crucial role in monitoring a patient's health parameters. Researchers developing health monitoring systems using different hardware platforms achieve the integration of various biomedical sensors, such as temperature and heart rate sensors, into a single system on a chip [10, 11]. This system continuously monitors the patient's heart rate and temperature readings.

The proposed study involves an intelligent system comprising multiple devices controlled by a microcontroller to monitor the patient's condition through various sensors, such as heart rate, blood pressure, and temperature sensors. This system ensures accurate signal readings, high efficiency, and faster processing. The collected signals are sent to the doctor via SMS to assess the patient's emergency status. The system, utilizing ATmega 16, has been successfully tested, confirming that each sensor effectively displays the patient's emergency situation, facilitating appropriate treatment.

Previously, numerous authors explored this concept using various methods [12]. Our developed system introduces a novel approach to healthcare monitoring by employing a volume oscillometric method and sensor network for continuous blood pressure and temperature measurement. The data is displayed on two seven-segment modules, offering better visibility. Additionally, the system allows setting upper and lower limits for temperature and heart rate. If the temperature exceeds the upper limit or falls below the lower limit, the buzzer sounds, and the load is turned off. Similarly, if the heartbeat sensor is disconnected, and the system detects a low heartbeat, the buzzer activates, and the load is switched off. This buzzer serves as an emergency signal for the patient's well-wishers. When the temperature and heart rate are within control, the bulb turns on, and the alarm deactivates.

In recent years, the healthcare industry has rapidly developed in terms of IoT technology. IoT can be utilized to track patient care and requirements effectively. Although IoT has various applications in healthcare, maintaining a high level of security is crucial. Applications include remote monitoring, integration of smart sensors and medical devices, activity trackers, wearable biometric sensors, blood glucose monitors, prescription dispensers, and smart beds. The Internet of IoMT is used to enhance patient diagnosis and treatment, with medical equipment companies developing connected devices for improved patient outcomes. IoT implementation can boost patient satisfaction and engagement by streamlining workflows, providing clarity for patient releases, and facilitating better communication between patients and doctors, as vital information can be easily transmitted through connected devices.

Support the use of connected devices to remotely monitor chronic disease patients with persistent diseases can benefit from remote examinations, mainly by using appropriate wearable clinical equipment. Patients who experience relapses of cardiovascular diseases can be provided with devices with the ability to inform the attending physician about the occurrence of the disease. Such devices will make it possible to plan places in hospitals in advance and treat patients using online recommendations. Such systems are able to monitor the work of medical personnel online, as well as the condition of patients. Improved versions of such systems can reduce costs and thus affect the economy of the whole country.

It is important to consider prevention as one of the main and major areas, since based on it, you can control the next stages of treatment and detection of diseases. The medical history of each patient in a digital and correct format can be used to generate a correct lifestyle regimen and predict diseases. The use of Internet of Things technologies can contribute to the improvement of methods and methods of treatment. In the insurance industry, there is a problem for physicians in providing companies with documentation of measures taken to improve the health of patients.

Online monitoring of the condition of patients can really support to reduce the material costs that were intended for inpatient monitoring. The widespread introduction of monitoring devices can not only reduce costs, but also respond in time to a patient's problem. According to the World Health Organization, heart disease is the leading cause of death in patients around the world [13]. Diseases of the cardiovascular and circulatory system are also common causes of death in our country: it is 24.2% of cases, or in numbers it is 18.6 thousand people. Among them, about 7 thousand people died from coronary heart disease, more than 6 thousand people from cerebrovascular disease, and more than 530 people from arterial hypertension. Acute myocardial infarction and angina pectoris are also considered common causes of premature death. Such unsatisfactory statistics are reflected not only in the healthcare sector of the country, but also in the economic and sociological development of the country [14, 15].

In Russia in 2008–2009, cardiovascular diseases caused a significant scale-economic loss of 1 trillion rubles, which in those years was 3 percent of Russia's gross domestic product. Such a loss to the national economy justifies such large investments in prevention programs and research programs aimed at reducing cardiovascular diseases, which will inevitably lead to a decrease in early disability and mortality. Therefore, one of the important tasks of health care is the prevention of the disease, the prevention of its causes, early preclinical diagnosis, control, prevention, and offering a detailed treatment of this disease.

2 Research Background

Two sensors were used in the [16] study: one was a temperature sensor (LM35) and the other was a heart rate sensor (AD 8232). A study was conducted by connecting both sensors to an Arduino. The received data is used as input data to the Arduino device. In case of values exceed the threshold, a notification is sent to the patient's relatives, and this information is stored in the cloud. Summarizing the results of the research, the authors concluded that the advantage of this prototype is that if the patient forgets to tell the doctor or misrepresents certain information, the doctor can access the correct information at any time, from any location. But according to the authors, this is still a very simple prototype. It has yet to be converted into a nanoscale product that integrates all sensors into a single chip core.

Researchers of [10] article used a data monitoring system with five components for monitoring: Arduino MEGA, Wi-Fi module ESP8266–01, fingerprint sensor, ECG sensor, respiration sensor. According to the authors, the advantage of this system is that the user can access the fingerprint sensor only with his fingerprint to enter the application for viewing data, which means that the security aspect is also considered. The proposed by [1] microcontroller-based system used the option of administering a predetermined dose of anesthesia to the patient at equal time intervals. The anesthesia dose must be known in advance because the preset value is programmed as an input value. Components used in software development: Arduino Uno is used for full control, LM35 is for measuring degree of heating, cordial rate sensor, infusion pump with a stepper motor for controlling the movement of the syringe, L293D is needed to drive a DC motor, and LSD display (LM016L) parameters required to display status.

This system does not need the physical presence of a doctor, but nevertheless is not inferior in determining and evaluating the exact diagnosis of the patient. The author [2] believes that the system still needs improvement in solving complex problems. For example, for eight different inputs, several tests were run to monitor the speed of the system during processing. The conducted research shows that the accuracy shown by the Arduino system is comparatively much higher than other systems. Also in reliability when monitoring the length and delay of transmitted signals, Arduino shows good results.

The biggest advantage of using Arduino technology is the availability of open source. It is important to note the fact that Arduino is very accessible and there is a lot of supporting material on the Internet for working with this device. The authors refer to the fact that high speed and expensive analog devices cannot boast of other super features over Arduino. Perhaps these super devices can work milliseconds faster and more accurately.

The authors of the article [3] conducted research on the capabilities of microcontrollers and microcomputers. Conducted research by measuring ECG, pulse measurement, respiration measurement, EMG measurement, EEG measurement, bioimpedance measurement, skin temperature measurement, humidity determination, sweat analysis, and other biosignals using Arduino and Raspberry boards. According to the results of the research, the advantage of single printed circuit boards when measuring signals is their convenience. That is, it allows us to make measurements that take a long time without disturbing the patient's comfort. According to the authors, the convenience of using microcontrollers and microcomputers is high, especially when it is necessary to collect certain data for a long time and to approve treatment measures based on it. But, according to the authors, in terms of low computing power and memory of single-circuit boards, disadvantages may be observed when compared with laptops and computers of the latest model.

In the proposed system of [9], an Arduino Uno-based system is used to administer the drug that controls the amount of anesthesia administered to the patient. The amount of anesthesia must be known in advance, that is, it is given as an input parameter for anesthesia control. And the Arduino Uno can be programmed to adjust this anesthesia dose. According to the results of the article, this system is very useful for anesthesiologists who monitor certain parameters of the patient and regulate anesthesia. The authors of this article [12] worked on a prototype consisting of a user interface, a control system, a central controller, and sensors. As a result, a health monitoring system that reads the frequency of pulse and body temperature has been successfully developed.

But, according to the authors, the main obstacle of this system is its cost. Implementation of the system is likely to suffer if a person is not motivated to manage their own health. Because the system is highly dependent on wide-area wireless communication infrastructure, access to the system is low in rural areas. In addition, the transmission or reception of this sensitive data over telecommunications networks may pose an information security problem. The authors of the article [13] studied a patient monitoring system consisting of Arduino Uno, temperature sensors, arterial sensor, pressure, heart rate sensor, motion sensors, buzzer, Bluetooth, Android phone, and power supply. According to the results of the study, the advantages of the system are that the system allows doctors to monitor the patient on the spot, monitor his vitals, and give them advice on first aid.

The authors of the article [17] used the Arduino Nano, programmed in Java, to control the servo motor as a research object. Thus, it was possible to perform operations written on Arduino without the help of any circuitry. The authors designed the robot in such a way that it can imitate the activity of a real human hand. The advantage of the robotic hand is that it allows a person to feel the actions of a real hand. However, instead of manually grounding the high-voltage system with the help of a robot-manipulator, it was concluded that the automatic connection of the high-voltage system could be dangerous.

The project of the authors [18] offered tools for automating the process of anesthesia administration using a syringe mechanism and an infusion set mechanism. The proposed system is a working prototype of the anesthesia delivery system. Also, the system consists of a database containing dosage values of drugs for various modes of operation. The automated system is ideal for both patients and doctors. But according to the authors, the biggest drawback is that if the operation time is too long, for example, in 5 hours, if it is not possible to introduce the full dose of anesthesia in one dose, it can lead to the death of the patient. The authors [19] individually investigated the various sensors connected to the Arduino boards. Heart rate sensor, temperature sensor, and ESP8266 tools connected everything to Arduino Uno to complete the research.

Studies have shown that the results were most accurate when the heat measurement was in the armpit or in the mouth. And heart rate data could be most accurately obtained if the receptor was located on the patient's finger or ear midge. Daily monitoring of patient data using such a system could give a good accumulated experience of knowledge and dataset, for further use in various situations, especially it would be indispensable in a pandemic. It is also important to note that very simple devices were involved in this study, which would not cope with very complex diseases in which more data on the patient's condition is needed.

The system proposed by the authors in the research work [20] implemented a system with a high level of efficiency, which serves to monitor the patient's life-critical medical data. They compare the newly obtained data with the previous ones using sensors. Also, one of the most useful aspects based on the study of the authors is that when it sends the above information to the patient to the nearest hospital, a notification is sent based on his location. According to the authors, this is noted in the fact that the system needs to be improved by adding temperature and ECG frequency sensors.

The authors [21] fully monitored the patient's heart frequency, the state of the arteries by monitoring the functionality of the ATmega328 microcontroller, as a result of which access to data from anywhere showed good results. In their opinion, monitoring the use of Wi-Fi concluded that the overlap of frequencies in wireless networks with different radio technologies can create a complex situation, and the resulting interference can reduce the reliability of communication.

In this research paper [22], Arduino and Android devices were used to control the patient's state. Here, information about the patient's condition is obtained and sent to 2 separate interfaces, which are to display the patient's data and store that data on a server, which doctors can monitor the patient's data through the application on their Android phone.

Telemedicine is one of the most important and very necessary industries in our time. However, the implementation of such devices so that they can work with smartwatches and devices is a requirement of the time. In this research [23], a patient health monitoring system is presented, which utilizes the Arduino microcontroller and the things board web server. Multiple individual metrics are taken into account and collected, such as temperature, humidity, and other variables. The data from various sensors, which contains information about the patient's health, is transmitted to a server accessible by doctors. Through this setup, medical professionals can continuously and remotely observe the patient's well-being.

Scientific researchers [24] reviewed several articles and investigated the connection of Arduino UNO input pins with other Arduino UNO output pins. As a result, specialists came to conclusion that in case of an emergency, patients can easily review their reports and come to an appropriate decision, give recommendations, such a system automatically generates a map and informs the doctor about changes in the body of the patient and the necessary News. It was concluded that cloud computing is also useful for keeping patient information up to date. Cloud computing is also useful for keeping patient updates. But, according to the authors, this proposed machine should be further improved.

The authors of the [25] article took into account the shortage of oxygen ventilators during the pandemic and proposed an electronic machine made with Arduino that works like an oxygen ventilator. According to the results of the study of the system, the system is suitable for medical use for patients who cannot breathe voluntarily or have difficulty breathing. It allows patients to be treated comfortably, however, as mentioned in the article, this machine is a portable system for emergency use only [25, 26]. proposed a smart sensor for measuring signals. The system is a prototype of advanced electronic components that use the national myRIO tool for intelligent data collection. Smart displays are designed as consumer products with smart sensors. In order to test the proposed monitoring system, four accuracy predictions of the physiological signals of the two users were calculated. In the experimental setting of the prototype, the average accuracy was obtained by 97.2%.

Studies [27, 28] consider the process of creating a system for use with patients with an intelligent module with an IOT element to monitor the patient's condition online using heart rate, temperature, ambient temperature, and other important data sensors. For each specific situation, the percentage of errors in the prediction chain is within a certain limit (<5%) [29] considered the details of the reliability and safety of this system, a model was proposed using an intelligent module for the medical field using big data.

The paper [30] in order to provide an auxiliary diagnostic solution using smart phones, Holter had developed two wearable IHD detection platforms based on smartphones, which can collect and display ECG in real time, extract labels, and classify data, combining the portability of the monitor with the real-time processing power of the most advanced ECG equipment [31] and developed Android applications, providing suitable watches of different levels. Electrode pads or telemetry belts without wireless sensors made it effective to use it in health and health plans provided through mobile phones and additional tests required to determine its use in exercise-related exercises.

The authors of this article [32] explored the impact of a system with virtual reality built into it with musical effects. Next, modules with musical elements were studied, which affect the reduction of stress and depression. In this virtual environment with elements of the three-dimensional space of the real world and the corresponding accompanying music, relaxation and emancipation of the test subjects were observed. This system was aimed at patients who were in a coma. The system has built-in sensors for temperature control, heart control, SpO2 sensors, an eye pupil movement control sensor, CO2 control based on Arduino boards with the ability to send patient data to the cloud [33] in their scientific work considered a solution to the problem using the example of mini robots designed for home security. The robot uses ATMEGA2560 as a microcontroller to provide high clock speed and high clock speed due to the large amount of RAM and flash memory. Therefore, compared with other microcontrollers, the implemented system can provide faster response [34] point out the importance of strengthening the integrated types of microcontrollers with big data. There is a large amount of research and related work in the field regarding the use of IoT in medicine. Another interesting application of microcontrollers in medicine is a device called AliveCor [35], which has a connection to a mobile device, with the ability to control an ECG, interpret an image, send a record to the attending physician, record anomalies that may be present in the image.

3 Materials and Methods

According to the Market Research Engine, the healthcare IoMT market will reach $158 billion by 2024. The IMT is being used in a wide variety of medical industries, where technology supports to remotely monitor patients and diagnose them more efficiently. People need convenient and useful digital technologies. In particular, according to Statista, user spending on the Internet of Things has doubled since 2017 and will grow another 6 times in the next five years. The big advantage of using this technology in the field of medicine is its wide prevalence and ease of use. Monitoring the condition of patients will probably always be an urgent problem all over the world. That is why the topic of remote control will also always be explored and studied with great enthusiasm. Even now, the modern development and research of this topic are gaining global momentum not only in the field of healthcare, but also in the field of IT.

The challenges of global health systems today, such as population aging and the rise of chronic and viral diseases, are forcing clinicians, healthcare providers, and governments to look to new technologies to deliver high-quality healthcare and reduce overall costs. Huge discoveries in the use of microcontrollers in healthcare, reduction of computing devices in size, improvement in the computing power of devices in medical installations every year lead to an increase in connected systems and sensors that can collect data, analyze the information received, process, transform, and broadcast them. The received data, together with sensors and microcontrollers, form a complete system of medical devices, software, and services. Microcontrollers are used as analogues of medical technology in the field of medicine. As a result, the efficiency of honey is growing. Personnel and processes in the workplace, especially in remote areas. The microcontroller is nothing new and has recently become increasingly relevant in industries such as energy, transportation, and healthcare. Taking advantage of connected healthcare solutions allows healthcare providers to monitor patients in real time by collecting, recording, and analyzing limitless information using microcontrollers. These are, in particular, patients whose physiological conditions requiring constant monitoring can be monitored using non-invasive monitoring controlled by a microcontroller. Thus, the use of sensors and microcontrollers reduces the workload of medical personnel who monitor the condition of patients, collect, analyze, and process data, and also provide a valuable opportunity not inherent in medical personnel, such as continuous monitoring.

Monitoring health status requires specific components, including an Arduino Uno board, ATmega328 microcontroller, Wi-Fi module ESP8266, LM35 temperature sensor, heart rate sensor, 10kΩ resistor, button, connecting wires, breadboard, and MicroSD card. The heart rate sensor, also known as a pulse sensor, is a user-friendly plug-and-play device that easily connects to the Arduino board. It can be worn on the fingertip or earlobe and comes with an open-source heart rate monitoring application capable of graphing real-time heart rate data.

The heart rate sensor has a heart-shaped logo on its skin-contacting side, which also features a small round hole for the LED light to shine through. Below the LED is a light sensor, similar to those found in cell phones and laptops, used to adjust screen brightness under different lighting conditions. This sensor emits light toward the capillary tissue in the fingertip, earlobe, or any other suitable body point, and the light sensor measures the reflected light to determine the heart rate. To ensure measurement accuracy and prevent short circuits caused by sweat, it's important to protect the exposed part of the sensor before use. The pulse sensor has three contacts: Signal (S) for the signal wire, Vcc (3–5 V) for the DC supply voltage, and GND (ground).

The LM35 temperature sensor is an analog linear sensor whose output is proportional to the temperature in degrees Celsius. It has an operating temperature range of −55 °C to 150 °C, and its output voltage changes by 10 mV per one-degree temperature change. The sensor can operate on both 5 V and 3.3 V supply voltage, and its rest current consumption is less than 60 μA. In this health monitoring setup, an ATmega328 microcontroller is used on the Arduino Uno board (Fig. 1). The ATmega328 is an 8-bit CMOS microcontroller based on the advanced AVR RISC architecture. The schematic diagram of the ATmega328 microcontroller is shown in Fig. 2 [36].

The microcontroller measures human data such as temperature, pulse, and pressure. All data is stored on a MicroSD card (Fig. 3). MicroSD card interface with Arduino board uses a microSD card module (SPI communication protocol). Six pins are used to connect the MicroSD card, and the interaction is carried out via the SPI interface. To connect the card, you need an ATmega328 microcontroller, a card module, and 6 wires. Arduino Uno data logging to MicroSD card is shown in Table 1.

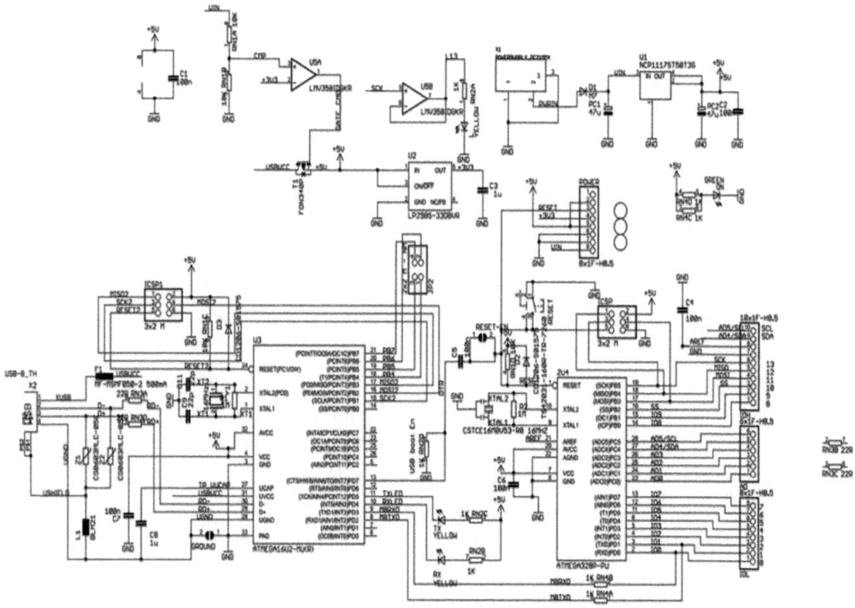

Fig. 1 ATmega328 microcontroller on Arduino Uno board [36]

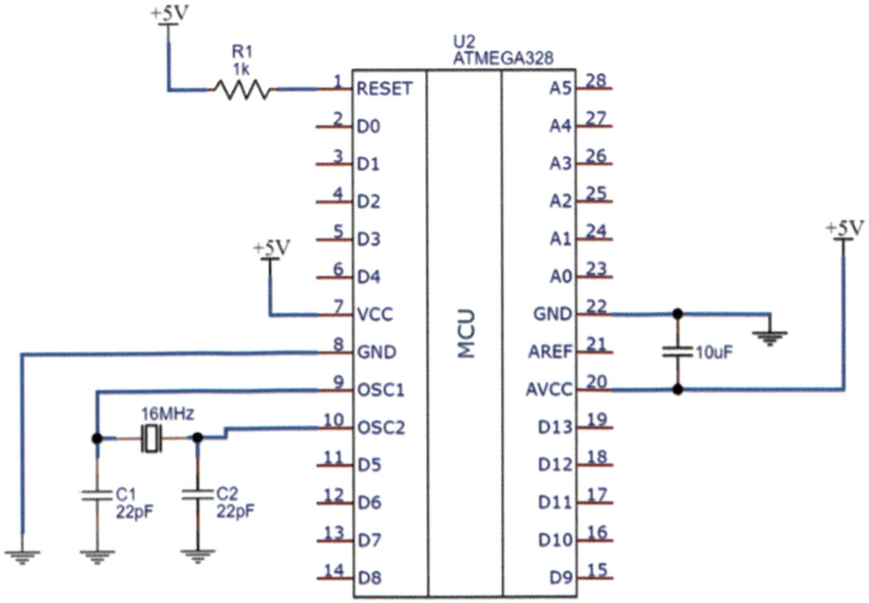

Fig. 2 Schematic diagram of the ATmega328 microcontroller

Fig. 3 MicroSD cards [33]

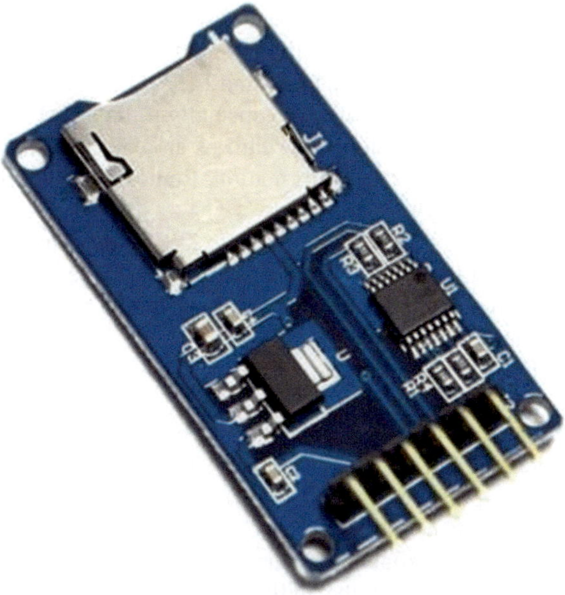

Table 1 Data logging Arduino Uno to MicroSD card module

MicroSD card	Vcc	GND	CS	SCK		MISO	MOSI
Arduino Uno	+5 V	GND	4	13	12	11	

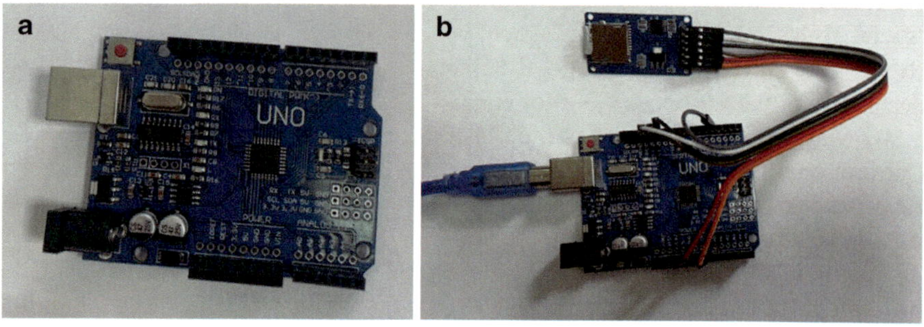

Fig. 4 MicroSD card module connects to the ATmega328 microcontroller

Digital I/O is connected as follows: MOSI and MISO pins on Arduino Uno board D11, SCK to D13, CS to 4, VCC to +5 V, GND to GND. The board has connectors connecting to 3.3 and 5 volts. The microSD card's power supply is 3.3 volts, so you need to use a microcontroller with the same power supply, otherwise voltage level converters are needed. SD and microSD cards (Fig. 4) can significantly expand the capabilities of Arduino projects that work with large amounts of data: data loggers, weather stations, and smart home systems. The Arduino boards are equipped with a relatively small internal memory, only up to 4 kilobytes, including both flash memory and EEPROM. This memory will not be enough to write large amounts of data, especially if the board is constantly turning off or off. Connecting an Arduino SD card as an external drive allows you to multiply the storage space for any information. Removable SD drives are cheap, easy to connect, and easy to use.

The diagram for writing data to a SD card using a microcontroller was implemented in the Fritzing software utility. The type of connection is a simple scheme since all modules were combined on 1 board. On the next Fig. 5 shows how this type of connection is implemented.

The ESP8266 microcontroller is used as a Wi-Fi, as it has a Wi-Fi technology module embedded in it (Fig. 6).

The scheme of the patient health control technology based on the Arduino board is presented in the following Fig. 7. The program uses a special library for working with the pulse sensor Pulse sensor Playground. Timer.h is also used to set the time interval between data readings. First of all, all used libraries must be connected to the program. Serial communication library (software serial) is used for interaction with esp8266. Next, the ability to use low-level interrupts to increase the accuracy of measurements and enable DEBUG to display incoming commands in the serial monitor window is initialized. Then in the program you need to enter the name of your Wi-Fi connection, the password to connect to it and the IP service.

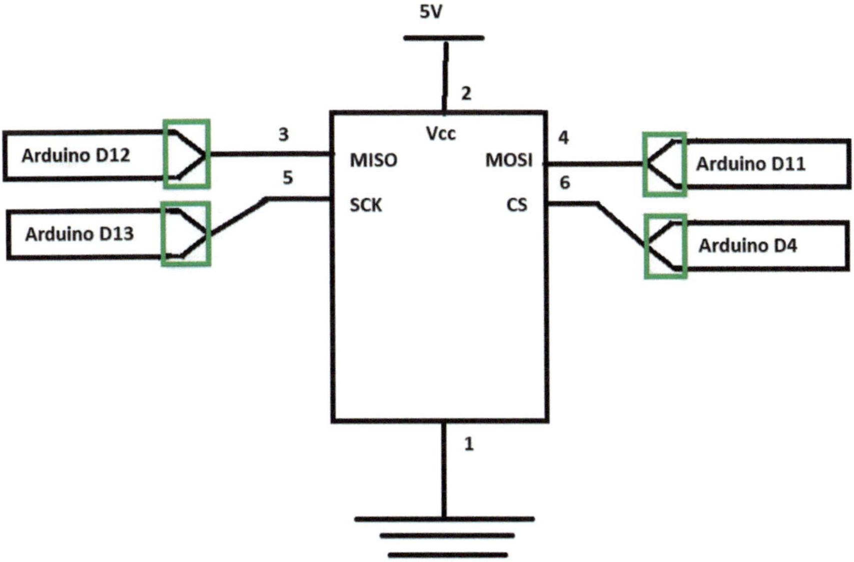

Fig. 5 ATmega328 microcontroller schematic diagram

Fig. 6 ESP8266 Wi-Fi module [33]

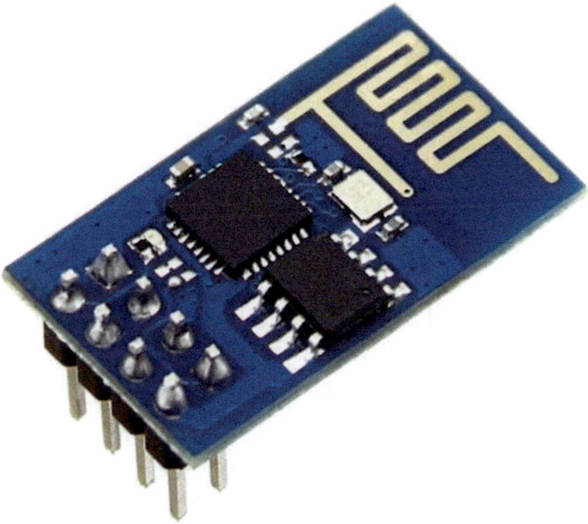

The setup function establishes the baud rate for serial communication between the Arduino serial monitor and the esp8266 module. To initiate the esp8266 module, we issue the appropriate command and connect it to the Wi-Fi network by calling the connectWiFi() function. Subsequently, we set up the timer by invoking the t.every(time_interval, do_this) function, which determines the interval for reading data from the sensor.

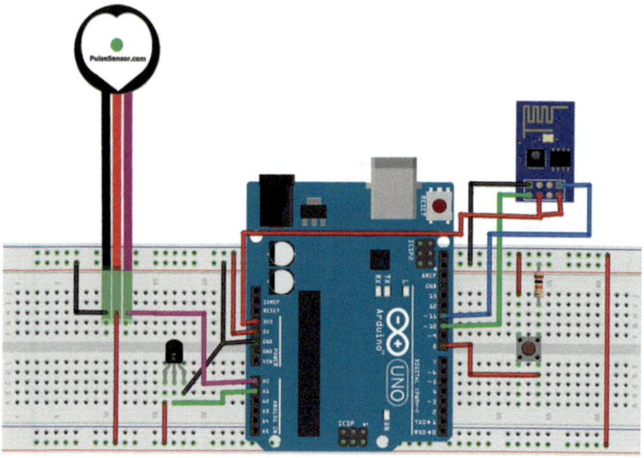

Fig. 7 Connection scheme [drawn in fritzing.org]

Additionally, within the program, we need to define the functions connectWiFi(), panic_button(), update_info(), and getReadings(). The connectWiFi() function returns a True or False value based on whether the module successfully connects to the Wi-Fi network. The command AT+CWJAP = 1 instructs the ESP8266 module to function in station mode, while the AT+CWJAP = \ command facilitates the connection to our Wi-Fi access point. The getReadings() function reads data from the pulse sensor and the temperature sensor LM35, converting them into strings using the dtostrf() function. To store BPM (beats per minute) and temperature values, we initialize a character array and then convert the sensor outputs into strings using the dtostrf() function [37].

3.1 *Project Testing*

To conduct the test, it is necessary to combine the physical details of this project, and then install the program on the board. To check and run the program, you need to open the display window.

In the scheme, it is necessary to make the following connections:

- Signal contact pulse sensor - > contact A0 board Arduino;
- Contact Vcc sensor pulse - > 5 V board Arduino;
- Contact GND sensor pulse - > GND board Arduino;
- Vout sensor LM35 - > contact A1 board Arduino;
- Tx module ESP8266 - > contact 10 board Arduino;
- Rx module ESP8266 - > contact 11 board Arduino;
- CH_PD and Vcc module ESP8266 - > 3.3 V board Arduino;
- GND module ESP8266 - > GND board Arduino.

Essential components for monitoring students' health status are saved in the MicroSd card module (Fig. 8).

Fig. 8 Patient information

G19

	A	B	C	D
1	Date and time		Pulse Rate (BPM)	Body Temp (F)
2	December 21, 2022 at 03:11 PM	Patient Info	217	51
3	December 21, 2022 at 03:15 PM	Patient Info	127	53
4	December 21, 2022 at 03:28 PM	Patient Info	220	50
5	December 21, 2022 at 04:10 PM	Patient Info	222	54
6	December 21, 2022 at 04:22 PM	Patient Info	209	64
7	December 21, 2022 at 04:35 PM	Patient Info	121	86,3
8	December 21, 2022 at 04:47 PM	Patient Info	103	83,9
9	December 21, 2022 at 04:55 PM	Patient Info	209	99,7
10	December 21, 2022 at 05:07 PM	Patient Info	212	83

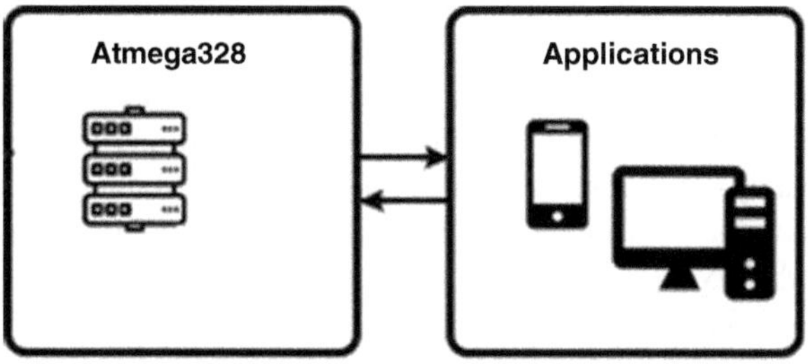

Fig. 9 Transfer of patient information to applications

The stored health data of patients on the MicroSD card connects via the COM port to the application. Students' health status can be viewed on the computer. Transfer of patient information to applications shows in Fig. 9.

4 Results

This paper describes the content of the experience of using the Arduino device and evaluates the effectiveness. Efficacy was assessed by a survey among patients using this intelligent system. Pre-processed and collected data from various sources make it possible to adequately evaluate the intelligent system in terms of the following parameters: patient satisfaction, reliability, usefulness.

In December 2022, patients using this intelligent system were asked to complete an online questionnaire through the google disk platform. The questionnaire was completed by 150 participants. 21.3% of participants—patients registered with cardiologists with severe forms of cardiovascular disease (n = 32), 12%—with signs of high blood pressure (n = 18), 46.6%—patients with chronic kidney disease (n = 70), and 20% are healthy patients. (n = 30). These study participants were registered at Polyclinic No. 30 in Almaty. Most of the participants were trained in the use of this device beforehand. Written consent for the use of these survey results for scientific purposes was obtained from all participants prior to completing the questionnaire. It was agreed that the empirical data collected would be used for research purposes only and that the questionnaire did not include any questions regarding patients' personal data, gender, age, and address. At the beginning of the questionnaire, information is given about the objectives of this study and a guarantee of anonymity. The first group of questions was aimed at finding out the knowledge of the use of this device, and how this device was useful to them. There was an item for patients to ask if they were not using the device for any purpose. If this question received an affirmative answer, the next question was on a Likert scale with an assessment of the usefulness of this device.

The second group of questions is devoted to assessing the patients' perception of the support of this device as an independent recommender device that can be used without a doctor. Participants used a 10-point scale to answer this question. The third group of questions contains 10 questions aimed at measuring patient satisfaction with this system. For each question, a 5-point assessment was used with responses ranging from "not satisfied at all" to "completely satisfied." In the last group of questions, patients had the opportunity to write their comments and opinions about the intellectual system, suggestions for improvement. To compare and analyze the results of the survey, we use parametric statistics. Parametric tests are commonly used on normally distributed data. Student's test and analysis of variance (ANOVA) is one of the most popular. Data normality was checked by kurtosis and skewness indices.

According to the data in Table 2, it can be seen that the deviation from the norm of asymmetry and kurtosis are small, it can be assumed that this distribution is close to normal.

Table 2 Rates of skewness and kurtosis of factors, scale validity using Cronbach's alpha for 150 data

	Parameter	Items	Asymmetry	Excess	Cronbach's alpha	Average dispersion	Reliability
Without a device with a doctor	Advisory and consulting support	3	−0.101	0.093	0.97	0.51	0.91
	Interaction and cooperation	2	−0.033	0.305	0.89	0.56	0.89
	Independence	1	−0.599	0.312	0.79	0.58	0.88
	Stress reduce effect	5	−0.425	0.218	0.82	0.50	0.88
With device	Advisory and consulting support	3	−0.203	−0.499	0.96	0.52	0.95
	Interaction and cooperation	2	0.100	−0.960	0.89	0.59	0.92
	Independence	1	−0.932	0.456	0.79	0.51	0.85
	Advisory and consulting support	4	0.203	−0.968	0.98	0.56	0.89
	Stress reduce effect	5	−0.94	0.512	0.86	0.55	0.98

The distribution skewness is the ratio of the central moment of the third order to the cube of the standard deviation:

$$\alpha s = \mu 3 / \sigma 3$$

The kurtosis (or kurtosis coefficient) of a random variable is a number:

$$\mathrm{es} = \mu 4 / \sigma 4 - 3$$

The number 3 is subtracted from the ratio because for the most common normal distribution, the ratio $\mu 4/\sigma 4 = 3$. In addition, the amount of statistical power increases due to the decrease in the size of the sampling error. The large sample size and the skewness and kurtosis indices make it possible to conclude that the data are normally distributed and suitable for parametric analysis. Each dimension, namely advisory support, interaction and collaboration, device autonomy, and patient satisfaction, was assessed for cohesion. Each questionnaire scale is represented by Cronbach's alpha coefficients. These coefficients fluctuate between 0.79 and 0.98, which is an excellent indicator. The mean variance and reliability index were also calculated. For each parameter, the average dispersion coefficient is higher than 0.50, and the reliability indicators are not lower than 0.85, which can be used to conclude that the presented scales are reliable.

To evaluate the advantages and disadvantages of the developed system, 150 responses from the participants in this experiment were analyzed. As shown in Fig. 10, the most useful module of the system is the availability of the device anywhere and at any time, this item was preferred by almost 28% of all respondents. Many patients noted that this factor plays a key role in reducing stress. One patient commented: "This system is available anytime, anywhere, no need to make an appointment and wait" (Availability anytime, anywhere). Another survey participant commented: "There is no need to go to the doctor and waste time on this" (Saving travel time). Another 50% of respondents noted: "There is no need to sit in line to see a doctor."

With regard to the convenience and ease of use of this device, 23 patients noted this factor as the most important. Also, the speed of work and the ability of the

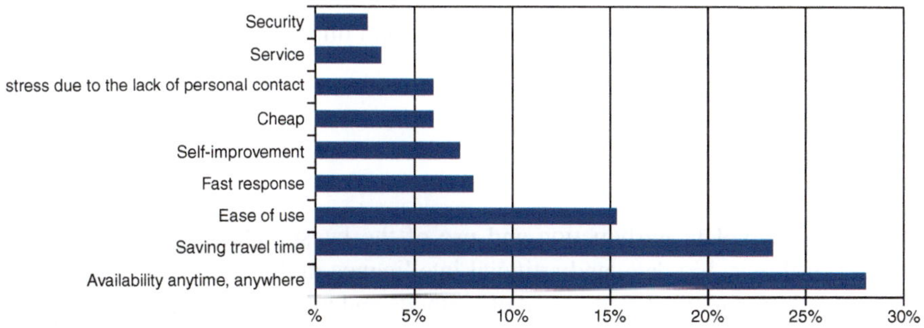

Fig. 10 Priority parameters for respondents

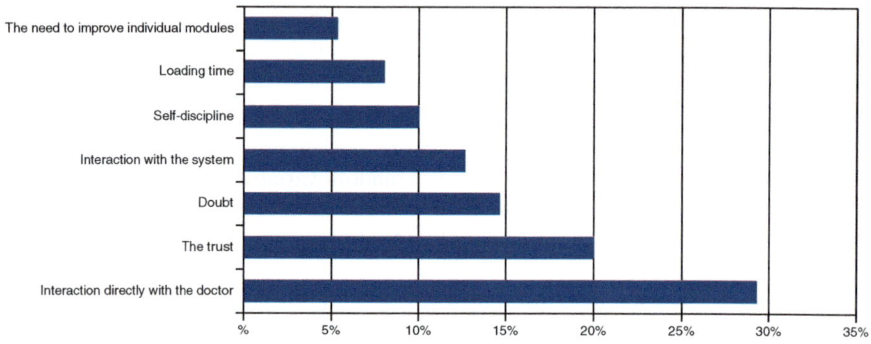

Fig. 11 Negative parameters for respondents

system to self-improve were noted by 12 and 11 respondents, respectively. 6% of respondents responded positively about the price. The absence of the need to communicate with other people and, accordingly, the possibility of avoiding stress in this way were noted by 9 patients. The security and maintenance of this system did not go unnoticed by the participants in this experiment, and 3% of the respondents noted these items as a priority.

The next Fig. 11 shows the negative aspects for the respondents.

More than 29% of the respondents expressed their unwillingness to interact directly with the doctor, although 10% of the respondents did not see anything of the kind in this and gave estimates in favor of this parameter. 20% and 15% expressed disbelief and doubts about the system, although these same participants noted the convenience, ease of use, safety, and stress reduction. 13% of respondents had problems directly interacting with the system, the main reasons for such problems were technical problems with the cable and microcontroller, communication interference. For the timely use of the device, self-discipline is also necessary, which 10% of the respondents could not show. Most of these 10% noted and recommended building a reminder module with a call or notification into the system. Boot and turn on time of the system usually did not take more than 15 seconds, however, 12 patients had problems with booting and this problem was again due to technical problems of the microcontroller, which were later corrected. A very small number of respondents, about 6%, recommend improving the system by integrating additional functions into it for recommendations and consultations, and improvements in design.

5 Conclusion

The almost complete introduction and use of the latest technologies such as the Internet of things, big data, and artificial intelligence in the healthcare sector have seen a revolution in the development of methods and methods of treatment, thereby developing medicine in a new direction. The covid period, which showed the importance of remote monitoring and treatment of people (IoMT) [38], developed these areas with unprecedented speed and zeal. Round-the-clock monitoring of the patient's condition and well-being without any special psychological and external influences and contacts at this time is also a problem requiring great attention. In this regard, the use of robotic systems simplifies the solution of this problem. Various devices developed on the Arduino platform help to automate the acquisition of data on the patient's condition such as measuring physical activity, heart rate, blood pressure, and online pulse pressure are very important for medical staff to quickly respond and take action. High-quality and prompt provision of medical care is always an urgent problem that requires special attention. With the advent of intelligent healthcare, doctors as well as patients can monitor, access, analyze data, and provide proper medication if any problem occurs from their location without the need to travel (R.Anandh, 2018). In the use of IoT technology, it is important to note the issue of security, which is important to always consider. Personal data hacking and information leakage from the cloud (G. Yamini, 2020) with medical data are especially dangerous for the medical profession.

In smart cities, intelligent healthcare systems extensively utilize IoMT sensors to monitor the health of patients. These sensors are designed for human use and include smart thermometers for tracking body temperature, Q-bands for assessing user mobility, and pacemakers integrated with medical alert systems to offer continuous monitoring and prompt alerts during cardiac emergencies. Moreover, proximity tracers are instrumental in identifying possible clusters of new contagious diseases. Additionally, temperature sensors are employed in hospitals to oversee plasma storage, providing valuable resources for future studies. These medical sensors exemplify some of the many devices accessible for monitoring citizens' well-being.

Implementation of data collection, a system module will be created that includes the following functions: data storage, anomaly fixation, receiving data from the Arduino sensor, smart watches and bracelets, sending signals to the treating staff, monitoring the patient's condition, and predicting the development of the disease. This article discusses the methodology for using an automated heart rate monitor for effective patient care and health monitoring. This system is very easy to use and designed with minimal hardware to be efficient.

Currently, one of the most pressing issues is the promotion of the innovative use of the Internet of things in medicine and healthcare and the acceleration of the integration of medicine and healthcare with information technology. With the help of innovative applications such as online data monitoring, sensor-based positioning, and monitoring, intelligent development is being achieved with high performance in areas such as medical management, telemedicine, and hierarchical diagnostics. The Medical Internet of Things helps to provide remote services to patients in real time and improve communication between them and healthcare facilities. As a result, the huge amount of data generated by the Internet of Things in the field of medicine and wellness provides an informational basis for the development of predictive, preventive, personalized, and participation-based drugs. Connected medical devices and the Medical Internet of Things can solve several challenges facing the global healthcare industry today. Despite rising treatment costs, turbulent regulatory environments, and changing reimbursement models, the Medical Internet of Things is still expected to improve patient care, improve healthcare outcomes, and reduce the cost of the entire system. This is why the healthcare industry urgently needs the Medical Internet of Things. The COVID-19 pandemic has doomed many to change their minds about the use and integration of information and communication technology tools under quarantine. In this study, the use of these funds was analyzed using a survey of participants who took part in this study, and these were patients of the clinic in Almaty (Kazakhstan). The responses to the survey made it possible to evaluate the pros and cons of using this system, identify future work`, and clarify improvements in the operation of this system.

References

1. Chandana R, Kaveen V, Gajalakshmi M, Manisha SJ. Automatic anesthesia control system. Int J Eng Appl Sci Technol. 2021;5(9):247–9.
2. D'Ausilio A. Arduino: a low-cost multipurpose lab equipment. Behav Res Methods. 2011;44:305–13.
3. Ehrmann G, Blachowicz T, Homburg SV, Ehrmann A. Measuring biosignals with single circuit boards. Bioengineering. 2022;9:84. https://doi.org/10.3390/bioengineering9020084.
4. Sundaram P. Patient monitoring system using android technology. Int J Comp Sci Mob Computing. 2013;5:191–201.
5. Rahimunnisa K, Atchaiya M. AI-based smart and intelligent wheelchair. J Appl Res Technol. 2020;18:362.
6. Lambat MM, Wagaj SC. Review: health monitoring system. Int J Sci Res. 2015;4:246–50.
7. Balakayeva GT, Darkenbayev D. The solution to the problem of processing big data using the example of assessing the solvency of borrowers. J Theor Appl Inf Technol. 2020;98(13):2659–70.
8. Balakayeva GT, Phillips C, Darkenbayev DK, Turdaliyev M. Using NoSQL for processing unstructured big data. News Natl Acad Sci Repub Kazakhstan Ser Geol Tech Sci. 2019;6(438):12–21. https://doi.org/10.32014/2019.2518-170X.151.
9. Gokilavani R, Gokulapriya M, Jasmine Christy AR, Jeeva R. Anesthesia control system with multi sensor using Arduino. Int J Innov Res Adv Eng. Mar 2019;6(03):86–90.
10. Aalan Santhosh B, Sujatha S. Securing and monitoring human health using Arduino Mega and sensors. Int J Electron Commun Technol. 2018;9(4):9–12.
11. Akhmed-Zaki DZh, Mukhambetzhanov ST, Nurmakhanova ZM, Abdiakhmetova ZM. Using wavelet transform and machine learning to predict heart fibrillation disease on ECG. SIST 2021–2021 IEEE international conference on smart information systems and technologies, 2021. https://doi.org/10.1109/SIST50301.2021.9465990.
12. Kale K, Dighe S, Dhakad T. Development of health monitoring system. Int J Eng Appl Sci Technol. 2019;4(6):72–6.
13. Keertirani, Ashwini S, Asha M, Aishwarya R, Sudharshan KM, Kumar CSA. Implementation of patient monitoring system using Arduino UNO. Int J Adv Res Sci Eng. 2018;07:118–23.
14. Oganov RG, Kontsevaya AV, Kalinina AM. Economic burden of cardiovascular disease in The Russian Federation. Cardiovasc Ther Prev. 2011;10(4):4–9. https://doi.org/10.15829/1728-8800-2011-4-4-9.
15. Kontsevaya AV, Balanova YA, Imaeva AE, Khudyakov MB, Karpov OI, Drapkina OM. "Economic burden of hypercholesterolemia in The Russian Federation", rational pharmacotherapy in cardiology. 2018;14(3):393–401. https://doi.org/10.20996/1819-6446-2018-14-3-393-401.
16. Anandh R, Indirani G. Real time health monitoring system using Arduino with cloud technology. Asian J Comput Sci Technol. 2018;7(S1):29–32.

17. Rajashekar K, Hanumantha R, Ruksar Begum TK, Begum S, Fathima SZ, Kauser S. Robotic arm control using Arduino. J Emerg Technol Innov Res. 2020;7(6):453–5.
18. Ramya T, Shajugeorge B. IoT based Anaesthesia injector. Int J Eng Sci Comput. 2020;10(3):24854–7.
19. Richa D, Kushwaha AK, Sreejeth M. An IoT based health monitoring system using Arduino Uno. Int J Eng Res Technol. 2021;10(03)
20. Sheta MAE, El-Adly RAE, ElAlfi AEE. Developing smart system for managing heart patients' crises. Res J Educ. 2022;67:313–46.
21. Sivasankari N, Parameswari M, Anbarasan K, Moses MB. Arduino based human health care monitoring and control system. IOSR J Electr Electron Eng. 2016;11(3):09–18.
22. Sneha Sravanti D, Srivalli M, Srilakshmi S, Sneha Mol PS. Personal health monitoring system using Arduino and android. Int J Eng Res Technol. 2016;4(22):1–5.
23. Sunehra D, Siddireddygari S. Patient health monitoring system using Arduino Mega 2560 and Thingsboard server. Int J Sci Technol Res. 2020;9(03):5020–6.
24. Unawane S, Jadhav S, Jagtap S. E patient monitoring system using Arduino. Int Res J Mod Eng Technol Sci. 2021;03(07):1498–505.
25. Pravin Yele S, Kaustubh Ahire B, Rakesh Nagpure R, Chetan Chaudhary P, Yogesh Chaudhari P. “Health monitoring system with ventilator using Arduino”, international journal of scientific research. Sci Technol. 2022;9(3):784–90.
26. Gulzat T, Lyazat N, Siladi V, Gulbakyt S, Maxatbek S. Research on predictive model based on classification with parameters of optimization. Neural Network World. 2020;30(5):295–308. https://doi.org/10.14311/NNW.2020.30.020.
27. Jeyaraj PR, Nadar ERS. Smart-monitor: patient monitoring system for IoT-based healthcare system using deep learning. IEEE J Res. 2019;68(2):1435–42.
28. Berdaly Z, Abdiakhmetova ZT. “Comparative machine-learning approach: study for heart diseases”. SIST 2022–2022 International conference on smart information systems and technologies, proceedings, 2022. https://doi.org/10.1109/SIST54437.2022.9945705.
29. Islam MM, Rahaman A, Islam MR. Development of smart healthcare monitoring system in IoT environment. SN Comput Sci. 2020;1:185.
30. Riazul Islam SM, Daehan Kwak MD, Kabir H, Hossain M. The internet of things for health care: a comprehensive survey. IEEE Access. 2015;3:678–708. https://doi.org/10.1109/Access.2015.2437951.
31. Joseph Oresko J, Jin Z, Cheng J, Huang S, Sun Y. A wearable smartphone-based platform for real-time cardiovascular disease detection via electrocardiogram processing. IEEE Trans Inf Technol Biomed. 2010;14(3):734–40. https://doi.org/10.1109/TITB.2010.2047865.
32. Matthew Gregoski J, Mueller M, Vertegel A, Alexey S, Brenda Jackson B. Development and validation of a smartphone heart rate acquisition application for health promotion and wellness telehealth applications. Int J Telemed Appl. 2012;2012:696324. https://doi.org/10.1155/2012/696324.
33. Lin X, Mahmud S, Jones E, Shaker A, Miskinis A, Kanan S, Kim J-H. Virtual reality-based musical therapy for mental health management. In: 2020 10th Annual computing and communication workshop and conference (CCWC). IEEE; 2020. p. 948–52.
34. Yaashuwanth C, Pachaiyappan P, Gopinath C. Smart home security surveillance robot using ATMega 2560 microcontroller. Int J Soft Comput. 2020;11(8):310–8.
35. Yin Y, Zeng Y, Chen X, Fan Y. The internet of things in healthcare: an overview. J Ind Inf Integr. 2018;1:03–13.
36. Temirbekova ZE, Pyrkova AY. Improving teachers’ skills to integrate the microcontroller technology in computer engineering education. Educ Inf Technol. 2022;27(6):8381–412. https://doi.org/10.1007/s10639-021-10875-8.
37. Temirbekova Z, Pyrkova A, Abdiakhmetova Z, Berdaly A. Library of fully homomorphic encryption on a microcontroller. SIST 2022–2022 International conference on smart information systems and technologies, proceedings, 2022. https://doi.org/10.1109/SIST54437.2022.9945722.
38. Pasluosta F, Gassner H, Winkler J, Klucken J, Eskofier BM. An emerging era in the management of Parkinson’s disease: Wearable technologies and the Internet of Things. IEEE J Biomed Health Inform. 2017;19(6):1873–81.

Predictive Measures to Tackle Mental Disorders During COVID-19

Syeda Hoor-Ul-Ain, Anwar Ahmed Khan, Shama Siddiqui, and Indrakshi Dey

Abstract The healthcare crisis emerged due to COVID-19 has escalated mental health predicaments ranging from several mental diseases and disorders. Mental illnesses triggered in the pandemic have shaped-up a challenging situation for the mental health practitioners to predict psychological distresses among the patients infected with COVID-19, healthcare practitioners/ workers, and a sizable population of the world who followed the strict SOPs of the pandemic. Social distancing and isolation are imperatives for the survival of mankind in the new normal. Contrarily, these two factors are identified as the supreme threats to the psychosocial well-being of the post pandemic population. The elderly population with known medical conditions suffered terribly during the global pandemic as psychological therapy and psychiatric services were halted across the world for a limited period. However, mental health practitioners were available online to provide the necessary therapy in a few developed countries. Advancements in medical science and computing technology have made it possible to predict the mental state of people by monitoring trends of their vital parameters. This chapter sheds light on some of the major predictive measures that may help managing the mental well-being during COVID-19. Primarily, detailed review has been presented focused on mental disorders. The technologies of Internet of Things, Machine Learning, mobile applications, big data analytics, assistive technologies, and federated learning have been

S. Hoor-Ul-Ain
Office of Research, Innovation, and Commercialization, University of Karachi, Karachi, Sindh, Pakistan

A. A. Khan
Department of Engineering and Computational Science, Millennium Institute of Technology and Entrepreneurship, Karachi, Sindh, Pakistan

S. Siddiqui (✉)
Department of Computer Science, DHA Suffa University, Karachi, Sindh, Pakistan

I. Dey
Walton Institute for Information and Communication Systems Science, South East Technological University, Waterford, Ireland
e-mail: indrakshi.dey@waltoninstitute.ie

G. Battineni et al. (eds.), *Computational Methods in Psychiatry*,
https://doi.org/10.1007/978-981-99-6637-0_4

discussed for their role in mental health management. Finally, the challenges associated with the use of computational technologies such as data acquisition, consent, confidentiality, lack of integration, and reliability issues have been discussed, and the solutions have been suggested.

Keywords COVID-19 · Psychology · Machine learning · IoT

1 Introduction

The outbreak of the novel human Coronavirus (COVID-19)[1] pandemic[2] has not only shaken the world but also stretched over an incertitude[3] of unprecedented healthcare crisis that has a colossal impact on mental health [1–3]. The novel disease has reckoned as the fifth documented pandemic of human pneumonia in the history of medicine since 1918 and declared as exponentially spreading disease through human-to-human transmission (HHT) [4]). The savage emergence of the global pandemic claimed many lives, triggered several mental illnesses, and amplified mental health predicaments ranging from several mental diseases and disorders [5, 6]. Mental health consists of psychosocial, emotional, behavioral, and cognitive well-being which denotes a positive aura of mental state and signifies absence of mental diseases and disorders. It falls under the ambit of all-inclusive allied disciplines of psychology and psychiatry. Conceptually, it focuses on a distinct aspect of positive feelings such as functioning happily and exhibiting prosocial behavior in personal and professional settings [7, 8]. Nevertheless, mental health conditions include mental diseases and disorders. Classifying mental illnesses into disorders and diseases has received significant attention in the literature over the last two decades. The terminologies are often used interchangeably but a clear demarcation can be drawn between the two in the light of nosology,[4] pathology,[5] radiology,[6] and

[1] COVID-19 was caused by severe acute respiratory syndrome (SARS)-CoV-2, has emerged as a global public health threat. It was first reported in Wuhan, China, and subsequently spread worldwide and later declared as a pandemic by WHO.

[2] A pandemic is an outbreak of an exponentially wide spreading infectious disease that affect substantial population locally, regionally, or globally.

[3] Incertitude is an unpredictable state of precariousness or uncertainty.

[4] Nosology is the branch of medical science that deals with the classification of diseases.

[5] Pathology is a branch of medical science that "involves the study and diagnosis of disease through the examination of surgically removed organs, tissues (biopsy samples), bodily fluids, and in some cases the whole body (autopsy). Pathology tests cover blood tests, and tests on urine, feces, and bodily tissues." (Source: https://www.mcgill.ca/pathology/about/definition)

[6] Radiology is a branch of medicine that uses imaging technology to diagnose and treat disease.

radiography[7] to use predictive measures to deal with mental illnesses [9, 10]. Mental diseases are akin on biological ailments, whereas mental disorders may also be diagnosed with the observable repeated patterns of behaviors. Mental diseases like Alzheimer, Amnesia, Huntington, Parkinson, etc., are either genetic or have biological reasons may be tested through pathological, radiological, radiographical tests, etc.. However, the majority of mental disorders are not categorized as medical diseases. No lab tests for chemical imbalance, X-rays, MRIs, or brain scans can verify the dependence of any mental disorder upon a physical/ biological condition [11, 12].

In psychiatry, the several mental disorders constructs led to much confusion over the years as all mental disorders were considered to be reducible to biological theory involving some form of dysfunction in brain circuitry. Contrarily, mental health scientists of Health Development Agency[8] (HDA) played a pivotal role in defining disease framework for establishing a foundation that identifies a set of mental disorders that are akin to medical diseases, whereas others are not [2, 13–15].

The medical phenomenon of the global pandemic affects the psychodynamics of human behavior and disrupted the social dynamics of human interactions in pre, during, and post pandemic challenges and its aftermath. Ultra-rapid human-to-human transmission of the novel coronavirus ensued lockdowns to restrain the exponential spread of the disease worldwide. World Health Organization's advisory confined people to stay indoors to break the chain of virus transmission. The restrictive measures include social distancing, wearing face masks, washing hands, and using sanitizers have forced the world's population to follow the prescribed SOPs stringently. Closure of the workplaces, educational institutions, recreational activities, picnic venues pushed people to stay in quarantine and self-isolation and worsened their mental health during the pandemic. The psychological impairment led to a negative impact on a community's social, emotional, physical, and professional well-being [16, 17]. The survivors of the coronavirus disease faced with the severity of stigma which is closely associated with mental illnesses [18].

The pandemic has triggered several mental health disorders that are not akin on medical diseases. Moreover, social distancing and isolation are imperatives for the survival of mankind in the new normal. Contrarily, these two factors are identified as the supreme threats to the psychosocial well-being of the post pandemic population. Social distancing and isolation have impacted many lives with the shockwave of xenophobia[9] that has resulted into psychosocial meltdown [1]. The impact of

[7] Radiography is a type of X-ray procedure, and it carries the same types of risks as other X-ray procedures. The radiation doses the patient receives vary depending on the individual procedure but is generally less than that received during fluoroscopy and computed tomography procedures. It includes computed tomography (Source: https://www.fda.gov/radiation-emitting-products/medical-x-ray-imaging/radiography#:~:text=Radiography%20is%20a%20type%20of,fluoroscopy%20and%20computed%20tomography%20procedures.).

[8] Health Development Agency is the UK's special health authority to raise the quality of public health function.

[9] Xenophobia is a metaphor used to define the fear of the unknown. It is a Greek word, where "phobos" means fear and "xenos" can mean stranger, foreigner, or outsider. The prefix "xeno" also signify strange or unprecedented occurrence of situations, circumstances, incidents, etc.

social distancing ranges from panic to serious anxiety disorders which may lead to the development of obsessive-compulsive disorders out of fear of novel viral infection and maintaining excessive personal hygiene [19]. Furthermore, repetitive bulletins about the pandemic on television and social media have aggravated the xenophobic state among the masses. Mental illnesses have shaped-up a challenging state of affairs for the mental health practitioners to predict psychological distresses among the patients infected with COVID-19, healthcare practitioners/ workers, and a sizable population of the world who followed the strict SOPs of the pandemic.

Brief psychotic disorder triggered due to psychosocial distress during the COVID-19 healthcare crisis that lasts less than a week's time as a result of acute stress [20]. However, the upsurgence to severe stress leads to anxiety and depression. Work from home (remote working with limitless working hours) is one of the causes of damaging physical, social, and emotional well-being of the isolated population. Limitless working hours are not only a precipitous[10] health hazard but also identified as a main cause of anxiety disorder. Setting work-life time fence for remote working model prevents obstacles in managing relationships, having work-life balance, and supporting community engagement initiatives. Comparatively, the isolated and quarantined COVID patients were more prone to depression as they were unsure about their recovery.

Many components of social distancing elicit more dangerous disorders such as paraphilic acts in public spaces. The terminology of "paraphilic attitude" is originated from paraphilia. In psychiatry, "paraphilia is defined as a mental disorder characterized by abnormal sexual desires, typically involving extreme or dangerous activities which may have social and legal consequences." [21, 22]. Several studies conducted during the pandemic affirm that the restraints and confinements of social distancing have caused anxiety among the sexual offenders with paraphilic disorders and increased their sexual desires of exhibitionism and touchrism that also fall under the ambit of deviant fantasies [23, 24]. The upswing in the prevalence of paraphilic disorder during the pandemic has been foreseen a significant and rising trend in healthcare expenditure with the expansion of "Global Paraphilia Disorder Treatment Market" in the post pandemic, i.e., from 2022 to 2029 [25, 26].

The pandemic has turned into an abysmal and drove people crazy as they were forced to work remotely for 24/7. Meeting crazy deadlines while being awake for the whole night set the irrational ethos for work from home such as "always on!" work culture [27]. Sleeplessness or sleep disturbance is a very common symptom of bipolar disorder which intensifies maniac episodes in the patients [28, 29]. COVID-19 stressors have not only disturbed the sleep patterns of the patients with known bipolar disorder but also triggered relapses in many patients [30]. Bipolar disorder has a high comorbidity with COVID-19 illness. Impairment in functioning has shown increased risk for severe manic episodes. Several cases have been reported with symptoms of mania in patients infected with COVID-19 who had no

[10] Precipitous health hazard means a dangerous health hazard which may steep to the unexpected levels such that its cure is unknown.

prior psychiatric history. Many studies have shown that a pre-existing medical condition of bipolar disorder may be triggered by COVID-19 [31, 32]. The novel virus has revealed an unknown condition of bipolar disorder in patients affected with COVID-19 who have no psychiatry history [33].

The elderly population with known medical conditions suffered terribly during the global pandemic as psychological therapy and psychiatric services were halted across the world for a limited period. However, mental health practitioners were available online to provide the necessary therapy in a few developed countries. Advancements in medical science and computing technology have made it possible to predict the mental state of people by monitoring trends of their vital parameters. This chapter sheds light on some of the major predictive measures that may help managing mental well-being with the help of computational technology.

1.1 Why Predictive Measures?

In the recent times of unprecedented healthcare crisis, detrimental lifestyle such as poor physical activity with observable repeated patterns of neuroticism[11] are the significant predictors of developing a mental disorder in the healthy populations of the pre-pandemic world.

Predictive measures help in identifying the mental disorder, whereas predictive metrics and analytics provide with the remedy and cure of mental illness [34]. Computational technology has developed digital predictive metrics to calculate the presence of identifiable mental disorders such as bipolar, paraphilic, depression, anxiety, and obsessive compulsion by using quantitative techniques to measure the behavioral intensity of mental illness with accuracy. Computer scientists have delivered upon the promises of supporting the field of psychiatry in predicting, diagnosing, monitoring, and providing with the intervention design of cure for these mental illnesses [35].

Predictive measures have received significant attention in the fields of psychiatry and computational technology to detect and prognosticate mental illnesses at an early stage so that the affected population may be treated without any delays. Technological advancements have played an important role in developing predictive models to improve e-mental health. Use of artificial intelligence, mobile technology, sensor devices, and machine learning has created new opportunities for mental healthcare practitioners to tackle mental illnesses more proficiently [36]. All requisite predictive measures are discussed in the subsequent sections.

[11] Neuroticism is the trait disposition to experience negative effects, including anger, anxiety, self-consciousness, irritability, emotional instability, and depression.

1.2 How May Technology Aid?

The global pandemic has brought the treatment of mental illnesses at the crossroads where psychologists and psychiatrists have joined hands with the technologists in paving the pathways of technological interventions as a mental health cure [37]. Technology has charted out new avenues for psychiatric treatment during the COVID-19 pandemic by means of digital health. It includes multifarious technological interventions such as mobile health, telehealth, and wearable medical devices [38]. Mobile health involves the use of mobile apps for healthy living which entails obtaining access to significant information pertinent to the identified mental illness. It also helps in establishing the clinical foundation and setting therapeutic goal as a mental healthcare solution. Mental Health Apps are convenient and cost-effective solution with personalized mental health treatment for patients [39]. Contrarily, telehealth interventions include home-based telemental health/ online mental health services provided by the psychiatrists to treat patients of post-traumatic stress disorder (PTSD), depression and anxiety disorders, bipolar disorder, etc., by means of telemedicine technologies in primary care [40]. Telemedicine methods such as telepsychiatry and teletherapy are widely used during the lockdown and helped several patients in recovering from their mental illnesses triggered by the xenophobic state of mind [38]. Furthermore, wearable sensors, electronic patches, and SMART devices attached to the skin monitor a patient's stress, depression, and anxiety levels via physiological changes. Wearable technology detects anomalies and treats mental health conditions [41, 42].

2 Mental Disorders that Can Be Dealt with Computational Technology

Mental disorders can wallop people of all ages irrespective of their genders [43]. According to the World Health Organization, "one in four people in the world will be affected by mental or neurological disorders at some point in their lives" [44]. An escalating trend in mental illnesses was inevitable during the pandemic where several populations struggled with their mental health since 2019 while others have managed the symptoms of their mental condition by means of technological aid.

Digital technology holds a great potential for improving the quality of mental health care. Most of the populations of the world had started shifting to the use of SMART Mobile Apps and other remote technologies for treatment and prevention of mental disorders in the pre-pandemic phase [45].

Nonetheless, computational psychiatry is a fast-growing advanced discipline of study that helps in prognostic diagnosis and better treatment for patients with mental illnesses by means of computational neuroscience and machine learning. It is founded on both data and theory driven principles for suggesting predictive measures associated with brain disorders. Innovative developments in the field of

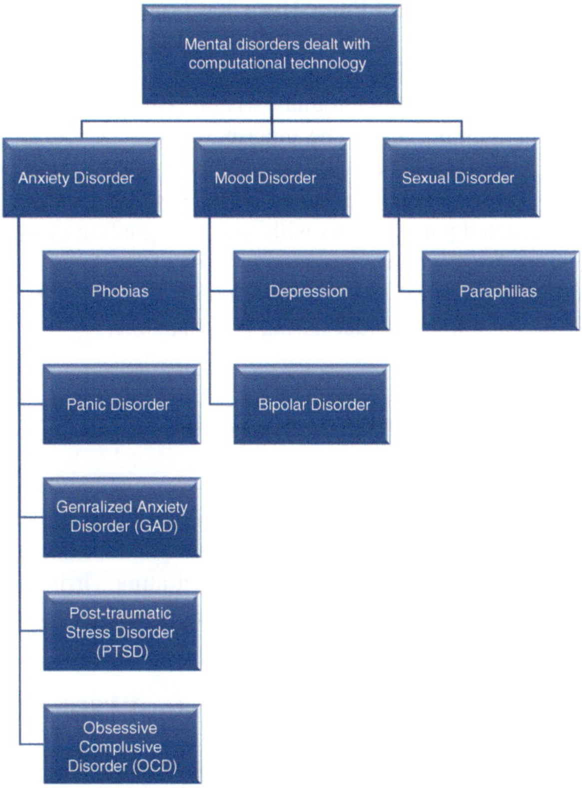

Fig. 1 Mental disorders triggered in COVID-19 and dealt with computational technology

computational technology are facilitating psychiatrists in diagnosing the right treatment of the prevalent mental illness [46]. The mental disorders that can be dealt with computational technology are as follows (Fig. 1).

2.1 *Anxiety Disorder*

Anxiety is a worrisome feeling of disquiet, such as unease which includes mild or severe emotions of disconcertment, tension, or fear. It is all about anticipating that something undesirable, unpleasant, unsavory, and irksome situation may occur. Baron [43], p. 484) defined anxiety as an "Increased arousal accompanied by generalized feelings of fear or apprehension." If the intensity of such sentiments become severe and last for an extended period of time then such distressful feelings cause anxiety disorder which includes panicking, post-traumatic stress disorder (PTSD), generalized anxiety disorder (GAD), and a few specific phobias. There are several types of anxiety disorders, but the relevant to the pandemic are focused here.

2.1.1 Phobia and Panic Disorder Triggered during the Pandemic

The outbreak of COVID-19 made people phobic which is an intense, irrational fear of the human-to-human transmission (HHT) of the novel coronavirus and massive deaths aggravated it. The intense xenophobic situation in the early phase of the pandemic caused panic disorder in most of the population of the world. Majority of the people experienced intense and terrifying anxiety pervaded by periodic and unexpected panic attacks with specific signaling symptoms of heart racing, pounding, and palpitations, sweating, nauseating feelings, fear of dying, insensibility, and chills or hot flashes. Akin panic attacks clubbed with anger flights became the hallmarks of panic disorder during the pandemic.

2.1.2 Generalized Anxiety Disorder (GAD)

It is a mental condition of exorbitant worry about daily/ routine issues without having no good reason and remain in the upsetting situation for at least 6 months [43, 47]. During the pandemic, the triggering symptoms include restlessness, agitation, impatience, fatigue, trouble concentrating, irritability and bad temperament, increased muscle tension, bodily cramps, and trouble sleeping [48, 49].

2.1.3 Post-Traumatic Stress Disorder (PTSD)

PTSD is an anxiety disorder in which people constantly and repetitively experience an episode of a past trauma in their thoughts/ dreams and keep reliving the event in their present. This mental health condition persists for more than a month where the patients get into the flashback of upsetting memories of the traumatic event such as re-experiencing it and occurring of repeated nightmares which completely disrupts their daily lives. Such patients usually avoid healthy interaction with people as they experience social anxiety as well [47]. The arousal level of reliving the past traumatic event causes chronic concentration issues that may result into an attention deficit. They often over-react and exhibit outbursts of anger to difficult situations in different settings. Feelings of hypervigilance, irritability, and sleeplessness are very common [50]. Patients who lost their loved ones during the pandemic and COVID survivors of all ages suffered through PTSD in the post pandemic phase [51, 52].

2.1.4 Obsessive-Compulsive Disorder (OCD)

People with this anxiety disorder have frequent repetitive thoughts (obsessions) that they cannot inhibit unless they perform specific learned behaviors (compulsions) that are resistant to extinction. Obsessive-Compulsive Disorder (OCD) is typified by conspicuous, intrusive, and uncontrollable thoughts or obtrusive urges that are followed by repetitive actions or compulsions that people feel determined to perform [43]. Compulsions are the actions people perform to offset their obsessions. Common symptoms of OCD are illustrated in Table 1.

A few captivating gender differences are observed in OCD patients which are influenced by sociocultural factors. Both genders are at equal risks to be the victim of this mental disorder. Women are much more likely to be "hygiene conscious and compulsive washers" than men. Comparatively, there are no gender differences observed in connection with other compulsive behaviors listed in Table 1. OCD patients engage themselves in performing repetitive religious rituals to reduce the anxiety levels and by doing so they keep themselves busy [47].

The exponential spread of COVID-19 has an enormous impact on the chain of obsessive thoughts and compulsive behaviors in OCD patients with contamination symptoms. As they love to live in their self-constructed-anxiety-ridden prisons, therefore a delivery of evidence-based treatments for OCD is a top priority concern to reduce this public health issue during the global pandemic. [53]. OCD cases were on the rise during pandemic as preventive measures of COVID-19 include repetitive hand washing and sanitizing actions which had worsened the mental condition of the population suffering from this anxiety disorder [19, 54, 55].

2.2 *Mood Disorder*

Experiences of extreme mood swings that destabilize one's emotional state for a prolonged period of time are known as mood disorders. These are triggered from gloomy, blue, and dejected feelings versus cheerful, elated, and thrilled emotions. Occasional mood swings are considered normal but rapid shifts in emotional states that are much more extreme and sustained for a longer period of time are categorized as psychological disorder that has physiological base of happiness and depressive hormonal secretion in the body. People who spend more time in these two

Table 1 Generic symptoms of obsessive-compulsive disorder

Obsessions	Compulsive actions
Cleaning and Hygiene	Repetitive hand washing, frequent bathing, cleaning bedrooms & restrooms, mopping with frequent intervals, excessive sanitizing habits, performing religious cleaning rituals higher than the required, etc.
Organizing and Maintaining Order	Maintaining symmetry and order such as rearranging books, flower vase, cutlery, or aligning wall pictures, bedsheets, pillows, and cushions, repeatedly.
Hoarding of old and useless objects	Collection of old newspapers, mails, outfits, tools, coins, and other objects for no obvious reason.
Anxiety of being safe and secured	Checking doors, windows, locks, water taps, or stove knobs repeatedly.
Repetitive counting and rechecking habit	Counting objects a precise number of times or repeating an action a specific number of times such as the number of steps on a staircase or number of lights in a corridor or on the roads. If they lose count, they go back and start again.

extreme states than other people are described as sufferer of mood disorders. Depressive and bipolar disorders are the most significant mood disorders that are as follows.

2.2.1 Depression

Depression is a serious mood disorder that adversely affects the patient's emotional state, cognitive processes, and daily routine. It may also be referred to as a human blight as it is a prolonged illness. Luckily, it is treatable but widely remained undiagnosed because of the stigma attached to it. Depression causes anxious distress, melancholy, and agitation in mood which results into several impulsive behaviors such as jiggling of legs, fidgeting with one's hands, excessive physical movements, etc. [56]. The types and symptoms of depression derived from Diagnostic and Statistical Manual (DSM) IV & V are defined in Table 2 [43, 57, 58].

Several risk factors are associated with depression such as biochemical imbalance in the brain may cause major or psychotic depression. It may run in the patients'

Table 2 Types and symptoms of depression

Types	Symptoms
Major Depression	Depressive episodes prolonged for at least 2 weeks that typically interfere with one's ability to work, sleep, study, and eat.
Persistent Depressive Disorder (dysthymia)	It includes less severe symptoms of depression that last much longer, typically for at least 2 years • Change in your appetite (not eating enough or overeating) • Sleeping too much or too little • Fatigue • Low self-esteem • Trouble concentrating or making decisions • Feeling hopeless
Perinatal Depression	It occurs when a woman experiences major depression during pregnancy or after delivery. Around 80 per cent of women get the 'baby blues' in the first few days after childbirth. You might feel tearful or overwhelmed, but this will pass in a few days with care and support. The baby blues happens because of changes in your hormones after your baby is born and doesn't mean you'll develop depression.
Seasonal Affective Disorder (SAD)	It comes and goes with the seasons, typically starting in late fall and early winter and going away during spring and summer. Patients affected with SAD experience following symptoms. • Lack of energy • Sleep too much • Overeat and gain weight • Crave for carbohydrates
Depression with symptoms of psychosis	People with psychotic depression have the symptoms of major depression along with "psychotic" symptoms, such as: • Hallucinations (seeing or hearing things that aren't there) • Delusions (false beliefs) • Paranoia (wrongly believing that others are trying to harm you)

genes and people with low self-esteem, introvert, and pessimistic personalities who stress out easily are more likely to experience depression. On the other hand, a variety of emotional distresses cause functional impairment in the personal and professional lives of the patients. Various environmental factors such as feeling of being neglected and exposure to violence or physical abuse also contribute to this mental illness. At times, poverty may put majority of the populations into vulnerable situations that cause depressive disorders *[59]*.

The shockwave of the pandemic jolted a sizable population of the world and left them in an intense depressive phase of worrisome and awful feelings of catching coronavirus through human-to-human transmission (HHT) [60]. The prevalence of stress, anxiety, and depression heightened with a progressive rate in the COVID survivors during the pandemic [61]. Cases of depression and anxiety disorders skyrocketed by 25% over the last 2 years [62].

2.2.2 Bipolar Disorder

Baron [43], defined bipolar disorder as "*a mood disorder in which individuals experience very wide swings in mood, from deep depression to wild elation.*" The definition explicates that depression and bipolar disorder may be identified as the "*emotional sinkhole and roller-coaster of life*," respectively. Furthermore, bipolar disorder is also known as manic depression that brings ultra-rapid mood swings, sleep disturbances, hyper- and hypoactivity in behavior, rapid speech, and racing thought, etc. Mood swings usually occur over a period of weeks, months, and it often stretches to several years that destroys the complete life span of an individual, if remain untreated.

Bipolar is also known as "manic-depressive disorder" as it is a severe mental illness in which people experience recurrent mood swings with lifetime prevalence of morbidity. The mortality rate of the patients with known mental illness is significantly higher than that of the general population [63]. Bipolar disorder is classified into the following three types.

Bipolar I Disorder

People with bipolar I disorder experience chronic and persistent manic episodes with an extreme boost in their energy levels or dangerously ill-tempered mood swings. If such condition continues for more than a week's time, then hospitalization is recommended. In contrast, some people with bipolar I disorder also experience mixed emotions of depressive and hypomanic episodes. Mild manic symptoms are noted in a hypomanic episode that persists for 4 days in a row, but people can perform their daily tasks without any functional impairment. Bipolar I patients are treated with lithium or antipsychotic drugs [64].

Bipolar II Disorder

People with bipolar II disorder experience depressive and hypomanic episodes simultaneously. Bipolar II disorder is very devastating and even more dangerous as it triggers symptoms of chronic depression. The depressive state stretched over several years that lasts for lifetime. Such mental condition provokes the risk of suicidal attempts in patients. People with bipolar II disorder are first treated with antidepressants and later with antipsychotic drugs to make them functional at work.

Cyclothymic Disorder (Cyclothymia)

People with cyclothymic disorder experience unstable mood state, i.e., mild depression and hypomania for at least 2 years in adults and 1 year in children/ teens. People with cyclothymia may have periodic phases of normal mood which lasts for less than 8 weeks.

The types and symptoms of bipolar disorder derived from Diagnostic and Statistical Manual (DSM) IV & V are defined in Table 3 [43, 57, 58].

Bipolar disorder is a chronic mental health disorder with significant morbidity and mortality that affects a sizeable population during pandemic [32, 65]). The successful treatment of coronavirus onsets psychotic mania and depression in a male patient of 44 years who had no psychiatry history [33]. Biochemical, genetic, and environmental factors may cause bipolar disorder to anyone, irrespective of genders. Usually, it onsets at the age of 25 years or at the later age that ranges from 40s to 50s. A few cases of early childhood are also found in literature. The genetic prevalence is significant in onsetting mood disorder at the early age as compared to the older age-groups. The early age onset has symptoms of manic and hypomanic episodes, whereas the later age onset experience elevated moods [65–67]. Lithium is recommended as the preventive treatment for bipolar disorder. On the other hand, prophylactic treatment consists of use of carbamazepine and valproate as a second choice [63].

2.3 Sexual Disorder

Difficulties and disturbances in attaining sexual arousal, orgasms, and conditions involving pain during sexual relations are classified as sexual dysfunctions in nosology. Such sexual dysfunctions cause sexual desire, arousal, and orgasm disorders that are studied psychology and psychiatry as well [68].

The confinement and social distancing measures of the global pandemic resulted into a paradoxical situation. The COVID-19 SOPs were meant to protect the masses, but it led to aggravate the feelings of anxiety, depression, physiological and psychological discomfort during isolation which resulted into several sexual dysfunctions [69, 70].

Table 3 Types and symptoms of bipolar disorder

Types	Symptoms
Bipolar I disorder	Signs and symptoms of a manic episode include: • Excessive happiness, hopefulness, and excitement • Sudden and severe changes in mood, such as going from being joyful to being angry and hostile • Restlessness, impulsive, rapid speech, and racing thoughts • Increased energy and less need for sleep • Making grand and unattainable plans • Reckless and risk-taking behavior, such as drug and alcohol misuse, rash driving, and having unsafe or unprotected sex • Feeling like you're unusually important, talented, or powerful • Psychosis - experiencing hallucinations and delusions (in the most severe manic episodes)
Bipolar II disorder	The symptoms of depressive episodes in bipolar disorder are the same as those of major depression. These include: • Overwhelming sadness, low energy, and fatigue • Lack of motivation and irritability • Feelings of hopelessness or worthlessness • Loss of enjoyment of things that were once pleasurable • Difficulty concentrating and making decisions • Uncontrollable crying • Insomnia or excessive sleep • A change in appetite, causing weight loss or gain • Thoughts of death or suicide (suicidal ideation)
Cyclothymic disorder	Cyclothymic disorder symptoms include the following: • For at least 2 years, many periods of hypomanic and depressive symptoms, but the symptoms do not meet the criteria for hypomanic or depressive episode • During the 2-year period, the symptoms (mood swings) have lasted for at least half the time and have never stopped for more than 2 months

Cybersex is one of the examples of deviant sexual behaviors that intensified sexual arousal levels in paraphilias which resulted into the spread of paraphilic disorder across the globe [24, 25].

2.3.1 Paraphilia Disorder

Paraphilic disorder involves recurrent sexual arousal that intensifies sexual urges, desires, fantasies and provokes publicly unacceptable behaviors that are marked by bizarre metaphors such as images or acts that are atypical in nature [43, 71, 72].

Paraphilic acts fall under the ambit of public order crime and such sexual disorders are diagnosed principally in forensic settings. Diagnostic and Statistical Manual (DSM) V has a huge emphasis on forensic implications for bringing significant changes in the definitions of paraphilic disorders as it involves legal ramification [73]. The types and symptoms of paraphilias derived from Diagnostic and Statistical Manual (DSM) IV & V are defined in Table 4 [43, 74].

Table 4 Types of paraphilias

Description	Symptoms
Exhibitionism	Sexual urges or arousing fantasies involving exposure of one's genitals to an unsuspecting stranger.
Voyeurism	Recurrent sexual urges or arousing fantasies involving the act of observing an unsuspecting person who is naked, disrobing, or engaging in sexual activity
Fetishism Sadism and Masochism	Sexual arousal or persistent fantasies about or actual use of nonliving objects. Sadism: Sexual arousal or fantasies about or from engaging in actions of dominating or beating another person. Masochism: Sexual arousal or fantasies about or from engaging in the act of being dominated, humiliated, or even beaten.
Transvestic Fetishism	Intense sexual urges and arousing fantasies involving cross-dressing (dressing in the clothing of the other sex)
Other Paraphilias	Frotteurism: Sexual urges involving touching or rubbing against a nonconsenting person Necrophilia: Sexual obsession with corpses Klismaphilia: Sexual excitement from having enemas Coprophilia: Sexual interest in feces Zoophilia: Sexual gratification from having sexual activity with animals

2.4 Traditional Predictive Measures in Psychology to Assess Mental Disorders

Baron [43] explained that psychologists usually adopt a mode of research for diagnosing and identifying the causes of the earlier discussed mental disorders. They ask pain and pleasure inducing questions during the research and use the following four traditional assessment tools to choose the right treatment for a specific patient.

2.4.1 Life History of Patients

Collecting life history of patients for the record purpose is one of the sources of fundamental information of the patients' past life (e.g., childhood and adolescence academic performance, criminal records, medical history, family relations, etc.). This information helps in diagnosing the root cause by indicating the origin of the mental illness, its duration till the date of assessment, and how it has affected the patients' life.

2.4.2 Assessment Interviews and Behavioral Observations

Patients' personal opinion about their existing problems, reacting behaviors, and interpersonal relations are gathered via assessment interviews to understand their personality set. Another tool is observing repeated patterns of behavior of patients in natural and standardized situations (e.g., at academia and work, behavioral interactions and verbal exchanges family and friends, reactions to a traumatic video or news bulletin, showcasing objects, exposing them to situation they strongly fear to detect phobias).

2.4.3 Psychological Tests

Psychological tests are used to collect information on cognitive functioning of the brain as a few mental disorders occurred due to brain damage or malfunctioning of the nervous system. To diagnose such damages neuropsychological test titled "*Halstead– Reitan Neuropsychological Battery* is conducted to test the auditory, visual, and psychomotor functioning (e.g., eye–hand coordination). The pattern of scores obtained by a given individual can point to the existence of specific forms of brain damage" [43].

2.4.4 Biological Predictive Measures for Mood, Anxiety, and Sexual Disorders

As discussed earlier in Sect. 1, the biological measures include neuroimaging techniques such as radiography and radiology to predict the existence of anxiety and mood disorders. In radiography, computerized tomography (CT) scans and positron emission tomography (PET) scans are used to identify any brain damage, whereas X-rays and magnetic resonance imaging (MRI) are applied as a radiographical tool to study the biological bases of nervous system disorders. Moreover, biological markers include changes in liver physiology. Such variation in standard enzyme secretion level indicates alcoholism in patients of anxiety disorders [75], whereas rise in heart rate, blood pressure, and muscle tension are other important signs as well [43, 47].

Contrarily, pathological tests are used as biological markers for sexual disorders such as paraphilia. Paraphilic disorder may also be identified through urine and blood pathology. Fisher and Marwaha [71] explained in their research that "the increased levels of serotonin and norepinephrine, with a decreased concentration of DOPAC (3,4-dihydroxyphenylacetic acid) in urine samples" is a biological indicator of paraphilic disorder. Moreover, high levels of androgen (male hormone) in the blood sample of the patients are another predictive measure in association with physical medical checkup which includes complete blood count (CBC), rapid plasma reagent (RPR), and thyroid-stimulating hormone (TSH) level or thyroid function test (TFT) [76]. Psychiatrists prescribe three main pharmacological agents, namely selective serotonin reuptake inhibitors (SSRIs), synthetic steroidal analogs, and antiandrogens for managing paraphilic disorders [71].

2.5 Use of Computational Technology as a Predictive Measure for Anxiety, Mood, and Sexual Disorders

Computational predictive measures have its roots in traditional/ biological predictive measures of anxiety, mood, and sexual disorders as these are dependent upon Patient Health Questionnaire (PHQ) and the Depression, Anxiety and Stress Scale (DASS) for screening the symptoms associated with these mental illnesses. During pandemic, mental disorder like anxiety, depression, and stress have badly damaged psychological health of the masses and can be predicted by using machine learning algorithms with absolute accuracy [77, 78]; for example, recurrent episodes of bipolar disorder can be monitored using predictive modeling [79]. Clinical prediction of bipolar disorders has been made easier by means of neuroimaging scans and machine learning [80]. Machine learning also added value to precision psychiatry for clinically informed psychiatric diagnosis by setting immunological, neuroanatomical, and cognitive biomarkers [81]. Moreover, smartphones are generally considered useful tool for detecting the symptoms of mental disorders, and various customized mobile applications have been developed. Computational chemoproteomics played a significant role in treating sexual disorders (paraphilias) using pharmacological agents [82–84]. Detailed aspects of such technologies are explained next.

3 Major Computing Technologies for Tackling Mental Disorders

3.1 Internet of Things (IoT)

IoT technology promises to reshape the healthcare service delivery, and its role has particularly been prominent during the pandemic. Due to the crucial requirements of social distancing, novel ways of using IoT sensors and wearable devices emerged to control the spread of COVID-19 [85, 86]. The linked devices powered by IoT technology do not only ensure improving physical health but also guarantee monitoring and managing mental health of populations. Timely indication about change in psychological and physiological parameters may alert the users as well as mental healthcare providers about developing methods to prevent more serious mental disorders.

It is to be noted that the IoT is best suited for the mental disorders that result in observable changes. So far, IoT systems have been developed for bipolar disorders, depression, anxiety, PSTD, and schizophrenia [87]. As previously discussed, bipolar disorders are characterized by mood changes that can be identified by varying energy levels of the patient. IoT sensors may be used for detecting behavioral changes and subsequently, appropriate level of medical or technology intervention (such as therapy) may be suggested. For example, monitoring of walking and movement patterns is often utilized for identifying physical impairments in people [88], but they may also indicate behavioral or lifestyle changes. Cameras, motion, and pulse rate sensors are mostly deployed for physical activity monitoring. Similarly, data about location, speech features, and interaction with devices such as smart phone, watches, and computers may also indicate the presence of expected mental disorders; for example, the voice features collected from mics embedded with smart phones or watches are known to correctly identify depression disorders.

The emerging domains of Ambient Assisted Living (AAL) and Activities of Daily Living (ADL) provide capability of monitoring behaviors of people in their own home or work environments [89]. ADLs help to monitor the behaviors related to various routine activities related to mobility, hygiene, eating, continence, and dressing. Since in most of the mental disorders, the aspect of self-maintenance is compromised, the IoT could provide a timely insight into the changing patterns which may be utilized for developing prevention strategies.

In addition to detecting mental disorders using IoT, several solutions have also been proposed to solve them. For example, a novel scheme of automated music therapy integrated with wearable sensors has been proposed [90], where the focus is on reducing anxiety by playing music of appropriate type. Moreover, the brain activity sensing headbands may be used to analyze the impact of music therapy and neurofeedback may be incorporated for improving the automated therapy experience [91].

3.2 *Emerging Mobile Applications*

The mental healthcare sector was overwhelmed during COVID-19 due to the existing shortage of mental healthcare professionals/therapists and also due to the restrictions on providing elective therapy services. Thus, there has been a surge in digital initiatives for mental health along with the development of various mobile apps. These apps target the mental health needs of the population and deliver cost-effective service while maintaining confidentiality. Majority of the mental health apps are free, with optional subscription-based components; here, it is to be noted that even the full version of apps is significantly lower in cost as compared to the conventional therapy services [92]. For the cultures, where mental disorders are still regarded as a taboo subject, these apps have particularly been useful [93]. Also, the perceived need about therapy is often low, even in the highly vulnerable population groups.

A wide variety of apps have been developed to track and treat anxiety, depression, and other mood disorders. A few to mention include, What'sMyM3 [94] for tracking mood disorders, Depression CBT [95] for keeping cognitive thought diary, Breathe2Relax [96] for stress management, Headspace [97] for reducing anxiety through meditation, Mood Track Diary [98] for tracking and visualizing mood cycles, and eMoods Charting [99] for tracking bipolar disorders.

3.3 Machine Learning/Deep Learning

Use of artificial intelligence, machine learning, and deep learning technologies brings numerous benefits to the mental health, some of these benefits include development of new and reliable methods of treatment, opportunities to excess far-off populations, better patient response, and ensuring a greater deal of work-life balance for the mental health professionals as there is already a severe shortage of these practitioners. Standard prediction modeling techniques of machine learning such as logistic regression are widely established for predicting mental health problems. For example, a machine learning approach has been applied particularly to identify anxiety and depression symptoms. The random forest approach has been employed for classifying major predictors of mental distress. Moreover, expert systems have also been used for identifying the sexual deviations that might have appeared in people due to COVID-19. A web-based system using Dempster Shafer method can be used to detect Paraphilia and other sexual disorders [100]. As previously discussed, it has been crucial in clinical psychology to be able to differentiate between different mental disorders in order to develop appropriate treatment strategies. Machine learning models have also been proposed to differentiate between closely resembling mental disorders, such as bipolar disorder (BD) and major depressive disorder (MDD) [101]. Moreover, healthy people and those with BD can be differentiated using neuroimaging scans coupled with a machine learning algorithm [102]. Schizophrenia has also been successfully identified using machine learning models. For such studies, the parameters of interest have been risky behavior, recklessness, grandiosity, and elevated mood.

During COVID-19, various machine learning models have been used to identify the behavior changes among the population. Since social media has been one of the major forums where people have been expressing/sharing their concerns and views, human-centered machine learning models have been developed to predict the mental health state of users. In this regard, Natural Language Processing (NLP) and opinion mining have been prominent technologies [103]. The major focus of these technologies has been on identifying extract symptoms, classifying severity of illness, providing psychopathological clues, comparing effectiveness of therapy, and challenging the current nosography. Moreover, NLP has often been used for confirming clinical hypotheses, rather than developing entirely new information. However, the unexplored data about lifestyles is extracted using machine learning and NLP. Similarly, social media population is the major category that has been the imprecise cohort for NLP.

Machine learning tools can even be used for detecting the impact of psychological interventions delivered via internet. For example, the behavior of people who receive internet-based cognitive behavioral therapy (CBT) may be analyzed using machine learning algorithms [104]. Similarly, the impact of mental health mobile apps can also be assessed using supervised machine learning models that are generally used for classification problems.

3.4 Big Data Analytics

IoT, AI, and big data are often combined for screening, prediction, and phenotyping of mental health problems. Data from various sources such as social media, ubiquitous sensors, and healthcare systems are merged to identify complex trends in population health data. During COVID-19, big data analytics algorithms may efficiently be used to collect user data and predict their mental disorder risk. Mainly, travel data has been combined with social media using big data algorithms to generate preventive alerts and track quarantine. Data collected at multiple points such as airports, checkpoints, community entrances, traffic entrances, and social media were combined to maintain the recommended level of social isolation.

Although the major trends of big data analytics during COVID-19 have been related to physical health, some solutions have also been developed for mental health. As previously mentioned, social media has been the major forum to collect information about sentiments and lifestyle changes of populations. In this context, Twitter corpus has been used to identify the emerging themes regarding mental health at the US during COVID-19. Various other insights have also been developed using big data techniques, such as changing patterns of social media usage during COVID-19 and sentiment change as a response to social isolation [105]. In some approaches, big data algorithms merge data from electronic health records and social media to assess the mental health risk. Similarly, social media big data has been used to study the impact of collectivism and fear on the public's preventive intention toward COVID-19. All these big data trends provided an opportunity to predict the mental health state. Since it has been a challenge to collect data about mental health due to restricted clinical visits, big data techniques provided a great deal of insight by collecting massive datasets.

Furthermore, big data analytics have been used to guide the policy making regarding lockdown and quarantine. Mental health was most affected due to social isolation and limited access of population to the community facilities, data collected about impact of policies were directly associated with mental health management. Therefore, data analytics was performed at different countries that practiced different levels of lockdown [106]. The effectiveness of different lockdown strategies was compared by collecting big data about number of cases reported in each country, the severity of those cases, the number of deaths, etc. Similarly, the prevalence of mental disorders among different regions has been identified using big data algorithms, and the impact of lockdown and isolation policies has been assessed. Moreover, big data analytics techniques may also help to understand the attributes of users of mental health services.

3.5 Assistive Technologies

As per the *Technology Related Assistance to Individuals with Disabilities Act of 1988*, "any item, piece of equipment or product system, whether acquired commercially off the shelf, modified or customized, that is used to increase, maintain or improve functional capabilities of individuals with disabilities," is referred to as an ***Assistive Technology*** (AT) [107]. Predominantly AT has been developed and used to help with different ailments of the body and physical disabilities, like hearing impairments, blindness, dumbness, etc. However, recently several digital platform-based ATs have been introduced to help with mental disorders like stress, anxiety, depression, especially during the spread of COVID-19. Social distancing, high mortality rate, financial lockdown resulted in an increased mental health concerns like increased depression and anxiety, predominantly among the elderlies. A few AT digital platforms have been developed over the past few years, both to deal with COVID-19-related and, in general, mental health issues.

In the following, we describe one such digital platform-based AT for real-time monitoring and self-assessment of individual's psychological health. The solution integrates wearable devices, computing platform, psychological intervention tools, and a mobile application called ***Stay Healthy*** [108]. Wearables record relevant psychological data from an individual and the individuals self-report their perceptions through two intervention tools suitable for elderlies, Geriatric Anxiety Scale (GAS) [109] and Geriatric Depression Scale (GDS) [110]. Both observations are collected through a mobile application of Stay Healthy, which, in turn, determines the range of anxiety and depression risk of the monitored individual at any particular point in time.

The functional overview of Stay Healthy is provided in Fig. 2, where the wearables report psychological parameters like pulse rate, SPO_2, temperature, and blood pressure and the individuals report their cognitive perception through GAS (30-items version) and GDS (15-items version). 4-point Likert scale (0 = not at all, to 3 = all of the time) is used in GAS involving three sub-scales: somatic, cognitive, and affective. Anxiety scores are leveled at, *0–7: No Anxiety*; *8–15: Mild Anxiety*; *16–25: Moderate Anxiety* and *25* indicates *severe level of anxiety*. GDS records yes/no with scores between 0 and 15; < *5: Normal*, *5–9: Mild* and > *9: Severe*

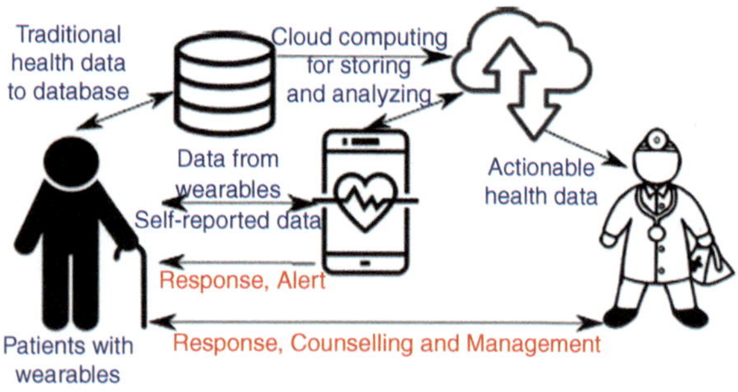

Fig. 2 Functional overview of stay healthy

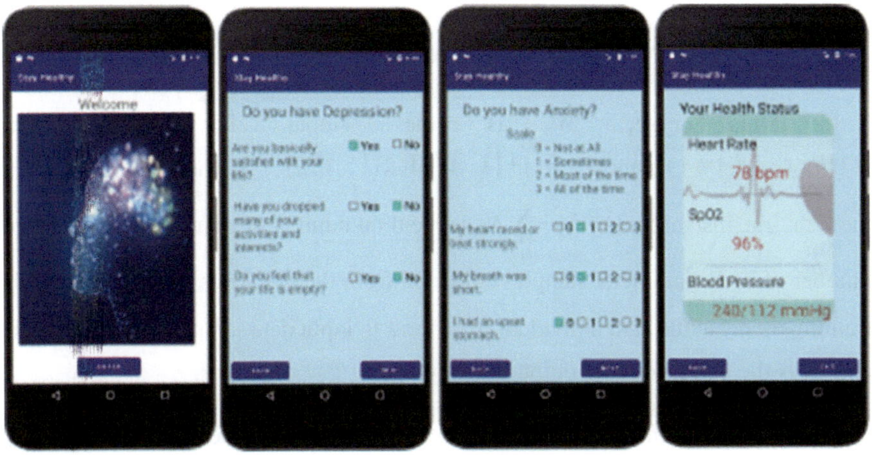

Fig. 3 Snapshot of stay healthy

Depression. Based on the recordings from both the wearable platform and the individual's perceptions, Stay Healthy can categorize the anxiety level of the individuals and generate alerts if the individual needs immediate attention from oneself and/or doctors and caregivers. A snapshot of Stay Healthy is provided in Fig. 3.

Stay Healthy could be extended to several application possibilities. It can be further developed to support multiple national and regional languages and integrate it with cloud hosting services. Stay Healthy can be deployed for clinical trials to assess user comfort level and improve outcomes for individuals as well as caregivers. Finally Stay Healthy can be integrated with an Artificial Intelligence (AI) platform for anxiety risk categorization and activating automated response.

3.6 Federated Learning

As AI and Machine Learning (ML) are pervading every walk of life in different forms, they are also finding applications in healthcare and remote health management. One of the most popular techniques that found its way to healthcare applications is Federated Learning (FL) owing to its capability of training multiple devices with data-handling capacity, preserving patient privacy and managing compliance with data protection acts. An FL algorithm is developed below to predict patient anxiety level in individuals using decentralized body parameters from the patients. These parameters include pulse rate, blood pressure and blood oxygen level, SPO_2, which are indicative of anxiety and stress level of individuals [90].

Let us consider there are M number of individuals that are monitored and their hand-held device (mobile phone, tablet, etc.) jointly execute the FL algorithm. The first step is the FL training process whose aim is to solve the minimization problem

$$\min_{w_1, w_2 \ldots\ldots w_M} \frac{1}{N} \sum_{m=1}^{M} \sum_{k=1}^{N_m} f\left(w_m, x_m^k, y_m^k\right) \text{ subject to } w_1, w_2 \ldots\ldots w_M = \boldsymbol{W} \tag{1}$$

In this case, $\boldsymbol{W}$ is the global FL model and $f\left(\boldsymbol{W}, x_m^k, y_m^k\right) = -y_m^k \log\left(x_m^{kT} \boldsymbol{W}\right) + \left(1 - y_m^k\right) \log\left(1 - x_m^{kT} \boldsymbol{W}\right)$ is the loss function at the T th time instant. In (1), $N = \sum_{m=1}^{M} N_m$ is the total number of training data, N_m is the number of body parameter samples collected from the m th user, w_m is the local FL training model at the m th individual, x_m^k is the k th input data sample of the m th user, and y_m^k is the corresponding output anxiety level.

In each FL iteration, each individual can exhibit his/her anxiety level in one of the four ranges: normal, moderate, severe, and extreme. Let the probability of each individual experiencing one of the anxiety levels at the t th time instant can be expressed as a vector

$$\boldsymbol{p}_{m,t} = \left[p_{m,t,0}, \ldots\ldots p_{m,t,4}\right]. \tag{2}$$

where $p_{m,\,t,\,0}$ is the probability that the individual experience current stress level, while $p_{m,\,t,\,1}$, $p_{m,\,t,\,2}$, $p_{m,\,t,\,3}$, $p_{m,\,t,\,4}$ are the probabilities with which the stress level changes to normal, moderate, severe, and extreme, respectively. Once the local FL models are collected, the next step is to formulate the global FL model for each iteration and the threshold time for waiting to update the global model is given by γ. The updated global FL model in this case can be formulated as

$$\boldsymbol{W} = \frac{\sum_{m=1}^{M} N_m w_{m,t} 1_{\{\tau_m \le \gamma\}}}{\sum_{m=1}^{M} N_m 1_{\{\tau_m \le \gamma\}}} \tag{3}$$

where τ_m is the waiting time for the m th individual, $1_{\{\tau_m \le \gamma\}}$ is the indicator function and is equal to 1 for the time taken by the local FL model to reach the global consensus. The next step is to train back the local FL models and update the local models using

$$w_{m,t+1} = \boldsymbol{W} - \frac{\lambda}{N_m} \sum_{k=1}^{N_m} \nabla f\left(\boldsymbol{W}, x_m^k, y_m^k\right). \tag{4}$$

where λ is the learning rate and $\nabla f\left(\boldsymbol{W}, x_m^k, y_m^k\right)$ is the gradient of $f\left(\boldsymbol{W}, x_m^k, y_m^k\right)$ with respect to $\boldsymbol{W}$**.** The updated local model is sent back to the platform to update the global FL model using

$$\boldsymbol{W}' = \frac{\sum_{m=1}^{M} N_m w_{m,t+1} 1_{\{\tau_m \le \gamma\}}}{\sum_{m=1}^{M} N_m 1_{\{\tau_m \le \gamma\}}} \tag{5}$$

Finally, W' is distributed back to the individuals to finalize their FL models. Using this procedure, it is possible to manage anxiety risk in real time whether arising due to COVID-19 or in general scenario.

4 Challenges Associated with Use of Computing for Mental Health Management

Although computing brings numerous benefits to the domain of mental health management, there are certain challenges that must be addressed to avail the full benefit. There are issues related to data acquisition, consent, privacy, organization of devices, service level agreements in addition to the possibility of bias and flaws in the computing solutions/automated services. In this section, we briefly look at such challenges.

4.1 Data Acquisition

It is vital for computing technologies to be able to acquire accurate data for preventing mental disorders. However, there are various limitations and challenges that must be efficiently dealt with. First, device limitations come into play in majority of the technical solutions developed toward mental health management, cameras and sensors are used for data collection. For the cases where cameras are used, the users are always assumed to be in a specific range and remain line-of-sight which is clearly not possible [88]. Therefore, wearable movement and other vital parameter sensors are used in integration to ensure continuous data collection regarding activity monitoring. Second, there are also constraints associated with malfunctioning or lack of precision in the sensing devices.

4.2 Consent

The ambitious claims made by technological proposals for mental health management are often constrained due to the ethical principles of protection of autonomy and consent. Although when population data is collected and analyzed using Big Data techniques, individual human subjects are not identified, yet it is not possible to ensure consent of the users. The data is not only accessed by the designated healthcare practitioners, but also by software and hardware developers and other third-party users. Therefore, there is a need to clearly define the access level of each user for the patients' data, and the consent for same must be obtained by the patients.

4.3 Confidentiality

Digital software and hardware have heavily been used by mental health professionals for communicating with patients and storing their information. Various computing tools including emails, text messages, mobile apps, cloud-based storage, electronic medical records are used for facilitating mental health monitoring and management processes. Although technology has empowered patients and medical professionals a lot, at the same time, there are serious concerns related to patient's confidentiality. For example, the apps developed for offering online CBT collect audio, video, text messaging, and activity data from patients' phones to assess the impact of CBT. Furthermore, the advanced apps also collect data from sensors and sleep monitors. Although such data would provide valuable insight to the treatment teams, at the same time, unauthorized users including device manufacturers, app developers, network operators, data storage, and data analytics companies present threat to the patients' privacy and security. Even the researchers and app developers may be using patients' data for testing their AI and other computing solutions, without considering the crucial requirements of ethics and privacy. Therefore, the risk for patients to face unintended breaches has been increasing and there must be effective security measures (such as encryption and cryptography) embedded within the computational systems associated with mental healthcare.

4.4 Lack of Legislation

It is a public health priority worldwide to protect health related data. Unauthorized access to sensitive health information may lead to various consequences including social stigma, embarrassment, social discrimination, etc., by insurers and employers. The use of computing technologies in the field of mental health is still in infancy stage and necessary legislations are yet to be made in most parts of the world. Similarly, guidance for the development, implementation of computing technologies, and underlying ethical principles are also not clearly stated. These constraints of technology often act as a major barrier for accessing treatments. Although there are laws such as Health Insurance Portability and Accountability Act of 1996 (HIPAA), their application is restricted to only certain applications and organizations. The wide scale deployments of computing solutions for mental health monitoring and management are not required to comply with the existing laws.

4.5 Reliability Issues

A major concern for using computational technology for healthcare in general and mental health in particular is the lack of reliability from both the software and hardware perspectives. This is particularly true for the patients suffering from elevated risks such as those having suicidal thoughts. In case the technology solution is not able to timely detect the mental health risk, life-threatening situations may occur. The hardware equipment (sensors, actuators, and similar) should be smart enough to timely communicate the risks; similarly, the software solutions (AI applications and others) must also be transparent.

In addition to technical reliability issues, there is also a lack of awareness in people regarding the use of computational technologies. For example, limited digital literacy acts as a major barrier for population to begin using mobile apps that could offer them accessibility to cost effective mental care. Similarly, due to the lack of trust on technology, people often refrain from accessing online therapy and other treatment services as they are afraid of becoming vulnerable to data breach. There is limited to no guidance provided to communities about choosing from thousands of available mental health apps. Hence, there is a need to develop reliable computational solutions targeted at mental healthcare needs; at the same time, community awareness needs to be created providing clear evidence of safety, possible risks, and benefits.

5 Summary

Advanced computing technologies are capable to offer predictive measures for monitoring and managing mental disorders under normal and pandemic situations. This chapter presented a detailed account of mental disorders that emerged during COVID-19 including phobias, anxiety, depression, bipolar disorders, and paraphilia. The role of Internet of Things, Machine Learning, Big Data analytics, Assistive Technologies, and Federated Learning has been discussed for reducing the mental healthcare services cost and delay. Multiple technologies are often combined to ensure timely assessment of mental health state of the patients, which subsequently helps the therapists to identify the risk levels and developed customized therapy/treatment plans. Despite promising revolution in mental healthcare, the use of computing technology for this domain still faces several constraints related to data acquisition, patient consent and confidentiality, and lack of legislation and reliability. Hence, there is a scope of future research for addressing gaps in regulatory and ethical framework to ensure safe access of computing technologies for improving mental health state.

References

1. Javed B, Sarwer A, Soto EB, Mashwani Z-U-R. The coronavirus (COVID-19) pandemic's impact on mental health. Int J Health Plann Manag. 2020;35:993–6.
2. World Health Organization. Mental disorders. 2022. https://www.who.int/news-room/fact-sheets/detail/mental-disorders.
3. World Health Organization. The impact of COVID-19 on mental health cannot be made light of. 2022. https://www.who.int/news-room/feature-stories/detail/the-impact-of-covid-19-on-mental-health-cannot-be-made-light-of.
4. Liu Y-C, Kuo R-L, Shih S-R. COVID-19: the first documented coronavirus pandemic in history. Biom J. 2020;43(4):328–33. https://doi.org/10.1016/j.bj.2020.04.007.
5. Bakkeli NZ. Predicting psychological distress during the COVID-19 pandemic: do socioeconomic factors matter? Soc Sci Comput Rev. 2022;41(4):1227–51. https://doi.org/10.1177/08944393211069622.
6. Murtaza M. COVID-19 and mental health challenges in Pakistan. Int J Social Psychaitry. 2021;67(3):303–4. https://doi.org/10.1177/0020764020954487.
7. Fountoulakis KN. Mental health. In: Fountoulakis KN, editor. Psychiatry. Cham: Springer; 2021. p. 385–8. https://doi.org/10.1007/978-3-030-86541-2_14.
8. Keyes CL. The mental health continuum: from languishing to flourishing in life. J Health Social. 2002;43(2):207–22. https://pubmed.ncbi.nlm.nih.gov/12096700/.
9. Henriques, G.. 2013. Mental disorders vs diseases (psychiatry is in crisis because it is committed to the "mental disease" model). https://www.psychologytoday.com/us/blog/theory-knowledge/201305/mental-disorders-vs-diseases.
10. Lane C. The NIMH withdraws support for DSM-5. Psychology Today; 2013. https://www.psychologytoday.com/us/blog/side-effects/201305/the-nimh-withdraws-support-dsm-5.
11. Brülde B, Radovic F. What is mental about mental disorder? Philosophy, Psychiatry and Psychology. 2006;13(2):99–116. https://muse.jhu.edu/article/209809.
12. Citizens Commission on Human Rights. Real Disease vs. Mental "Disorder". Citizens Commission on Human Rights (Watchdog investigating and exposing psychiatric human rights violations). n.d.. https://www.cchr.org/quick-facts/real-disease-vs-mental-disorder.html.
13. Henriques G. The harmful dysfunction analysis and the differentiation between mental disorder and disease. Sci Rev Ment Health Prac. 2002;1(2):157–73. http://www.srmhp.org/0102/dysfunction-analysis.html.
14. McVey D. The new health development agency. Health. 2005;Variations(5):3. https://www.lancaster.ac.uk/fass/projects/hvp/pdf/nl5art2.pdf.
15. Mental Health Center of America. Alphabetical list of mental disorders. Mental Health Center of America; n.d.. https://mentalhealthcenter.com/alphabetical-list-of-mental-disorders/.
16. Chen R, Wang Y. Mental health impacts of COVID-19. Globalization and Health; 2021. https://www.biomedcentral.com/collections/MentalHealthCOVID19.
17. Su Z, McDonnell D, Roth S, Li Q, Šegalo S, Shi F, Wagers S. Mental health impacts of COVID-19. Glob Health. 2021;17(67):1–11. https://doi.org/10.1186/s12992-021-00710-7.
18. Yuan Y, Zhao Y-J, Zhang Q-E, Zhang L, Cheung T, Jackson T, Xiang Y-T. COVID-19-related stigma and its sociodemographic correlates: a comparative study. Glob Health. 2021;17(54):1–9. https://doi.org/10.1186/s12992-021-00705-4.
19. Prestia D, Pozza A, Olcese M, Escelsior A, Dettore D, Amore M. The impact of the COVID-19 pandemic on patients with OCD: effects of contamination symptoms and remission state before the quarantine in a preliminary naturalistic study. Psychiatry Res. 2020;291:113213. https://doi.org/10.1016/j.psychres.2020.113213.
20. Valdés-Florido M, López-Díaz Á, Palermo-Zeballos FJ, et al. Clinical characterization of brief psychotic disorders triggered by the COVID-19 pandemic: a multicenter observational study. Eur Arch Psychiatry Clin Neurosci. 2022;272:5–15. https://doi.org/10.1007/s00406-021-01256-w.

21. American Psychiatric Association. Paraphilic disorder. American Psychiatric Association; 2013. https://www.psychiatry.org/File%20Library/Psychiatrists/Practice/DSM/APA_DSM-5-Paraphilic-Disorders.pdf.
22. Moulden H, Bradford J. Coping with COVID-19: pandemic life and problematic sexual behaviour. Int J Risk Recovery. 2021;4(2):1–3. https://doi.org/10.15173/ijrr.v4i2.5012.
23. Mumm J-N, Vilsmaier T, Schuetz JM, Rodler S, Zehni A, Bauer R, Batz F. How the COVID-19 pandemic affects sexual behavior of hetero-, homo-, and bisexual males in Germany. Sex Med. 2021;9(4):100380. https://doi.org/10.1016/j.esxm.2021.100380.
24. US National Library of Medicine (NIH). Covid-19 lockdown and deviant sexual fantasies. ClinicalTrials.gov - US National Library of Medicine (NIH); 2020. https://clinicaltrials.gov/ct2/show/NCT04448405.
25. Banerjee D, Rao T. "#intimacy" at times of COVID-19: the renewed impetus behind cybersex. J Psychosexual Health. 2021;3(1):13–7. https://doi.org/10.1177/26318318211004397.
26. CDN Newswire. (2022). Paraphilia disorder treatment market Covid-19 impact analysis, opportunities, threats, drivers, restraints, trends, applications, and growth forecast to 2029. https://www.digitaljournal.com/pr/paraphilia-disorder-treatment-market-covid-19-impact-analysis-opportunities-threats-drivers-restraints-trends-applications-and-growth-forecast-to-2029.
27. Khan KS, Mamun MA, Griffiths MD, Ullah I. The mental health impact of the COVID-19 pandemic across different cohorts. Int J Ment Heal Addict. 2020;1-7:380. https://doi.org/10.1007/s11469-020-00367-0.
28. Harvey AG, Talbot L, Gershon A. Sleep disturbance in bipolar disorder across the lifespan. Clin Psychol (New York). 2009;16(2):256–77. https://doi.org/10.1111/j.1468-2850.2009.01164.x.
29. Stuart A, Nazario B. Bipolar Disorder and Sleep Problems. WebMD; 2022. https://www.webmd.com/bipolar-disorder/guide/bipolar-disorder-and-sleep-problems
30. Fellendorf FT, Reininghaus EZ, Ratzenhofer M, Lenger M, Maget A, Platzer M, Dalkner N. COVID-19-related fears and information frequency predict sleep behavior in bipolar disorder. Brain and Behavior. 2021;11(9):e02182. https://doi.org/10.1002/brb3.2182.
31. Casale AD, Modesti MN, Rapisarda L, Girardi P, Tambelli R. Clinical aspects of manic episodes after SARS-CoV-2 contagion or COVID-19. Front Psychol. 2022;13:926084. https://doi.org/10.3389/fpsyt.2022.926084.
32. Spelber D, Strakowski SM. Expert opinion in bipolar disorder: impact of COVID-19 on outcomes and treatment of bipolar disorder. Pers Med Psychiatry. 2021;27:100074. https://doi.org/10.1016/j.pmip.2021.100074.
33. Kurczewska E, Nawojczyk M, Ferensztajn-Rochowiak E, Jaracz J, Rybakowski F. Onset of bipolar disorder induced by treated COVID-19 infection in a 44-year-old man with no psychiatric history. Bipolar Disord. 2022;24(2):214–6. https://doi.org/10.1111/bdi.13173.
34. Beard JR, Heathcote K, Brooks R, Earnest A, Kelly B. Predictors of mental disorders and their outcome in a community based cohort. Soc Psychiatry Psychiatr Epidemiol. 2007;42(8):623–30. https://doi.org/10.1007/s00127-007-0182-3.
35. Chancellor S, Choudhury MD. Methods in predictive techniques for mental health status on social media: a critical review. NPJ Digital Medicine. 2020;3(43):1–11. https://doi.org/10.1038/s41746-020-0233-7.
36. Becker D, Breda WV, Funk B, Hoogendoorn M, Ruwaard J, Ripercd H. Predictive modeling in e-mental health: a common language framework. Internet Interv. 2018;12:57–67. https://doi.org/10.1016/j.invent.2018.03.002.
37. American Psychiatric Association. Paraphilic Disorder. American Psychiatric Association; 2019. https://www.psychiatry.org/psychiatrists/practice/mental-health-apps/app-evaluation-model. Accessed 18 Dec 2022.
38. Hategan A, Giroux C, Bourgeois JA. Digital technology adoption in psychiatric care: an overview of the contemporary shift from technology to opportunity. J Technol Behav Sci. 2019;4:171–7. https://doi.org/10.1007/s41347-019-00086-x.

39. U.S. Food & Drug Administration. *Digital Health Center of Excellence*. U.S. Food & Drug Administration; 2022. https://www.fda.gov/medical-devices/digital-health-center-excellence. Accessed 18 Dec 2022.
40. Bashshur RL, Howell JD, Krupinski EA, Harms KM, Bashshur N, Doarn CR. The empirical foundations of telemedicine interventions in primary care. Telemed J E Health. 2016;22(5):342–75. https://doi.org/10.1089/tmj.2016.0045.
41. Elgendi M, Menon C. Assessing anxiety disorders using wearable devices: challenges and future directions. Brain Sci. 2019;9(3):50. https://doi.org/10.3390/brainsci9030050.
42. Hickey, B. A., Chalmers, T., Newton, P., Lin, C.-T., Sibbritt, D., McLachlan, C. S., . . . Lal, S. (2021). Smart devices and wearable technologies to detect and monitor mental health conditions and stress: a systematic review. Sensors, 21(10), 3461. doi:https://doi.org/10.3390/s21103461.
43. Baron RA. Psychology. 5th ed. Noida: Dorling Kindersley; 2009.
44. World Health Organization. (2001). The world health report 2001: mental disorders affect one in four people. https://www.who.int/news-room/detail/28-09-2001-the-world-health-report-2001-mental-disorders-affect-one-in-four-people.
45. Naslund JA, Aschbrenner KA, Araya R, Marsch LA, Unützer J, Patel V, Bartels SJ. Digital technology for treating and preventing mental disorders in low-income and middle-income countries: a narrative review of the literature. Lancet Psychiatry. 2017;4(6):486–500. https://doi.org/10.1016/S2215-0366(17)30096-2.
46. Huys Q, Browning M, Paulus M, Frank M. Advances in the computational understanding of mental illness. Neuropsychopharmacology. 2021;46(1):3–19. https://doi.org/10.1038/s41386-020-0746-4.
47. Baron RA, Branscombe NR, Byrne D, Bhardwaj G. Social psychology. 10th ed. Noida: Dorling Kindersley; 2010.
48. John Hopkins Medicine. Generalized Anxiety Disorder (GAD). n.d.. https://www.hopkinsmedicine.org/health/conditions-and-diseases/generalized-anxiety-disorder#:~:text=Generalized%20anxiety%20disorder%20is%20a,muscle%20tension%2C%20and%20trouble%20sleeping.
49. National Institute of Mental Health (NIMH). Anxiety disorders. National Institute of Mental Health (NIMH); 2022. https://www.nimh.nih.gov/health/topics/anxiety-disorders.
50. Mao, J., Wang, C., Teng, C., Wang, M., Zhou, S., Zhao, K., . . . Wang, Y. (2022). Prevalence and associated factors of PTSD symptoms after the COVID-19 epidemic outbreak in an online survey in China: the age and gender differences matter. Neuropsychiatr Dis Treat, 18, 761—771. https://doi.org/10.2147/NDT.S351042.
51. Pasquale CD, Conti D, Dinaro C, D'Antoni RA. The COVID-19 pandemic and posttraumatic stress disorder: emotional impact on healthcare professions. Front Psychol. 2022;13:832843. https://doi.org/10.3389/fpsyt.2022.832843.
52. Tu Y, Zhang Y, Li Y, Zhao Q, Bi Y, Lu X, Wang L. Post-traumatic stress symptoms in COVID-19 survivors: a self-report and brain imaging follow-up study. Mol Psychiatry. 2021;26(12):7475–80. https://doi.org/10.1038/s41380-021-01223-w.
53. Guzick AG, Candelari A, Wiese AD, Schneider SC, Goodman WK, Storch EA. Obsessive–compulsive disorder during the COVID-19 pandemic: a systematic review. Curr Psychiatry Rep. 2021;23(71):1–10. https://doi.org/10.1007/s11920-021-01284-2.
54. Cunning C, Hodes M. The COVID-19 pandemic and obsessive–compulsive disorder in young people: systematic review. Clin Child Psychol Psychiatry. 2021;27(1):18–34. https://doi.org/10.1177/13591045211028169.
55. Wheaton MG, Ward HE, Silber A, McIngvale E, Björgvinsson T. How is the COVID-19 pandemic affecting individuals with obsessive-compulsive disorder (OCD) symptoms? J Anxiety Disord. 2021;81:102410. https://doi.org/10.1016/j.janxdis.2021.102410.
56. Smith K. Mental health: a world of depression. Nature. 2014;515:180–1. https://doi.org/10.1038/515180a.

57. Beyond Blue. Types of depression. Beyond Blue; n.d.. https://www.beyondblue.org.au/the-facts/depression/types-of-depression.
58. Bruce DF. 2021. Types of depression. https://www.webmd.com/depression/guide/depression-types. Accessed 01 Dec 2022.
59. Torres F. What is depression? American Psychiatric Association; 2020. https://www.psychiatry.org/patients-families/depression/what-is-depression.
60. Renaud-Charest O, Lui LM, Eskander S, Ceban F, Ho R, Di Vincenzo JD, McIntyre RS. Onset and frequency of depression in post-COVID-19 syndrome: a systematic review. J Psychiatr Res. 2021;144:129–37. https://doi.org/10.1016/j.jpsychires.2021.09.054.
61. Salari N, Hosseinian-Far A, Jalali R, Vaisi-Raygani A, Rasoulpoor S, Mohammadi M, Khale-Paveh B. Prevalence of stress, anxiety, depression among the general population during the COVID-19 pandemic: a systematic review and meta-analysis. Glob Health. 2020;16(57):1–11. https://doi.org/10.1186/s12992-020-00589-w.
62. United Nations. (2022). COVID-19: depression, anxiety soared 25 per cent in a year. https://news.un.org/en/story/2022/03/1113162.
63. Müller-Oerlinghausen B, Berghöfer A, Bauer M. Bipolar disorder. Lancet. 2002;359(9302):241–7. https://doi.org/10.1016/S0140-6736(02)07450-0.
64. Carvalho AF, Firth J, Vieta E. Bipolar Disorder. N Engl J Med. 2020;383:58–66. https://doi.org/10.1056/NEJMra1906193.
65. Bolton S, Warner J, Harriss E, Geddes J, Saunders KE. Bipolar disorder: Trimodal age-at-onset distribution. Bipolar Disord. 2021;23(4):341–56. https://doi.org/10.1111/bdi.13016.
66. Baldessarini, R. J., Tondo, L., Vazquez, G. H., Undurraga, J., Bolzani, L., Yildiz, A.,. Mauricio, T. (2012). Age at onset versus family history and clinical outcomes in 1,665 international bipolar-I disorder patients. World Psychiatry, 11(1), 40–46. doi:https://doi.org/10.1016/j.wpsyc.2012.01.006.
67. Soni A, Singh P, Kumar S, Shah R, Batra L, Verma M. Role of age at onset in the clinical presentation of bipolar disorder in Indian population. Ind Psychiatry J. 2021;30(1):41–6. https://doi.org/10.4103/ipj.ipj_8_20.
68. Rowland DL, Cooper DL, Slob AK. Genital and psychoaffective response to erotic stimulation in sexually functional and dysfunctional men. J Abnorm Psychol. 1996;105:194–203.
69. Banerjee D, Rao TS. Sexuality, sexual well being, and intimacy during COVID-19 pandemic: an advocacy perspective. Indian J Psychiatry. 2020;62(4):418–26. https://doi.org/10.4103/psychiatry.IndianJPsychiatry_484_20.
70. Masoudi M, Maasoumi R, Bragazzi NL. Effects of the COVID-19 pandemic on sexual functioning and activity: a systematic review and meta-analysis. BMC Public Health. 2022;22(189):1–18. https://doi.org/10.1186/s12889-021-12390-4.
71. Fisher KA, Marwaha R. Paraphilia. In: StatPearls. Treasure Island (FL): StatPearls Publishing LLC; 2022. https://www.ncbi.nlm.nih.gov/books/NBK554425/. Accessed 20 Dec 2022.
72. Yakeley J, Wood H. Paraphilias and paraphilic disorders: diagnosis, assessment and management. Adv Psychiatr Treat. 2018;20(3):202–13. https://doi.org/10.1192/apt.bp.113.011197.
73. First MB. DSM-5 and paraphilic disorders. J Am Acad Psychiatry Law. 2014;42(2):191–201. https://jaapl.org/content/42/2/191
74. Baron RA, Misra G. Psychology. Uttar Pradesh: Pearson India Education Services Pvt. Ltd; 2016.
75. Allen JP, Litten RZ. Psychometric and laboratory measures to assist in the treatment of alcoholism. Clin Psychol Rev. 1993;13:223–40.
76. Reardon CL. Paraphilic Disorders Workup. Medscape; 2020. https://emedicine.medscape.com/article/291419-workup.
77. Albagmi FM, Alansari A, Al Shawan DS, AlNujaidi HY. Prediction of generalized anxiety levels during the Covid-19 pandemic: a machine learning-based modeling approach. Inform Med Unlocked. 2022;28:100854. https://doi.org/10.1016/j.imu.2022.100854.

78. Priya A, Garg S, Tigga NP. Predicting anxiety, depression and stress in modern life using machine learning algorithms. Procedia Computer Science. 2020;167:1258–67. https://doi.org/10.1016/j.procs.2020.03.442.
79. Antosik-Wójcińska, A. Z., Dominiakb, M., Chojnacka, M., Kaczmarek-Majer, K., Opara, K. R., Radziszewska, W., . . . Święcicki, Ł. (2020). Smartphone as a monitoring tool for bipolar disorder: a systematic review including data analysis, machine learning algorithms and predictive modelling. Int J Med Inform, 138, 104131. https://doi.org/10.1016/j.ijmedinf.2020.104131.
80. Wu M-J, Mwangi B, Bauer IE, Passos IC, Sanches M, Zunta-Soares GB, Soares JC. Identification and individualized prediction of clinical phenotypes in bipolar disorders using neurocognitive data, neuroimaging scans and machine learning. NeuroImage. 2017;145(B):254–64. https://doi.org/10.1016/j.neuroimage.2016.02.016.
81. Fernandes, B. S., Karmakar, C., Tamouza, R., Tran, T., Yearwood, J., Hamdani, N., . . . Leboyer, M. (2020). Precision psychiatry with immunological and cognitive biomarkers: a multi-domain prediction for the diagnosis of bipolar disorder or schizophrenia using machine learning. Transl Psychiatry, 10(162), 1–13. https://doi.org/10.1038/s41398-020-0836-4.
82. Fine J, Lackner R, Samudrala R, Chopra G. Computational chemoproteomics to understand the role of selected psychoactives in treating mental health indications. Sci Rep. 2019;9(13155):1–15. https://doi.org/10.1038/s41598-019-49515-0.
83. Hingorani M, Pise N. Detection of mental illness using machine learning and deep learning. In: Proceedings of the international conference on industrial engineering and operations management. Monterrey, Mexico: IEOM society international; 2021. p. 2272–8. http://ieomsociety.org/proceedings/2021monterrey/403.pdf. Accessed 26 Dec 2022.
84. Thubaut F, Cosyns P, Fedoroff JP, Briken P, Goethls K, Bradford JM. The world Federation of Societies of biological psychiatry (WFSBP) 2020 guidelines for the pharmacological treatment of paraphilic disorders. World J Biol Psychiatry. 2020;21(6):412–90. https://doi.org/10.1080/15622975.2020.1744723.
85. Siddiqui S, Khan AA, Dev K, Dey I. Integrating federated learning with IoMT for managing obesity in smart city. In: Proceedings of the 1st workshop on artificial intelligence and Blockchain Technologies for Smart Cities with 6G. ACM; 2021.
86. Siddiqui S, Khan AA, Nait-Abdesselam F, Dey I. Anxiety and depression management for elderly using internet of things and symphonic melodies. In: IEEE International Conference on Communications; 2021b.
87. de la Torre Díez I, Alonso SG, Hamrioui S, Cruz EM, Nozaleda LM, Franco MA. IoT-based services and applications for mental health in the literature. J Med Syst. 2019;43:1–6.
88. Rodrigues J, Mariana OP, Cercas F. Physiological and behavior monitoring systems for smart healthcare environments: a review, vol. 20. Sensors; 2020.
89. Andò B, Baglio S, Castorina S, Crispino R, Marletta., V. Advanced sensing solutions for ambient assisted living: the NATIFLife framework. IEEE Ind Electron Mag. 2020;23:33–40.
90. Siddiqui S, Shakir MZ, Khan AA, Dey., I. Internet of things (IoT) enabled architecture for social distancing during pandemic. Front commun netw. 2021c;2:614166.
91. Khrisna BM, Jhansi VC, Shama PS, Leelambika AB, Prakash C, Manikanta., B. V. Novel solution to improve mental health by integrating music and IoT with neural feedback. J of Computl Inform Sys. 2019;15(3):234–9.
92. Stein DJ, Fineberg NA, Chamberlain SR. Mental health in a digital world. Academic Press; 2021.
93. Marcu G, Ondersma SJ, Spiller AN, Broderick BM, Kadri R, Buis., L. R. The perceived benefits of digital interventions for behavioral health: qualitative interview study. J Med Internet Res. 2022;24:e34300.
94. Checklist M. Take control of your mental health. 2022. Retrieved from M3 Checklist with Mooditude: https://whatsmym3.com/
95. Healthline. Cognitive behavioral therapy for depression. n.d.. https://www.healthline.com/health/depression/cognitive-behavioral-therapy.

96. Breathe2Relax. 2022. https://www.my-therappy.co.uk/app/breathe-2-relax.
97. Headspace. Make it your year with Headspace. 2022. https://www.headspace.com/.
98. Moodtrack. Track and graph your moods, anytime, anywhere. Moodtrack; 2022. http://www.moodtrack.com/.
99. eMoods. The easiest way to track your moods online or offline. 2022. https://emoodtracker.com/.
100. Gulo NR. Xpert system for diagnosis of sexual diseases (paraphilia) using method Dempster Shafer. J Intell Decision Support Syst. 2022;5:28–36.
101. Resnik P, Choudhury MD, Schafer KM, Coppersmith G. Bibliometric studies and the discipline of social media mental Health Research. Comment on machine learning for mental health in social media: bibliometric study. J Med Internet Res. 2021;23(6):e28990.
102. Mwangi B, Wu M-J, Cao B, Passos IC, Lavagnino L, Keser Z, Soares JC. Individualized prediction and clinical staging of bipolar disorders using neuroanatomical biomarkers. Biol Psychiatry Cogn Neurosci Neuroimaging. 2016;1(2):186–94.
103. Le Glaz A, Haralambous Y, Kim-Dufor D-H, Lenca P, Billot R, Ryan TC, Marsh J. Machine learning and natural language processing in mental health: systematic review. J Med Internet Res. 2021;23(5):e15708.
104. Chien I, Enrique A, Palacios J, Regan T, Keegan D, Carter D, Tschiatschek S. A machine learning approach to understanding patterns of engagement with internet-delivered mental health interventions. JAMA Netw Open. 2020;3(7):–e2010791.
105. Valdez D, Thij MT, Bathina K, Rutter LA, Bollen., J. Social media insights into US mental health during the COVID-19 pandemic: longitudinal analysis of twitter data. J Med Internet Res. 2020;22:e21418.
106. Massaad E, Cherfan., P. Social media data analytics on telehealth during the COVID-19 pandemic, vol. 12. Cureus; 2020. p. e7838.
107. Congress.gov. S.2561—Technology-Related Assistance for Individuals With Disabilities Act of 1988. n.d.. Congress.gov: https://www.congress.gov/bill/100th-congress/senate-bill/2561#:~:text=passed%20Senate%2C%20amended)-,Technology%2DRelated%20Assistance%20for%20Individuals%20With%20Disabilities%20Act%20of%201988,of%20all%20ages%20with%20disabilities.
108. Siddiqui S, Nesbitt R, Shakir MZ, Khan AA, Khan AA, Khan KK, Ramzan N. Artificial neural network (ann) enabled internet of things (iot) architecture for music therapy. Electronics. 2020;9(12):2019.
109. Segal DL, Granier KL, Pifer MA, Stone., L. E. Geriatric anxiety scale. In: Encyclopedia of gerontology and population aging. Basingstoke: Springer Nature; 2019.
110. Wongpakaran N, Wongpakaran T, Kuntawong P. Evaluating hierarchical items of the geriatric depression scale through factor analysis and item response theory, vol. 5. Heliyon; 2019. p. e02300.

Intelligent Digital Monitoring of the Levels of Stress

Amandeep Kaur, Manish Kumar, and Rajesh Kumar Bhatia

Abstract The human body is regulated by a variety of glands that produce hormones, which are responsible for making us feel good or bad. Cortisol is a hormone that falls under the category of feel-bad hormones as it increases stress levels in the body. Stress can come in different forms such as acute, episodic acute, and chronic and can have adverse effects on a person's physical, mental, and emotional health. It can lead to the development of diseases such as diabetes, heart ailments, depression, asthma, obesity, Alzheimer's disease, gastrointestinal problems, and anxiety, among others. Early diagnosis and prevention of such diseases can be aided by monitoring and predicting stress levels. Various techniques are reported in the literature to measure stress, including wearable devices, behavioural coding, self-reporting, physiological measuring tools, heart rate variability analysis, psychosocial approach, perceived stress scale, and measuring salivary and hair cortisol. This chapter focuses on digital monitoring techniques for measuring stress levels, such as using intelligent wireless sensor systems, personal digital assistants, mobile applications, bioelectronics, digital signal processing, and other such technologies. The role of recent computational techniques such as machine learning, deep learning, and the Internet of Things in real-time stress detection has also been discussed, highlighting potential directions for further research in this area.

Keywords Episodic acute stress · Chronic stress · Bioelectronics · Deep learning · Real-time stress detection

A. Kaur (✉) · M. Kumar · R. K. Bhatia
Department of Computer Science and Engineering, Punjab Engineering College (Deemed to be University), Chandigarh, India
e-mail: amandeepkaur@pec.edu.in

G. Battineni et al. (eds.), *Computational Methods in Psychiatry*,
https://doi.org/10.1007/978-981-99-6637-0_5

1 Introduction

Human thought and behaviour are influenced by various factors, including stress management. Stress was originally defined by Hans Selye in 1936 as a non-specific response of the body to any demand [1]. Stress is a reaction of the body towards different situations and circumstances which the mind finds complex to process or handle. Multitasking can often become physically and mentally exhausting for the body's processes, inducing stress. The secretion of hormones by various glands regulates these bodily processes. Cortisol, a feel-bad hormone, is responsible for increasing stress levels in the body. This primary stress hormone releases glucose in the bloodstream and has various effects on different parts of the body. Health risks, bad habits, and diseases can further increase stress levels. Figure.1 displays some parameters that affect stress levels.

There are many types of stress such as acute stress, episodic acute stress, chronic stress, etc. which can affect a person's physical, mental, and emotional well-being. The types of stress are tabulated in Table 1. This can also induce illnesses and disorders leading to several diseases such as diabetes, heart ailments, depression, asthma, obesity, Alzheimer's disease, gastrointestinal problems, anxiety, etc. Stress has huge impact on the neurological processes as well as other physical and emotional processes of human body and is a game-changer in making or breaking a person. Therefore, the management of stress levels becomes a very important factor

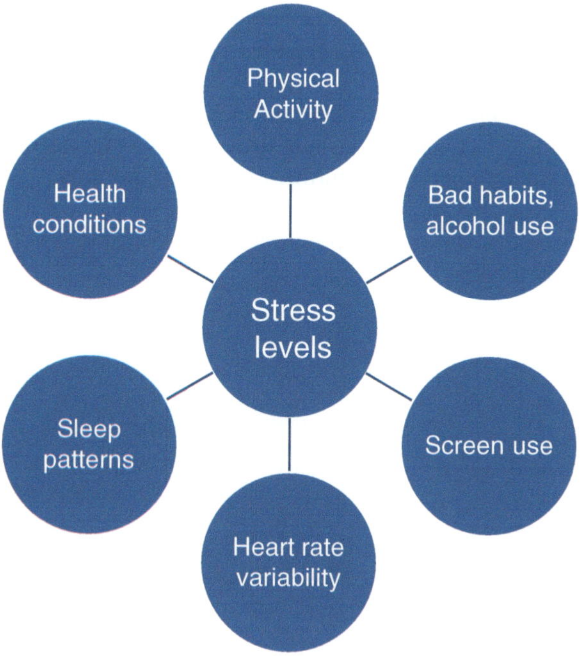

Fig. 1 Parameters affecting stress levels

Table 1 Types of stress

Sr. No.	Types of stress	Characteristics
1.	Acute stress	• Body's reaction towards a relatively new and challenging circumstance • Severe acute stress could result from post-traumatic stress disorders • Reactions towards life threatening situations can cause severe acute stress
2.	Episodic acute stress	• Frequent episodes of acute stress cause this type of stress • Anxiousness and worries in routine activities
3.	Chronic stress	• When stress levels remain high for a significant period of time, chronic stress is induced in body • Causes various disorders, headaches, changes in sleeping patterns, eating patterns, etc.

for the overall well-being of a person. Onus lies on the research community to find out technological ways to measure the levels of stress in human body so that appropriate methods for stress management may be devised.

This chapter discusses various techniques that are reported in the literature to measure stress levels such as wearable devices, behavioural coding, self-reporting, physiological measuring tools, heart rate variability analysis, psychosocial approach, perceived stress scale, measuring salivary and hair cortisol, etc. [2].

This chapter also focuses on the techniques involving digital monitoring of stress levels, for example, using intelligent wireless sensor systems, personal digital assistants, mobile applications, bioelectronics, digital signal processing, etc. The role of recent computational techniques like machine learning, deep learning, and the Internet of Things in real-time stress detection has also been discussed.

2 Measurement of Stress Levels

Various physical, behavioural, situational, emotional, and psychological factors lead to the rise in levels of stress. Quantitative indication of stress by observation of these factors can help in the management of stress. For instance, human facial expressions can indicate the presence of stress. According to the facial action coding system developed by Ekman and Friesen, seven basic emotions anger, disgust, neutral, fear, happiness, sadness, and surprise are innate and universal to humans and these can be used for indication of stress levels. Digital techniques to measure stress levels are gaining popularity due to their non-invasive and convenient nature. In this section, we discuss various techniques which can help in the measurement of stress levels in the human body.

2.1 Wearable Devices

In the rapidly emerging field of stress monitoring, real-time cortisol-sensing wearable devices are being developed. Wearable cortisol aptasensors and cortisol sweat-sensing devices [3] significantly collect stress-related information which can be used for monitoring and measurement. Objective stress monitoring systems are also being designed which can measure stress based on electrocardiograms (ECG), photoplethysmography (PPG), and galvanic skin response. The wearable sensors used for the above-said technique are Shimmer3 ECG, Shimmer3 GSR+, and Empatica E4 [4].

Wearable devices which involve the audio signal and heart rate monitoring for stress detection provide effective solutions in a real-world scenario. Machine learning is applied to test the accuracy of these frameworks so that these can be employed in the real world for the safety of people especially children [5]. A list of currently available wearable devices which monitor stress and related parameters is given in Table 2.

The wearable devices provide lot of benefits but face several challenges as well. Accuracy of these devices needs further research elaboration. COVID-19 pandemic has brought a change in the lifestyle of people. More dependency on digital devices has added to the stress parameters in human body and also affects the overall well-being by introducing habitual changes.

Therefore, the use of wearable devices should be planned with care and consideration, while not affecting the very spirit of natural bodily processes. Figure.2 shows a graphical abstract of stress detection using wearable devices, where the data is collected by the wearable sensors [6]. The collected data is then pre-processed using various data cleaning approaches. From the data that is now put in format by

Table 2 Wearable devices for stress monitoring

Name of the device	Characteristics
Fitbit Sense2	Scans the body for the presence of stress, notifies the user, asks for feedback, and provides suggestions on coping mechanisms
Garmin watch	Provides stress tracking by taking into consideration heart rate variability measurements and also monitors sleep, guides into breathing exercises
Samsung smartwatches	Heart rate monitoring, stress tracking, heart rate variability measurement, mindfulness, meditation,
Apple watch series 8 and watch SE	Third-party apple watch apps may provide stress monitoring features by taking into consideration the heart rate variability
Google Wear OS smartwatches	Heart rate monitoring, breathing exercises, monitoring stressful moments
Apollo neuro	Haptic technology for skin vibrations, various modes such as energy, wakeup, clear, focussed, sleep, and renew
Muse2	Uses seven electroencephalogram sensors along the scalp, real-time brain activity measurement, calming exercises, monitoring body movements and breathing, heart rate rhythm tracks using the pulse oximeter

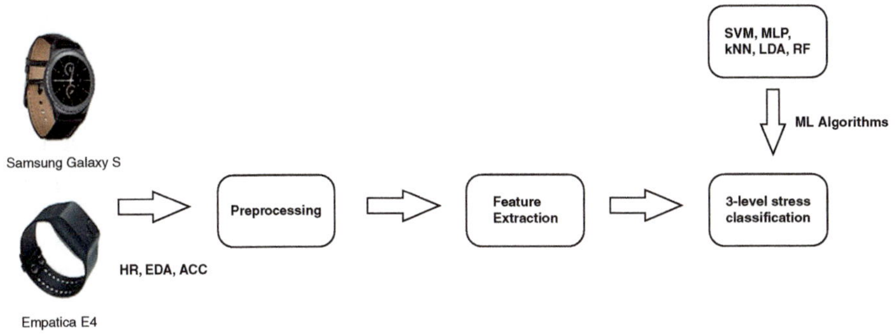

Fig. 2 Graphical abstract of stress detection using wearables [6]

Table 3 Various behaviours of stress management

Stress management behaviours	
Positive behaviours	Deep breathing, exercising, mindfulness, yoga, listening to calming music, connecting with the community, finding time for yourself, walking, travelling
Negative behaviours	Alcohol use, smoking, addiction towards screens, absence of physical activities, junk eating

pre-processing, relevant features are extracted. Then, classification techniques of machine learning are implemented to get 3-level stress classification.

2.2 *Behavioural Coding*

The behavioural coding focusses towards the stereotypical behaviours of people under stress. The parental monitoring and psychological controls during adolescence years also affect the cognition and stress handling capabilities of the individual. The development of stereotypes during the early years affects thought and behaviour, which in turn affects the ways of managing stress by the body of that individual.

Electronic monitoring of the stress-inducing parameters plays a significant role in stress management. Intellectual physical disabilities also introduce stress levels at the unprecedented situations. The coding of all such behaviours under given circumstances is very important to design stress monitoring solutions for individuals with different backgrounds and abilities. Various stress management behaviours are listed in Table 3.

2.2.1 Self-Reporting

Self-reporting is a powerful tool for managing stress as it allows individuals to monitor their own stress levels and identify triggers for stress. Self-reporting involves tracking and recording one's thoughts, emotions, and behaviours over time to gain insights into patterns and trends. One of the primary benefits of self-reporting for stress management is that it empowers individuals to take control of their own well-being. By tracking their stress levels and identifying triggers, individuals can develop strategies to manage stress proactively. For example, if an individual notices that they feel particularly stressed after a certain activity or in response to a specific situation, they can take steps to avoid or minimize those triggers. Self-reporting can take many forms, including keeping a journal, using mobile apps, or participating in online support groups. Mobile apps, in particular, have become increasingly popular for self-reporting stress management. These apps often include features such as mood tracking, stress tracking, and goal setting, enabling individuals to monitor their progress and stay motivated.

While self-reporting is a powerful tool for stress management, it also has some limitations. Self-reported data may be subject to bias or inaccuracies, as individuals may not always accurately recall or report their emotions and behaviours. Additionally, self-reporting may not be sufficient for individuals with severe or chronic stress, as they may require more intensive interventions such as therapy or medication. Self-reporting can be an effective tool for managing stress, particularly for individuals with mild to moderate stress. By tracking and monitoring their stress levels, individuals can gain insights into their own well-being and develop strategies to manage stress proactively.

Self-reporting is a way of managing stress by being vocal about it. Listing the issues that cause stress helps in finding ways to alleviate these. Wearable sensors provide a personalized stress monitoring mechanism in order to measure self-reported stress. The ways of reporting include developing a mood adjective checklist, filling up questionnaires and surveys, getting yourself tested through remote applications via web browsers or mobile phone interface. During the stages of pregnancy, the hormonal changes introduce several mood related issues which can be monitored via self-reporting and stress can be categorised accordingly. This makes it possible to assess the risks during pregnancy through self-reported stress.

2.2.2 Physiological Measuring Tools

There are various studies to find out accurate algorithms to measure the stress levels of users. One such study is about inconspicuous stress monitoring system that makes use of physiological sensors [7]. In this system, around 50 participants were included in the experimentation through a mobile application interface. Three physiological signals were taken into consideration, viz. heart rate, galvanic skin response, and skin temperature, in order to classify the stress-related data and produce distributions. The algorithms of support vector machines and K means-clustering were deployed to carry out the classification and monitoring tasks. This system gave an accuracy of about 91.26 and is able to assist people in alleviating their stress significantly.

Another study considering the wearable physiological sensors to monitor stress in the working environments was developed as an integrated system using biological markers [11]. ECG, EDA, and EEG parameters were used to identify the stress in humans and correlate the detected stress with cortisol levels of salivary glands. The statistical analysis was majorly carried out using support vector machine classification algorithm. This system was able to test human stress and carry out the quantification of the stress levels. The results obtained from this study are further encouraging the design of portable and remotely controlled systems.

2.2.3 Heart Rate Variability Analysis

Heart rate variability (HRV) analysis is a technique that refers to the beat-to-beat fluctuations of the rate of heart [8]. The various factors that affect the heart rate are further instrumental in causing a rise in the stress levels. Therefore, the analysis of heart rate variability becomes paramount. There is various software which are capable to do this analysis. One such software is Kubios HRV [9] which is considered an advanced and easy-to-use software for HRV analysis. There are various data formats which can be supported by this software to process ECG and beat-to-beat data. The algorithm used in this software is QRS detection algorithm, and there are number of tools for analysis sample selection, trend removal, and artefact correction in order to complete the analysis task. The software can compute the time domain as well as frequency domain parameters of HRV and many other non-linear parameters as well. Various settings are there which are adjustable and optimum for different types of data. The results are available in different formats so that further processing can be done on different platforms and software. Heart rate variability analysis can be performed using HRV analysis software [10] which is available for Windows and MAC operating systems. It is ideal for human as well as animal cardiovascular studies. It displays the time domain, frequency domain as well non-linear parameters associated with beat-to-beat analysis. HRV software utilizes algorithms and mathematical calculations to process and analyse heart rate data obtained from wearable devices, such as heart rate monitors or electrocardiogram (ECG) devices. These software applications can transform the raw heart rate data into meaningful metrics and provide comprehensive reports for further analysis.

HRV software can receive heart rate data from various sources, including wearable devices, fitness trackers, ECG monitors, or data files stored in compatible formats. The software may include data pre-processing capabilities to clean and filter the heart rate data, removing any artefacts or outliers that may interfere with accurate HRV analysis. It applies mathematical algorithms, such as time domain, frequency domain, and non-linear analysis methods, to extract relevant HRV metrics. These metrics include measures of overall HRV, sympathetic and parasympathetic activity, stress levels, and cardiovascular health markers. This software generates detailed reports and visualizations, presenting HRV metrics in an understandable format. This enables users to track their HRV trends over time and identify patterns or changes in their autonomic function. It may also integrate with other health and fitness platforms, allowing users to synchronize and analyse their HRV data alongside other health parameters, such as physical activity, sleep patterns, and nutrition.

2.2.4 Psychosocial Approach

Psychosocial stress occurs when the individual is fearful of the social threats and situations such as feeling excluded from the society, fearing failures, fearing being evaluated by the society as per the set parameters. People having certain disorders like inflammatory bowel diseases, bipolar disorders, metabolic syndromes, etc. also encounter such challenges due to their health conditions. It is even observed that people with severe ailments such as cancer are being affected by the psychosocial stress with their weakening immune systems. Therefore, an approach to analyse this kind of stress and develop ways to manage it is the need of the hour.

One approach to monitor acute stress after a traumatic experience has been developed, which basically integrates the available evidence for behaviour therapy of cognition and recently found neuroscience results [11]. This approach signifies the importance of fear reduction learning which can be increased by modulation of glutamatergic systems, which are the major excitatory neurotransmitter systems in the nervous system. The integration of neurological findings with the digital technologies can be further explored in order to develop psychosocial approaches to monitor stress levels.

2.2.5 Perceived Stress Scale

Perceived stress scale is a psychological instrument which is helpful in finding out the perception of stress. It measures the degree which tells about the situations and circumstances that make the life of a person stressful. A study on the review of perceived stress scale was conducted, and it was found that reliability of internal consistency, factorial validity, and hypothesis validity of the perceived stress scale (PSS) was reported significantly by various research articles [12]. Questionnaires were quite helpful to measure the PSS and identify the stressful situations. However, there is a lack of computational methods to measure PSS and correlate it with other parameters which induce stress. Based on perceived stress scale tests, brain wave stress patterns can be generated and analysed. Various region-specific studies on PSS have also been made in Greece, Turkey, Spain, Germany, etc.

2.2.6 Measuring Salivary and Hair Cortisol

In today's world, the effects of stress on human health and overall well-being are well recognized. Therefore, establishment of biomarkers to measure the levels of stress over a period of time is critically required [13]. Saliva, urine, and hair cortisol are some of the hormones which can complement the real-time monitoring of stress levels. Hair cortisol as a parameter to assess stress is being used widely in the clinical studies. There are many studies which are focussing on these parameters individually, but there is a scope of exploring digital solutions which assess the levels of stress based on all of these three parameters to have a comprehensive analysis.

A smartphone-based technique has been developed to measure psychological stress based on salivary cortisol [14]. This technique involved the development of a mobile application which will measure the different concentrations of cortisol using images. The statistical analysis is then carried out and validation is done with the smartphone by using actual human saliva to evaluate the system.

2.2.7 Pupil Dilation Measurement

Pupil dilation measurement is a non-invasive digital technique used to measure stress levels. The size of the pupil changes as a result of the activity of the autonomic nervous system, which is responsible for the body's response to stress. The sympathetic nervous system activates the "Figureht or flight" response, causing the pupils to dilate, while the parasympathetic nervous system activates the "rest and digest" response, causing the pupils to constrict.

By measuring changes in the size of the pupils, researchers can infer the activity of the autonomic nervous system and estimate stress levels. Pupil dilation measurement can be done using a digital pupillometer, which is a small device that shines a light into the eye and measures the amount of light that is reflected back. The device can provide objective and accurate measurements of pupil size, which can be used to assess stress levels in various contexts, such as during cognitive tasks, emotional situations, or physical activity. However, it is important to note that other factors, such as lighting conditions, medication use, and individual differences, can also affect pupil size, so results should be interpreted with caution and in combination with other measures of stress.

2.2.8 Electroencephalography

EEG (electroencephalography) is a non-invasive technique used to record and measure the electrical activity of the brain. EEG can be used to measure stress levels by detecting changes in brainwave patterns that are associated with stress. When a person is under stress, there is an increase in the beta wave frequency in the frontal region of the brain and a decrease in the alpha wave frequency in the parietal and occipital regions of the brain.

In studies, participants who underwent stress-inducing tasks showed an increase in beta waves, particularly in the frontal area, and a decrease in alpha waves in the parietal and occipital regions. These changes in the brainwave pattern can be detected and analysed using EEG to indicate the level of stress.

Moreover, EEG can also be used to identify different stages of stress. For example, when a person is initially exposed to a stressful situation, there is an increase in the beta wave frequency in the frontal region. As the stress continues, the alpha wave frequency in the parietal and occipital regions also decreases. By analysing these changes in brainwave patterns, it is possible to differentiate between different stages of stress and provide early intervention. However, it is important to note that EEG is not a standalone method for measuring stress levels, and it should be used in combination with other techniques such as self-report questionnaires or behavioural observations.

Additionally, EEG requires specialized equipment and trained professionals to perform the analysis and interpretation of the results, which can make it more challenging to implement on a large scale.

2.2.9 Speech Analysis

Speech analysis is another digital technique used to detect stress levels. Stress affects the way we speak, altering the pitch, tone, and rhythm of our speech. Therefore, speech analysis can be a non-invasive, low-cost, and easy-to-use technique for detecting stress.

Several studies have investigated the use of speech analysis for stress detection. For example, researchers have used various features of speech, such as pitch, energy, and speech rate, to develop stress detection models. These models have been trained on speech samples collected from individuals under various stress conditions, such as public speaking, mental arithmetic, and cognitive tasks.

One study used automatic speech recognition (ASR) technology to transcribe speech and extract features such as the fundamental frequency (F0), spectral centroid, and formant frequencies. The study showed that speech features could be used to detect stress with an accuracy of up to 80%. Another study focused on the analysis of speech prosody, which includes features such as pitch, loudness, and rhythm. The study found that speech prosody can be used to detect stress with an accuracy of up to 85%.

Overall, speech analysis can be a promising digital technique for detecting stress levels. However, the accuracy of the technique depends on various factors, such as the quality of the speech signal, the type of stressor, and the individual differences in speech patterns. Further research is needed to develop reliable and accurate stress detection models based on speech analysis.

2.2.10 Computer Mouse Usage

Computer mouse usage can be used as a proxy for stress detection. When a person experiences stress, their movements can become more erratic and jittery, which can be reflected in the patterns of mouse movement. This has led to the development of software applications that can track mouse movements and use them as a means of detecting stress. These applications typically use machine learning algorithms to analyse the patterns of mouse movement and identify when they deviate significantly from the user's normal behaviour. However, it's important to note that mouse movement is just one potential indicator of stress and should be used in conjunction with other measures for more accurate results.

3 Digital Monitoring of Stress Levels

The digital monitoring of stress levels includes the use of intelligent wireless sensor systems, personal digital assistants, mobile applications, bioelectronics, digital signal processing, machine learning, etc. This section discusses such techniques which would be helpful in monitoring the stress levels efficiently.

3.1 Intelligent Wireless Sensor Systems

Intelligent Wireless Sensor Systems (IWSS) can be used for stress monitoring in a variety of applications, including healthcare, sports, and workplace safety. These systems use advanced sensors to detect and monitor physiological signals associated with stress, such as heart rate variability, electrodermal activity, and respiration rate.

The data collected by these sensors can be transmitted wirelessly to a central monitoring system, where it can be analysed and used to identify patterns of stress and potential triggers. This information can be used to help individuals manage their stress levels, as well as to inform organizational policies and interventions aimed at reducing workplace stress.

In addition to physiological sensors, IWSS can also incorporate other types of sensors, such as environmental sensors, to provide a more comprehensive understanding of the factors contributing to stress. For example, temperature, noise, and lighting can all have an impact on stress levels, and incorporating these data into IWSS can help identify potential stressors and inform interventions aimed at reducing them.

IWSS have the potential to revolutionize stress monitoring by providing real-time, objective data that can be used to inform personalized interventions aimed at improving mental health and well-being. Wireless sensor systems make use of sensing devices to carry out the task at hand. Various smartwatches and fitness trackers which monitor the daily routine and bodily processes of individuals are proving to be quite effective in monitoring the levels of stress during different intervals of time. Salivary sensors and sweat cortisol sensors are becoming the front runners in measuring the stress levels effectively.

A device named SKINTRONICS [13] has been created to determine the stress levels by using electrodermal sensing of skin galvanic response. Personal health monitors using wireless intelligent sensor systems are being developed to monitor a group of people and identify their stress levels [15]. In order to accomplish these tasks, high precision computational instrumentation is required.

3.2 Personal Digital Assistance

Personal digital assistants are a way of breaking the barriers of social stigma to report, analyse and monitor personal health issues. A non-intrusive stress monitoring system has been developed based on the personal digital assistants. Sensing and estimation of stress is done in two phases in this system. The sensing phase consists of measurement of heart rate, skin temperature variation, and electrodermal activities. All these parameters are acquired from the finger without causing any comfort issue to the individual [16]. The benefits of personal digital assistants in healthcare domain are multi-fold, therefore steps are being taken to make use of these for stress monitoring.

3.3 Mobile Applications

Mobile applications pave the way to make digital assistance convenient and friendly for the users. The following Table 4 lists some of the mobile applications which are helpful in stress management.

3.4 Bioelectronics and Digital Signal Processing

For continuous stress monitoring over a period of time, wearable bioelectronics are quite significant. Emotion recognition systems based on non-intrusive and intrusive sensors have been developed [18]. There are three stages in this system: setting up experiments for physiological sensing, feature extraction using pre-processing of signals, and recognition using learning-based system. Four signals are monitored and analysed to find out the stages of stress. These signals are blood volume pulse, pupil diameter, skin temperature, and galvanic skin response. Support vector machines are used to classify the states of stress and provide information about the emotional changes in the person.

Table 4 Mobile applications for stress management [17]

Sr. No.	Name	Features
1	Breathe2Relax	Breathing exercises and instructions, documentation on stress management, information on the harmful effects of stress
2	Pacifia	Deep breathing and muscle relaxation guided exercises, anti-anxiety experiments, mood tracking, analysis of thinking patterns, and anxiety triggers
3	GPS for the soul	Stress level identification, meditation tools, calming pictures, and music
4	Happify	Brain training, activities to get rid of stress, anxiety, and negativity
5	Stress doctor	Stress busting deep breathing exercises, heart rate monitoring, etc.
6	Headspace	Guided meditation sessions, mindfulness training
7	Personal Zen	Games based on clinical findings, reducing anxiety levels
8	My mood tracker	Helping you to feel good and manage your moods
9	Squeeze and shake	Anger management
10	Pocket yoga	Yoga techniques for relaxation, range of yoga styles from beginner to difficulty level
11	Finding optimism	Recording symptoms and triggers, data visualization tools, information on wellness strategies
12	The Mindfulness app	Guided meditation, calming music, natural sounds
13	Pay it forward	Stress reduction with kindness, connecting with the community

3.5 Cognitive Behavioural Therapy and Conversational Chatbots

Cognitive behavioural therapy (CBT) is a technique of assessing human thought and behaviour to manage the problems faced by an individual. It has proven to treat acute stress disorders by monitoring and managing anxiety levels and stress reactions. If acute stress disorder is not treated timely, it may lead to severe post-traumatic stress disorders (PTSD). Since, CBT is a talk therapy, it makes it difficult for people with social issues to connect with their medical health counsellor. Therefore, techniques are being evolved to prepare chatbots who can counsel the subjects using cognitive behavioural therapy techniques. Connecting with a chatbot is much convenient for such people as they no longer have the fear of being judged while discussing about their mental health issues. The terminology used for such chatbots is therapy chatbots, which aim to have conversations with the patient in order to help them with anger, anxiety, and depression issues.

Table 5 provides a list of some chatbots which are helping people in managing stress.

Table 5 Chatbots for stress management [19]

Sr. No.	Name	Features
1	Woebot	Mood monitoring, cognitive behavioural therapy, therapeutic conversations
2	Moodkits	Depression monitoring, cognitive behavioural therapy, activity tools
3	MoodNotes	Categorizes user's thought patterns, records their emotions, identify thinking errors
4	Wysa	AI based, emotionally intelligent chatbot, dialectical behaviour therapy, guided meditation, evidence-based CBT
5	Youper	Monitors and improves emotional health, personalized conversations, mindfulness techniques

4 Role of Recent Technological Trends in Real-Time Stress Detection

Real-time stress detection involves the collection of data in real time using various sensors and then sending it to a processing unit through some mobile interface. The processed information is relayed back to the user to detect the levels of stress at the given time. The processing unit capable to carry out this task has a number of technologies running in its background such as database systems, machine learning, deep learning, and Internet of Things. This section discusses the role of such recent computational techniques employed for detection of stress in real time.

4.1 Machine Learning

Machine learning (ML) has a significant role to play in stress detection and monitoring. ML algorithms can analyse large volumes of physiological and environmental data collected by sensors to identify patterns and predict future stress events [20]. Here are some ways in which ML can be used for stress detection and monitoring:

- Feature extraction: Machine learning algorithms can automatically identify relevant features from physiological signals, such as heart rate variability, electrodermal activity, and respiration rate, that are associated with stress. These features can then be used as inputs to predict stress levels.
- Pattern recognition: ML can be used to identify patterns in physiological and environmental data that are associated with stress, such as changes in heart rate, respiration rate, and skin conductance. This can help in the early detection of stress and provide an opportunity for timely interventions.
- Personalization: ML algorithms can be trained on individual data to develop personalized stress models. This can help in providing tailored interventions and support to individuals, based on their unique stress patterns.
- Predictive analytics: ML can be used to develop predictive models that can identify individuals who are at risk of developing stress, based on their past stress

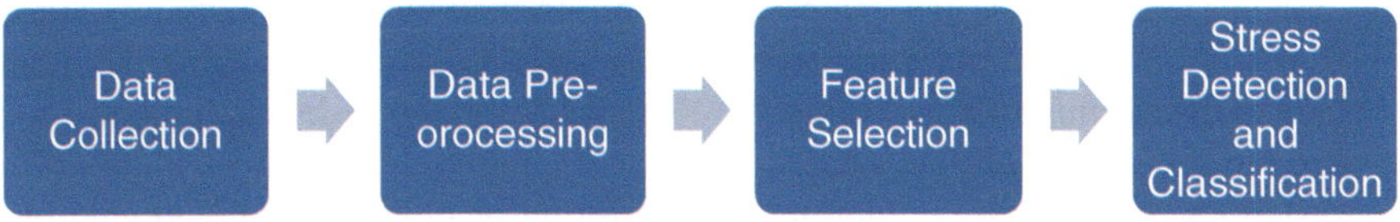

Fig. 3 Process of stress detection using machine learning

patterns, environmental factors, and other relevant data. This can help in preventing stress-related illnesses and promoting early interventions.

- Real-time monitoring: ML can be used to develop real-time stress monitoring systems that can provide continuous monitoring of physiological and environmental signals. This can enable timely interventions and support for individuals who are experiencing high levels of stress.

Machine learning has the potential to revolutionize stress detection and monitoring by providing real-time objective data that can be used to inform personalized interventions aimed at improving mental health and well-being. ML-based stress detection and monitoring systems can be used in a variety of settings, such as healthcare, sports, and workplace safety, to help individuals and organizations manage stress and promote well-being. The general process of using machine learning to detect and classify stress levels is shown in Fig. 3.

For instance, if we are developing a system that uses social media analysis to identify stress. One method would be to collect the social media posts pertaining to the user by using various data collection methods. Next step would require the cleaning and pre-processing of the data. The dataset is organized in a way so that feature selection could be possible. And after that the machine learning model is trained and accordingly the results for stress detection and classification are generated [21].

4.2 *Deep Learning*

Deep learning (DL) has emerged as a powerful tool for stress detection and monitoring. DL algorithms can learn complex representations of physiological and environmental data, which can be used to accurately predict stress levels and identify potential triggers. Here are some ways in which DL can be used for stress detection and monitoring:

- Multimodal data integration: DL algorithms can integrate data from multiple sensors, including physiological sensors (such as heart rate variability, electrodermal activity, and respiration rate) and environmental sensors (such as temperature, noise, and lighting), to develop a more comprehensive understanding of the factors contributing to stress.

- Transfer learning: DL algorithms can use pre-trained models to extract features from physiological and environmental signals that are relevant to stress. This can help in developing more accurate stress models, even when data is limited.
- Real-time monitoring: DL can be used to develop real-time stress monitoring systems that can provide continuous monitoring of physiological and environmental signals. This can enable timely interventions and support for individuals who are experiencing high levels of stress.
- Personalization: DL can be used to develop personalized stress models, based on individual data. This can help in providing tailored interventions and support to individuals, based on their unique stress patterns.
- Deep reinforcement learning: DL algorithms can be used to develop adaptive stress interventions, based on real-time stress monitoring. This can enable personalized interventions that are tailored to an individual's unique stress patterns.

Deep learning has the potential to revolutionize stress detection and monitoring by providing real-time, objective data that can be used to inform personalized interventions aimed at improving mental health and well-being. DL-based stress detection and monitoring systems can be used in a variety of settings, such as healthcare, sports, and workplace safety, to help individuals and organizations manage stress and promote well-being. Machine learning techniques require hand-crafted manually generated features in order to detect stress. This drawback can be eliminated by the use of deep convolutional neural networks. One such architecture has been proposed by researchers where all the parameters obtained from different sensors are processed individually in different 1D convolutional blocks [22]. These different set of features are then concatenated and processed further using deep learning models. Deep learning models are proving to provide much better accuracy by use of deep neural networks and address the issue of manual feature generation.

4.3 Internet of Things

Internet of Things paradigm provides opportunities to manage and monitor stress levels by making use of sensors and transmitting that information directly to the processing units. Real-time stress monitoring can be done using Internet of Things concepts. The parameters like heart rate, blood pressure, and body temperature are captured using sensors. The collected information is then pre-processed and sent to the processing units or devices through the internet, and the real-time results can be displayed or visualized using high end monitoring systems [23].

A cloud server and Internet of Things based stress monitoring assistance system has been proposed recently, which aims to detect stress in real time [23]. This system has the capability to provide personal assistance to people in stress. Galvanic skin response is taken as the input parameter to measure stress by the stress device. The threshold value is identified after due analysis on MATLAB software and then the interfacing of the stress device with the cloud server is done to log real data.

Following are some more ways in which IoT can be used for stress detection and monitoring:

- Wearable devices: IoT-enabled wearable devices, such as smartwatches and fitness trackers, can collect physiological data (such as heart rate and skin conductance) and environmental data (such as temperature and noise) to provide a comprehensive understanding of an individual's stress levels.
- Smart home devices: IoT-enabled smart home devices, such as smart thermostats and lighting systems, can collect data on environmental factors that can impact stress levels, such as temperature and lighting. This can provide a more comprehensive understanding of the factors contributing to stress.
- Real-time monitoring: IoT-enabled devices can collect and transmit data in real time, allowing for continuous monitoring of physiological and environmental signals. This can enable timely interventions and support for individuals who are experiencing high levels of stress.
- Data analytics: IoT can be used to collect and analyse large volumes of data, which can be used to develop predictive models and identify patterns that are associated with stress. This can help in the early detection of stress and provide an opportunity for timely interventions.
- Personalization: IoT can be used to develop personalized stress models, based on individual data. This can help in providing tailored interventions and support to individuals, based on their unique stress patterns.

IoT-based stress detection and monitoring systems can be used in a variety of settings, such as healthcare, sports, and workplace safety, to help individuals and organizations manage stress and promote well-being [24].

4.4 Brain-Inspired Computing

Brain-inspired computing, also known as neuromorphic computing, is an emerging field that draws inspiration from the structure and function of the human brain to design computing systems. This technology has the potential to revolutionize stress detection by leveraging the power of artificial neural networks to process large amounts of data in real time. One of the primary advantages of brain-inspired computing is its ability to process data in a parallel, distributed manner, similar to the way in which the human brain processes information. This allows for the efficient processing of large amounts of data, making it well-suited for stress detection and monitoring applications.

Brain-inspired computing can be used to detect stress by analysing physiological signals such as heart rate variability, electroencephalography (EEG) signals, and skin conductance. By modelling the way in which the human brain processes these signals, artificial neural networks can be trained to detect patterns and identify signs of stress. Brain-inspired computing can also be used to develop personalized stress detection models based on individual data. By training the neural networks on individual physiological and environmental data, the models can be tailored to each individual's unique stress patterns, allowing for more accurate and effective stress detection.

However, the use of brain-inspired computing for stress detection also poses some challenges. One of the significant challenges is the need for large amounts of data to train the neural networks effectively. Additionally, the interpretability of the models can be challenging, making it difficult to understand the factors that contribute to stress. Overall, brain-inspired computing holds significant promise for stress detection and monitoring, offering a powerful tool for processing and analysing large amounts of data in real time. Further research in this area has the potential to lead to the development of more accurate and effective stress detection models, enabling individuals to take timely action to manage stress and improve their overall well-being.

4.5 Natural Language Processing

Natural Language Processing (NLP) is a subfield of artificial intelligence that focuses on the interaction between computers and human language. NLP has the potential to revolutionize stress detection and monitoring by analysing textual data such as social media posts, chat messages, and emails to detect patterns and identify signs of stress. One of the primary advantages of NLP is its ability to analyse unstructured data, enabling the detection of stress in natural language expressions. By analysing linguistic features such as sentiment, tone, and lexical patterns, NLP algorithms can detect stress and other emotional states in text.

NLP can also be used to monitor stress over time, enabling the detection of patterns and changes in stress levels. By analysing longitudinal data, NLP algorithms can identify stress triggers, monitor the effectiveness of stress management interventions, and provide personalized recommendations for stress management. However, the use of NLP for stress detection and monitoring also poses some challenges. One of the significant challenges is the need for large amounts of data to train the NLP models effectively. Additionally, NLP algorithms may have difficulty understanding sarcasm, irony, and other nuances of language that can affect the interpretation of emotional states.

NLP holds significant promise for stress detection and monitoring, offering a powerful tool for analysing natural language expressions to identify signs of stress. Further research in this area has the potential to lead to the development of more accurate and effective NLP models, enabling individuals to take timely action to manage stress and improve their overall well-being.

5 Conclusions and Future Research Directions

This chapter offers a comprehensive overview of digital monitoring and detection techniques that can be effectively utilized for stress management. The recent advancements in digital technologies, such as the Internet of Things, machine learning, deep learning, and brain-inspired computing, have led to a surge in studies exploring these techniques for real-time stress detection. However, despite these technological advancements, there are numerous challenges that must be addressed. Firstly, the presence of a digital divide can create barriers in effectively utilizing these digital techniques. Secondly, testing and validating these techniques to establish their accuracy in various scenarios are significant challenges. Additionally, it is essential to consider the unique circumstances and situations of individuals experiencing stress, which can significantly complicate the problem. Thus, a comprehensive analysis of all parameters affecting stress levels is necessary to establish correlations and develop integrated digital solutions. This chapter not only discusses various digital techniques of stress monitoring but also presents a literature review in this area, shedding light on potential avenues for future research. There are several potential future research directions that could be explored to improve stress detection and monitoring techniques. Some of these include the following:

- Developing digital tools that can overcome the digital divide: One of the primary challenges in utilizing digital techniques for stress monitoring is the presence of a digital divide. Future research could explore ways to bridge this divide and develop digital tools that are accessible and user-friendly for all individuals, regardless of their technological expertise.
- Exploring the use of augmented reality and virtual reality: Augmented reality (AR) and virtual reality (VR) technologies could offer innovative ways to monitor stress levels in real time. For example, AR or VR environments could simulate stress-inducing situations, allowing individuals to practice stress management techniques in a controlled setting.
- Utilizing wearable technology for stress monitoring: Wearable technology, such as smartwatches and fitness trackers, could offer a non-invasive way to monitor stress levels in real time. Future research could explore ways to improve the accuracy of wearable sensors and integrate them with other digital tools for more comprehensive stress monitoring.
- Examining the role of social media in stress monitoring: Social media platforms have become increasingly popular for individuals to express their emotions and share their experiences. Future research could explore ways to utilize social media data for stress monitoring, such as analysing language patterns and sentiment analysis.
- Developing personalized stress management solutions: As mentioned in the paragraph, it is essential to consider the unique circumstances and situations of individuals experiencing stress. Future research could explore ways to develop personalized stress management solutions that are tailored to an individual's specific needs and circumstances. This could involve combining multiple digital

techniques, such as machine learning and brain-inspired computing, to develop comprehensive solutions.

References

1. Rochette L, Vergely C. Hans Selye and the stress response: 80 years after his 'letter' to the editor of nature. Annal de Cardiol et d'Angeiol. 2017;66:181–3. https://doi.org/10.1016/j.ancard.2017.04.017.
2. Choi Y, Jeon YM, Wang L, Kim K. A biological signal-based stress monitoring framework for children using wearable devices. Sensors. 2017;17(9):1936.
3. Samson C, Koh A. Stress monitoring and recent advancements in wearable biosensors. Front Bioeng Biotechnol. 2020;8:1037.
4. Han HJ, Labbaf S, Borelli JL, Dutt N, Rahmani AM. Objective stress monitoring based on wearable sensors in everyday settings. J Med Eng Technol. 2020;44(4):177–89.
5. Salafi T, Kah JCY. Design of unobtrusive wearable mental stress monitoring device using physiological sensor. In: 7th WACBE World Congress on Bioengineering, vol. 2015. Cham: Springer; 2015. p. 11–4.
6. Can YS, Arnrich B, Ersoy C. Stress detection in daily life scenarios using smart phones and wearable sensors: a survey. J Biomed Inform. 2019;92:103139.
7. Padmaja N, Anusha A, Manaswi DVS, Kumar BS. IOT based stress detection and health monitoring system. Int J—"Helix - The Scientific Explorer". 2020;10(2):161–7.
8. Hejjel L, Gál I. Heart rate variability analysis. Acta Physiol Hung. 2001;88(3–4):219–30.
9. Tarvainen MP, Niskanen JP, Lipponen JA, Ranta-Aho PO, Karjalainen PA. Kubios HRV—heart rate variability analysis software. Comput Methods Prog Biomed. 2014;113(1):210–20. https://doi.org/10.1016/j.cmpb.2013.07.024.
10. ADInstruments. "Heart Rate Variability Analysis Software," 2021. https://www.adinstruments.com/products/hrv.
11. Setterlind, Larsson G. The stress profile: a psychosocial approach to measuring stress. Stress Med. 1995;11(1):85–92.
12. Lee EH. Review of the psychometric evidence of the perceived stress scale. Asian Nurs Res. 2012;6(4):121–7.
13. Russell E, Koren G, Rieder M, Van Uum S. Hair cortisol as a biological marker of chronic stress: current status, future directions and unanswered questions. Psychoneuroendocrinology. 2012;37(5):589–601.
14. Choi S, Kim S, Yang JS, Lee JH, Joo C, Jung HI. Real-time measurement of human salivary cortisol for the assessment of psychological stress using a smartphone. Sensing Bio-Sensing Res. 2014;2:8–11.
15. Jovanov E, O'Donnell Lords A, Raskovic D, Cox PG, Adhami R, Andrasik F. Stress monitoring using a distributed wireless intelligent sensor system. IEEE Eng Med Biol Mag. 2003;22(3):49–55.
16. Lee MH, Yang G, Lee HK, Bang S. Development stress monitoring system based on personal digital assistant (PDA). In: The 26th Annual International Conference of the IEEE Engineering in Medicine and Biology Society; 2004. p. 2364–7.
17. L Daskal. 13 of the best apps to manage stress, Inc, 2018. https://www.inc.com/lolly-daskal/13-of-the-best-apps-to-manage-stress.html.
18. Zhai J, Barreto A. Stress detection in computer users based on digital signal processing of noninvasive physiological variables. In: Conf Proc IEEE Eng Med Biol Soc.; 2006. p. 1355–8.
19. AIM Blog. 5 Great Mental Health Chatbots, 2021. https://www.aimblog.io/2021/03/02/these-chatbots-are-helping-with-mental-health-right-now/.

20. Vos G, Trinh K, Sarnyai Z, Azghadi MR. Machine learning for stress monitoring from wearable devices: a systematic literature review. 2022. arXiv preprint arXiv:2209.15137.
21. Stress wearables: best devices that monitor stress and how they work. Wareable. 2022. https://www.wareable.com/health-and-wellbeing/stress-monitoring-wearables-explained-7969#:~:text=At%20the%20heart%20of%20how,bpms%20(beats%20per%20minute).
22. Li R, Liu Z. Stress detection using deep neural networks. BMC Med Inform Decis Mak. 2020;20(suppl. 11):285.
23. Singh R, Gehlot A, Rashid M, Saxena R, Akram SV, Alshamrani SS, AlGhamdi AS. Cloud server and internet of things assisted system for stress monitoring. Electronics. 2021;10(24):3133. https://doi.org/10.3390/electronics10243133.
24. Kim S, Kim S. User preference for an IoT healthcare application for lifestyle disease management. Telecommun Policy. 2018;42:304–14.

Consequences of Brain Health in the Digital Era

Manish Kumar, Vaibhav Shamrao Ingale, Amandeep Kaur, and Kashish Bhatia

Abstract Recent scientific evidence suggests that frequent use of digital technology, such as problematic mobile use (PMU), has both negative and positive effects on brain function and behavior. Excessive screen time and technology use can lead to attention deficit symptoms, impairments in emotional and social intelligence, technology addiction, social isolation, impaired brain development, and sleep disturbances. Moreover, the COVID-19 pandemic has further increased screen time for both adults and children due to virtual classrooms. This has harmed brain health, as individuals have been attending their classes and working online without interaction with peers. However, certain online games and apps can improve neural activity in the brain. Additionally, numerous apps and digital tools are available to manage mental health issues, such as self-management, monitoring, skill training, and enhancing mood and behavior. In this digital era, we are akin to sailors without rudders, being driven by digital stimuli rather than our deliberate direction in the ocean. This chapter explores the various consequences for brain health in this digital era.

Keywords Brain health · Emotional and social intelligence · Skill training · Digital apps

1 Introduction

In the past, our great-grandparents were not exposed to the digital life that exists today. They relied solely on interpersonal communication and a few other sources for their information. However, in contemporary times, people of all ages are consuming and processing vast amounts of data from the digital world. Moreover, they are not just consuming data, but also generating large quantities of it in their daily

M. Kumar (✉) · V. S. Ingale · A. Kaur · K. Bhatia
Department of Computer Science and Engineering, Punjab Engineering College (Deemed to be University), Chandigarh, India
e-mail: manishkumar@pec.edu.in

G. Battineni et al. (eds.), *Computational Methods in Psychiatry*,
https://doi.org/10.1007/978-981-99-6637-0_6

lives. The number of internet users worldwide (in millions) from 2006 to 2020 is displayed in Fig. 1 (Source: FinancesOnline).

Over the past 3 years, people, especially the younger generation, have become more at ease with the digital world than the physical one. They spend the majority of their time online, and this shift toward an online existence has created a new field of study for neuroscientists [1]. They can now investigate how digital technology is changing the functioning of our brains and our behavior. However, as with most things, there are both positive and negative impacts. Neuroscientific data indicates that the digital era is affecting the brain in both negative and positive ways. For example, an elderly individual who can maintain their independence by using various digital apps is a positive outcome. Scientists use Magnetic Resonance Imaging (MRI) to track brain health and neural activity to measure the effect of the digital era on the brain. This chapter will cover all of the impacts that the digital era has had on the human brain.

The COVID-19 pandemic has had various impacts on children, particularly on their personality and brain health. Schools are supposed to shape children's personalities and brains with a positive approach, but unfortunately, the system often restricts them to a rat race, leading to anxiety, depression, and other mental illnesses at an early stage. With the pandemic, children have become more reliant on the internet for education and leisure activities. Additionally, the neglect of mental health issues has further exacerbated these problems. To understand how twenty-first century children have been affected, four main themes need to be taken into consideration as shown in Fig. 2 [2].

The digital era has brought about numerous benefits to society, but it has also resulted in potentially harmful effects on brain health. Some of the harmful effects have been discussed in further sections.

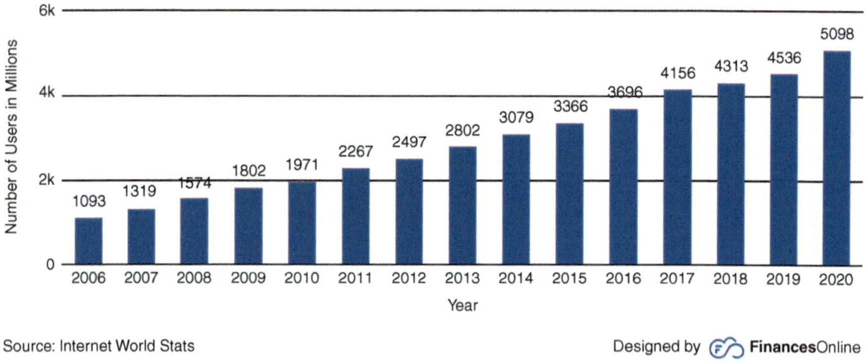

Fig. 1 Number of internet users worldwide (in millions) from 2006 to 2020

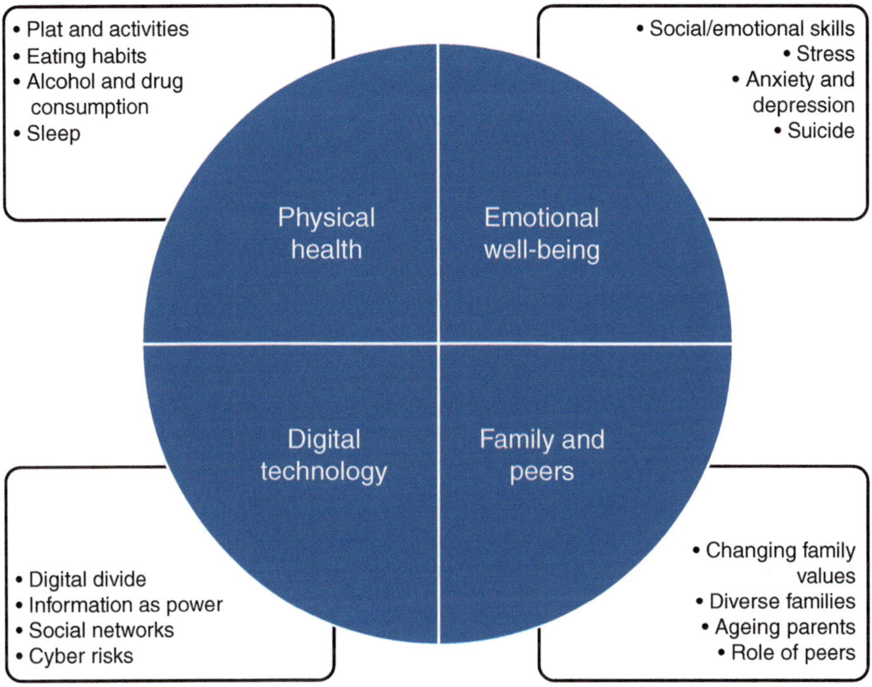

Fig. 2 Four main themes for analysis of twenty-first century children issues [2]

1.1 Attention Deficit Disorders

Many studies have shown a link between screen time on computers, mobile, or tablets and symptoms of Attention Deficit Hyperactivity Disorder (ADHD). Scientists have found a close association between excessive usage of digital media and symptoms of ADHD. Also, when people are online often they get less time to interact offline and reset their brains [3]. ADHD is a neurodevelopmental disorder that affects both children and adults. It is characterized by symptoms of inattention, hyperactivity, and impulsivity. People with ADHD may struggle with staying focused, paying attention, completing tasks, organizing themselves, and controlling their impulses.

The exact cause of ADHD is not fully understood, but it is believed to be a combination of genetic and environmental factors. Some of the common risk factors for ADHD include genetics, brain structure, and function, exposure to toxins, premature birth or low birth weight, and maternal smoking during pregnancy.

ADHD can be diagnosed by a healthcare professional based on the symptoms, medical history, and behavioral assessments. Treatment for ADHD may include medication, behavioral therapy, and lifestyle modifications. Medications such as stimulants and non-stimulants can help improve attention and reduce hyperactivity and impulsivity. Behavioral therapy can help individuals with ADHD develop coping strategies and improve their social skills, organization, and time management.

It is important to note that ADHD can impact people in different ways and that each individual's experience with the disorder is unique. With the right treatment and support, individuals with ADHD can learn to manage their symptoms and lead fulfilling lives.

1.2 Impairments in Emotional and Social Intelligence

The amount of time children spend online has significantly increased as everything becomes digital, but it is recommended by the American Academy of Pediatrics that screen time for children aged 2 years or younger should be limited due to the brain's heightened malleability at that age.

Spending excessive time online can reduce opportunities for face-to-face communication, and Kirsh and Mounts [4] hypothesized that playing video games can interfere with the ability to recognize human emotions. They studied the effects of playing video games on the recognition of facial expressions of emotions in 197 students and discovered that participants who had played violent video games before viewing a calm face were unable to recognize the emotion. Some of the bad effects of technology are displayed in Fig. 3.

Problematic mobile use (PMU) refers to a pattern of excessive and compulsive use of mobile devices, such as smartphones and tablets, that leads to negative consequences for the user. PMU is sometimes also referred to as mobile phone addiction, smartphone addiction, or nomophobia (fear of being without a mobile phone).

PMU is characterized by a range of symptoms, including the following:

- Spending an excessive amount of time on mobile devices, often at the expense of other important activities such as work, school, or socializing with others.
- Feeling a compulsive need to check one's mobile device regularly, even when it is not necessary or appropriate.
- Experiencing anxiety or distress when separated from one's mobile device or unable to use it for some time.
- Neglecting personal hygiene or self-care in favor of using a mobile device.
- Experiencing negative consequences as a result of PMU, such as poor academic or work performance, social isolation, relationship problems, or physical health issues.

PMU is a growing concern in today's society, as mobile devices have become an integral part of many people's daily lives. While the majority of mobile device users do not experience PMU, for those who do, it can have a significant impact on their well-being and quality of life. Treatments for PMU typically involve cognitive-behavioral therapy, which focuses on changing problematic behaviors and thought patterns related to mobile device use.

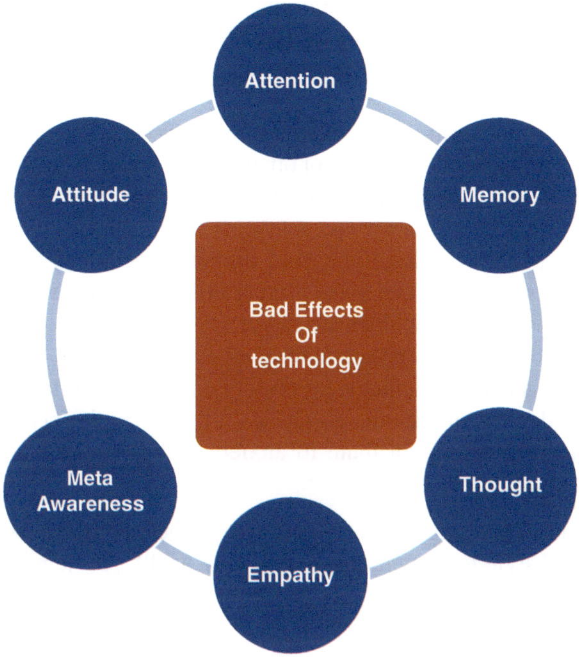

Fig. 3 Bad effects of technology in different ways

1.3 Physical Effects

Physical effects are the most easily quantifiable of other negative effects of technologies on the brain. Metabolic disease can be a very common cause of the use of technologies in daily life. As we sit with a digital device, it indirectly reduces the movement of the body. Movement of the body is required to stay healthy. Therefore, screen time and digital usage not only affect the brain but the entire body.

Prolonged and excessive use of screens can cause several health problems, including eye strain, headaches, neck and shoulder pain, back pain, and sleep disturbances. Here are some more diseases and conditions that can be associated with severe screen use:

- Computer vision syndrome (CVS): This condition includes a range of vision-related problems, such as eye strain, dry eyes, blurred vision, double vision, and headaches. CVS is often caused by the prolonged use of digital devices, especially computers.
- Carpal tunnel syndrome: This is a condition that causes numbness, tingling, and weakness in the hand and wrist. It is caused by pressure on the median nerve, which runs through the wrist. Repetitive use of a keyboard or mouse can increase the risk of developing carpal tunnel syndrome.

- Tennis elbow: Also known as lateral epicondylitis, tennis elbow is a condition that causes pain and inflammation in the elbow. It is often caused by repetitive use of the forearm muscles and tendons, such as when using a computer mouse or typing on a keyboard.
- Text neck: This is a term used to describe the neck pain and stiffness caused by constantly looking down at a phone or other digital device. The posture associated with this behavior can strain the neck muscles and lead to long-term neck problems.
- Insomnia: Exposure to blue light from digital devices can interfere with the body's natural sleep cycle and make it more difficult to fall asleep. This can lead to insomnia and other sleep disorders.
- Obesity: Spending too much time in front of screens can lead to a sedentary lifestyle, which is a major risk factor for obesity and other health problems.
- Anxiety and depression: Studies have shown that excessive screen use, particularly social media, can contribute to anxiety and depression in both children and adults.

It's important to take breaks from screen use, practice good posture, and maintain a healthy lifestyle to prevent these and other health problems associated with excessive screen use.

1.3.1 Mental Health

One of the major problems associated with the digital era is addiction, which can have detrimental effects on mental health, social life, and family bonds. Additionally, chronic smartphone stress has been identified as a newly discovered effect on health. Children who overuse technology are at a higher risk of developing serious mental health issues, including reduced attention and thinking power, delayed language, social and emotional development, and addiction to technology. Teenagers aged 15 to 16 years have been found to use digital media for longer periods, increasing the likelihood of creating symptoms of attention deficit hyperactivity disorder (ADHD). Furthermore, there are several other mental health issues associated with the digital era as mentioned below and as detailed in [5].

- Addiction.
- Anxiety and depression.
- Attention deficit hyperactivity disorder (ADHD).
- Decreased attention span.
- Poor sleep quality and insomnia.
- Impaired cognitive function.
- Decreased social skills and increased social isolation.
- Cyberbullying and online harassment.
- Low self-esteem.
- Body image issues.
- FOMO (fear of missing out).

- Online gaming addiction.

It's important to note that these issues may not affect every individual who uses digital media excessively, and the severity and prevalence of these issues can vary from person to person. However, it's still important to be aware of these potential risks and to use digital media in moderation to promote overall well-being.

1.3.2 Social Health

Social health is affected to a great extent due to the dependency on digital devices. A connection with the community is lost. For instance, earlier people used to visit banks physically and were patient enough to wait in queues to get their work done and there was a usual social connection. But with the advent of Internet banking facilities, the banks are now at a single click of our finger and the interaction with the community is lost [6]. Following are some of the one-liners which deprecate the effects of the digital era on human health.

- "Digital technologies have made it more difficult for me to say on task and devote sustained attention. This interferes with my work productivity."
- "I can't seem to get my brain to calm down and focus. It is all over the place. I can't concentrate. I just start thinking about what I'm going to do next."
- "Increased isolation is a negative effect I feel in my life; the time I spend using digital technologies could well be spent in other more creative and productive ways."
- "I am becoming increasingly aware of the way constant access to digital forms of communication can be overwhelming."
- "It has become an ever-present overhang on all aspects of life. There is no escape."
- "The rise of hatred, the manipulation of politics, and so on – these are not distant events with no personal impact."
- "Digital life has tipped the balance in favor of John Stuart Mill's 'lower pleasures' and has made engaging in higher-order pleasures more difficult."
- "One major impact is the overall decrease in short-term memory, and … what was the question?"
- "Real-life relationships are less bearable; everyone is so much less interested with the spoiling of technology."
- "Digital technology radically increases expectations for instantaneous responses. This is unhealthy."
- "It has become harder to take your eyes off a screen to enjoy life as it's happening."
- "Technology is being driven by business across all areas for money, money, money. Greed has taken over."

1.3.3 Impact on Cognitive and Brain Development

The use of screens has the potential to negatively affect cognitive and brain health, as shown in research [7]. Previous studies have revealed that children under the age of two spent approximately 1 h per day on screens, but this number increased to 3 h per day by the age of three. For infants aged between 6 and 12 months, excessive screen time has been linked to poorer early language development and behavioral problems.

Although digital media can aid in active learning in preschool and older children, it should be accompanied by parent–child interaction. However, excessive screen time and a lack of reading time have been linked to decreased brain connectivity in the areas of the brain responsible for word recognition, language, and cognitive control in children aged eight to twelve. This reduced connectivity can negatively impact reading skills, which highlights the detrimental impact of screen time on brain development. Given the increasing prevalence of screen use among very young children, whose brains are highly plastic, there is growing concern about the cognitive and brain development of children exposed to screens, which warrants further study.

1.3.4 Sleeping Patterns

Recent research suggests that screen time can negatively affect sleep, which in turn can impact cognition and behavior. Studies have shown that daily touch-screen use is associated with sleep disturbances such as reduced duration and increased night-time awakenings in infants and toddlers. Spending more time on mobile phones and touch screens is linked to more sleep disruptions, while tablet use is associated with poor sleep quality and more awakenings after sleep onset. Poor sleep quality can lead to brain changes, including decreased functional connectivity and gray matter volume, and increase the risk of age-related cognitive impairment and Alzheimer's disease.

Although it is unclear whether looking at screens or watching media content disrupts sleep, it is well established that the wavelength of light exposure affects circadian rhythms, and light-emitting diode (LED) screens on computers and phones emit slow-wave blue light that can disrupt these rhythms. Exposure to LED screens has been shown to alter melatonin levels and sleeping quality and reduce cognitive performance. Therefore, it is crucial to recognize the effects of screen time on sleep as a moderator of multiple negative impacts on memory and brain function.

1.3.5 Effects on Brain Functions

In a study, functional MRI was used to record neural activity in the brains of 12 participants who had never used the internet before and 12 who had, while performing simulated internet search tasks. It was hypothesized that the net-naive group would show increased activation in their frontal lobe network after internet training, whereas the net-savvy group would either show no change or a reduction in activation due to increased cognitive efficiency after training. During their initial scan, the net-naive group recruited a neural network that included various regions of the brain, and only this group showed additional activation in the middle and inferior frontal gyri during their second scan as shown in Fig. 4.

The net-savvy group initially displayed more extensive activation in a cortical system that controls mental activities involved in internet search tasks, but they showed a trend of reduced activation following the training, which is consistent with the hypothesis that the brain becomes more efficient and habituates to the task over time. These findings suggest that even short periods of internet browsing can alter brain activity patterns in middle-aged and older adults.

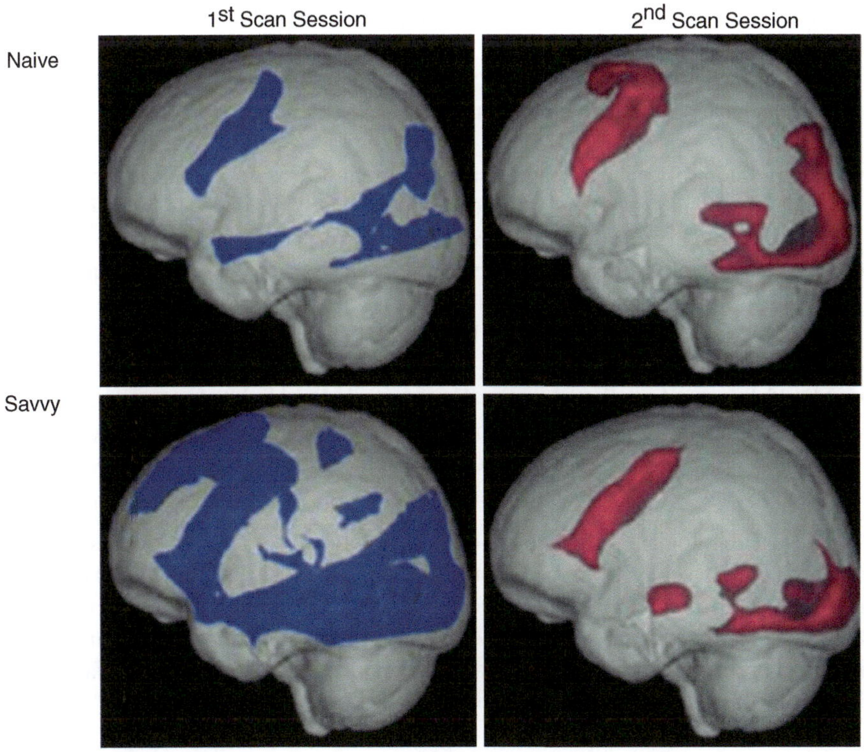

Fig. 4 Comparison between internet searching tasks before and after training

Several other research teams have studied how internet search training affects brain function and structure. One study [8] utilized diffusion tensor imaging to explore the impact of brief internet search training on the microstructure of white matter. They found that after just 6 days of training, the 59 participants (average age of 21) had an increased fractional anisotropy in the right superior longitudinal fasciculus and a reduced radial diffusivity in that area. These results imply that short-term internet search training can improve the integrity of white matter in the right superior longitudinal fasciculus, perhaps due to increased myelination.

2 Technological Interventions to Monitor and Protect from the Harmful Effects on Brain Health in a Digital Era

Several technological interventions can be used to monitor and protect individuals from the harmful effects of excessive screen time:

- Screen time tracking apps: These apps help individuals track and monitor their screen time and set usage limits. Some examples of screen time tracking apps include Moment, Screen Time, and Freedom.
- Blue light filters: These filters can be applied to digital devices, such as smartphones and tablets, to reduce the amount of blue light emitted. Blue light has been shown to disrupt circadian rhythms and negatively affect sleep. Some devices have built-in blue light filters, or users can download software that adds the filter.
- Parental controls: These features allow parents to set limits on their children's screen time and restrict access to certain apps and websites. Many devices have built-in parental controls, and there are also third-party apps available.
- Digital detox programs: These programs are designed to help individuals take a break from digital devices and reduce their screen time. Some examples of digital detox programs include the 30-Day Digital Detox Challenge and the National Day of Unplugging.
- Mindfulness and meditation apps: These apps help individuals practice mindfulness and meditation, which have been shown to reduce stress and improve mental well-being. Some examples of mindfulness and meditation apps include Headspace, Calm, and Insight Timer.

These technological interventions can be effective in helping individuals monitor and protect themselves from the harmful effects of excessive screen time. However, it's important to remember that reducing screen time and practicing other healthy habits, such as exercising and socializing in person, are also important for maintaining good brain health in the digital era. Some more techniques involving brain training have been discussed in this section.

2.1 Method of Cognitive Training to Improve Brain Health

Cognitive training refers to a set of activities or exercises designed to improve cognitive functions such as attention, memory, and problem-solving. Cognitive training has been studied as a potential intervention to improve brain health and cognitive abilities in older adults and individuals with neurological disorders.

Several methods of cognitive training have been developed to improve brain health, and some of them are discussed below:

- Computerized cognitive training: This method involves the use of computer-based programs designed to improve cognitive functions. These programs typically involve a series of exercises that challenge various cognitive skills, such as working memory, attention, and processing speed. The exercises can be adjusted in difficulty and intensity to suit individual needs.
- Cognitive stimulation therapy: This method involves engaging individuals in group activities that stimulate cognitive functions, such as discussion, reminiscence, and problem-solving. The activities are designed to be enjoyable and engaging to encourage participation.
- Mindfulness training: This method involves the practice of mindfulness meditation, which is aimed at improving attention and emotional regulation. Mindfulness training typically involves focused breathing and attention to the present moment.
- Physical exercise: Physical exercise has been shown to improve cognitive functions, particularly executive functions such as planning, decision-making, and working memory. Exercise may improve brain health through increased blood flow and neuroplasticity.
- Cognitive-behavioral therapy: This method is a type of psychotherapy that focuses on changing negative thinking patterns and behaviors that may be contributing to cognitive problems. Cognitive-behavioral therapy may involve problem-solving exercises, cognitive restructuring, and behavioral activation.

Overall, the goal of cognitive training is to improve cognitive function and promote brain health. The specific method of cognitive training used may depend on individual needs, preferences, and cognitive strengths and weaknesses. Cognitive training involves exercising the brain rigorously using intense mental exercises. Many applications can keep your brain busy as listed in Table 1.

Many other applications can help to keep the brain active and healthy while using digital devices. However, it is suggested to try and adopt natural cognitive training methods by taking a leave from the digital world for a short while. Following are some of the benefits of cognitive training which encourage taking care of the brain.

Table 1 Mobile apps to keep the brain active [9]

N	Name of the app	Features
1.	Lumosity	Improvement in memory and focus, concentration, mindfulness, cognitive ability
2.	Duolingo	Lessons in over 35 languages, language learning, and practicing tools
3.	Calm	Reduces anxiety, meditation, music, sleep stories, self-care
4.	Psychology compass	Cognition coach, weekly lessons to automate habits
5.	Headspace	Sleep-aiding tools, guided meditations, music
6.	Ten percent happier	Topic-specific meditations
7.	Insight timer	Workshops, guided meditations, music, etc.
8.	TED	Inspire me feature, many languages supported, world-class thinkers
9.	Forest	Virtual forests creation to view habitual changes, reminders, targets, and routines
10.	Words with friends	Build vocabulary, words with friends feature, challenges, games
11.	Chess—play and learn	Puzzles, brain games

2.2 *Cognitive Behavioral Therapy*

Cognitive-behavioral therapy (CBT) is a type of psychotherapy that aims to help individuals improve their mental health by changing negative thought patterns and behaviors. It is a goal-oriented, problem-solving approach that is based on the idea that thoughts, feelings, and behaviors are interconnected.

CBT is effective in treating a wide range of mental health conditions, including anxiety disorders, depression, post-traumatic stress disorder (PTSD), obsessive-compulsive disorder (OCD), and eating disorders. It is also used as a complementary therapy for individuals with chronic pain, sleep disorders, and substance abuse.

The basic principles of CBT include the following:

- Cognitive restructuring: This involves identifying and challenging negative thought patterns that may be contributing to mental health problems. The therapist helps the individual to replace negative thoughts with more positive, realistic ones.
- Behavioral activation: This involves identifying and changing negative behaviors that may be contributing to mental health problems. The therapist helps the individual to develop new, positive behaviors that promote mental health.
- Exposure therapy: This involves gradually exposing individuals to situations that trigger anxiety or fear, to reduce their sensitivity to these triggers.
- Relaxation techniques: This involves teaching individuals relaxation techniques such as deep breathing, progressive muscle relaxation, and visualization to help reduce anxiety and stress.
- Homework assignments: Individuals are often given homework assignments to practice the skills learned in therapy, such as challenging negative thoughts or practicing relaxation techniques.

CBT is typically a short-term therapy, lasting between 12 and 20 sessions. However, the length of therapy may vary depending on the individual and the severity of their mental health condition. CBT can be delivered in various formats, including individual therapy, group therapy, and online therapy. The therapy can also be adapted for children and adolescents. Overall, CBT is a structured, evidence-based therapy that can help individuals improve their mental health by changing negative thought patterns and behaviors. It is a highly effective treatment option for a range of mental health conditions and can be tailored to individual needs and preferences.

2.3 *Meditation Apps*

Meditation apps have become increasingly popular in the digital era as a way to improve brain health. These apps offer a convenient and accessible way to practice mindfulness meditation, which has been shown to have numerous benefits for mental and physical health. Meditation apps typically offer guided meditations, which can be tailored to different levels of experience and different goals. For example, some apps offer meditations for stress reduction, while others offer meditations for sleep or anxiety.

There are several benefits of using meditation apps for brain health, including the following:

- Stress reduction: Mindfulness meditation has been shown to reduce stress and anxiety, which can have a positive impact on brain health. Studies have found that regular meditation practice can reduce the size of the amygdala, which is part of the brain that is responsible for the Fight-or-flight response.
- Improved cognitive functions: Regular mindfulness meditation practice has been shown to improve cognitive functions such as attention, memory, and executive function. Studies have found that meditation can increase gray matter volume in the prefrontal cortex, which is part of the brain that is responsible for decision-making and planning.
- Improved emotional regulation: Mindfulness meditation can improve emotional regulation by helping individuals become more aware of their thoughts and emotions. Studies have found that regular meditation practice can reduce symptoms of depression and anxiety.
- Better sleep: Mindfulness meditation can improve sleep quality by reducing stress and promoting relaxation. Studies have found that meditation can improve sleep duration and reduce the time it takes to fall asleep.

Some popular meditation apps include Headspace, Calm, and Insight Timer. These apps offer guided meditations of varying lengths and can be accessed on a smartphone or tablet. Some apps also offer features such as progress tracking and personalized recommendations. Overall, meditation apps can be a useful tool for improving brain health in the digital era. However, it is important to remember that meditation is a practice that requires regular and consistent effort. Like any form of exercise, the benefits of meditation come with regular practice over time.

2.4 Wearable Technology

Wearable technologies have become increasingly popular in the digital era as a way to improve brain health. These technologies include devices such as fitness trackers and smartwatches, which can track physical activity, sleep patterns, and heart rate, among other metrics. These data can provide valuable insights into the overall health and can be used to inform lifestyle changes that can have a positive impact on brain health.

Some of the ways in which wearable technologies can improve brain health are as follows:

- Encouraging physical activity: Regular physical activity has been shown to have numerous benefits for brain health. Wearable fitness trackers can help individuals monitor their activity levels and provide feedback on progress toward activity goals.
- Improving sleep: Sleep is critical for brain health, and poor sleep has been linked to a range of cognitive and emotional problems. Wearable technologies that track sleep patterns can provide individuals with valuable information about their sleep quality, which can be used to make lifestyle changes that improve sleep.
- Reducing stress: Wearable devices such as smartwatches can provide feedback on stress levels and offer features such as guided breathing exercises to help individuals manage stress.
- Monitoring heart health: Heart health is closely linked to brain health, and wearable devices can track metrics such as heart rate variability, which is an indicator of overall cardiovascular health. Improving heart health can have a positive impact on brain health by improving blood flow to the brain.
- Providing feedback on cognitive performance: Some wearable technologies offer cognitive performance tracking, which can provide individuals with feedback on cognitive functions such as attention, memory, and executive function. This feedback can be used to inform lifestyle changes that improve cognitive performance.

Wearable technologies have the potential to be a valuable tool for improving brain health in the digital era. However, it is important to use these technologies in conjunction with other lifestyle changes such as regular physical exercise, healthy diet, and social connection. Additionally, it is important to use these technologies in moderation and to seek professional advice before making significant changes to lifestyle or starting any new exercise or health program.

2.5 Virtual Reality Technology

Virtual reality (VR) technology has emerged as a promising tool for improving brain health in the digital era. VR technology creates a simulated environment that can be experienced through a VR headset, allowing users to engage in activities and experiences that can have a positive impact on brain health.

Some of the ways in which VR technology can improve brain health are as follows:

- Stress reduction: VR technology can create immersive environments that can help users relax and reduce stress. For example, VR-guided meditations can create a calming environment that can promote relaxation and reduce stress levels.
- Cognitive training: VR technology can be used to create cognitive training programs that can help improve cognitive functions such as attention, memory, and executive function. VR cognitive training programs can provide a more engaging and immersive experience than traditional cognitive training methods, which can increase motivation and adherence to the program.
- Rehabilitation: VR technology can be used in rehabilitation settings to help individuals recover from brain injuries and improve motor function. For example, VR games can be used to improve hand-eye coordination and balance.
- Exposure therapy: VR technology can be used to create simulated environments that can help individuals overcome fears and phobias through exposure therapy. For example, VR exposure therapy can be used to help individuals overcome their fear of heights or fear of flying.
- Social connection: VR technology can be used to create virtual social environments that can help combat loneliness and social isolation, which are risk factors for cognitive decline and dementia.

While VR technology has the potential to improve brain health in numerous ways, it is important to use this technology in moderation and under the guidance of a trained professional. Additionally, VR technology is not suitable for everyone and may not be appropriate for individuals with certain medical conditions. As with any new technology or treatment approach, it is important to consult with a healthcare professional before incorporating VR technology into a brain health program.

2.6 Brain Stimulation Devices

Brain stimulation devices have become increasingly popular as a way to improve brain health in the digital era. These devices use electrical or magnetic stimulation to alter brain activity and have been used to treat a range of neurological and psychiatric conditions. They can also be used for non-medical purposes to enhance cognitive function, memory, and mood.

Some of the brain stimulation devices that are commonly used for improving brain health are as follows:

- Transcranial Magnetic Stimulation (TMS): TMS is a non-invasive brain stimulation technique that uses magnetic fields to stimulate nerve cells in the brain. It has been approved by the FDA for the treatment of depression and has also been used for the treatment of anxiety, chronic pain, and other conditions.
- Transcranial Direct Current Stimulation (tDCS): tDCS is a non-invasive brain stimulation technique that uses a low-level electrical current to stimulate the brain. It has been used for the treatment of depression, anxiety, and chronic pain and has also been shown to improve cognitive function and memory.
- Deep Brain Stimulation (DBS): DBS is a surgical procedure that involves implanting electrodes into specific areas of the brain to stimulate or inhibit activity. It has been used to treat a range of neurological and psychiatric conditions, including Parkinson's disease, obsessive-compulsive disorder, and depression.
- Vagus Nerve Stimulation (VNS): VNS involves implanting a device that delivers electrical impulses to the vagus nerve, which connects the brain to the rest of the body. It has been used for the treatment of epilepsy and depression and has also been used for the treatment of chronic pain and other conditions.

While brain stimulation devices have the potential to improve brain health in numerous ways, they should be used under the guidance of a trained healthcare professional. These devices can have side effects and are not appropriate for everyone. Additionally, they should be used in conjunction with other lifestyle changes such as regular exercise, healthy diet, and social connection, as these factors also play an important role in brain health. It is important to consult with a healthcare professional before incorporating brain stimulation devices into a brain health program.

2.7 *Online Therapy Platforms*

Online therapy platforms have become increasingly popular as a way to improve brain health in the digital era. These platforms provide individuals with access to licensed therapists and mental health professionals via the internet, making it more convenient and accessible for individuals to seek treatment for mental health conditions and improve their overall brain health. Some of the benefits of using online therapy platforms for improving brain health are as follows:

- Accessibility: Online therapy platforms make it easier for individuals to access mental health care, particularly for those who may live in remote areas or have limited mobility.
- Convenience: Online therapy sessions can be conducted from the comfort of one's own home, which can be particularly beneficial for individuals with busy schedules or those who have difficulty leaving the house.

- Privacy: Online therapy sessions offer a level of privacy and anonymity that may not be possible in traditional in-person therapy settings.
- Affordability: Online therapy platforms may be more affordable than traditional in-person therapy sessions, particularly for individuals who do not have insurance coverage for mental health care.
- Variety of services: Online therapy platforms offer a range of services, including individual therapy, group therapy, and specialized treatment programs for specific mental health conditions.

Online therapy platforms have numerous benefits, but it is important to choose a platform that is reputable and employs licensed therapists and mental health professionals. It is also important to ensure that the platform is secure and protects personal information. Additionally, online therapy may not be appropriate for everyone and may not be effective for certain mental health conditions. It is important to consult with a healthcare professional to determine if online therapy is a suitable option for improving brain health.

3 Benefits of the Digital Era on Brain Health

The digital era has brought about many benefits for brain health, particularly in terms of accessibility and convenience. However, it is important to use technology in moderation and to consult with healthcare professionals to ensure that technology is being used safely and effectively. Following are some benefits of the digital era on brain health.

3.1 Neural Exercises

The internet and digital era have provided many opportunities for neural exercise, allowing individuals to engage in activities that challenge and stimulate the brain from the comfort of their own homes. Here are some examples of neural exercises using the internet and digital tools. However, it is important to use these tools in moderation and to engage in a variety of neural exercises for optimal brain health.

- Brain training apps: There are many brain training apps available for smartphones and tablets that offer exercises and games designed to improve cognitive function, memory, and attention.
- Online learning platforms: Online learning platforms, such as Coursera and Udemy, offer a wide range of courses and tutorials that allow individuals to learn new skills and challenge their brains.
- Brain games and puzzles: Some many websites and apps offer brain games and puzzles, such as Sudoku, crossword puzzles, and memory games.

- Meditation apps: Meditation apps, such as Headspace and Calm, offer guided meditations that can improve attention and reduce stress.
- Virtual reality games: Virtual reality games offer a unique opportunity to challenge the brain in a new and immersive way, allowing individuals to improve cognitive function and memory.
- Online discussion forums: Engaging in online discussion forums can stimulate the brain and improve cognitive function by exposing individuals to new ideas and perspectives.

3.2 Access to Information

The internet and digital era have made it easier than ever to access information about brain health. Here are some ways that the internet and digital tools have improved access to information about brain health:

- Online resources: There are many online resources available that provide information about brain health, including websites, blogs, and forums. These resources offer a wealth of information on topics such as brain function, mental health, and neuroplasticity.
- Health and wellness apps: There are many health and wellness apps available that offer information and guidance on brain health. These apps may include features such as mindfulness exercises, brain training games, and sleep-tracking tools.
- Social media: Social media platforms can be used to access information about brain health, including posts from experts, research studies, and news articles. Users can follow accounts and pages that share information on brain health to stay informed on the latest news and trends.
- Online courses and webinars: Online courses and webinars offer access to information on brain health, including topics such as meditation, mindfulness, and cognitive-behavioral therapy. Many of these courses and webinars are led by experts in the field and offer a convenient way to learn about brain health from the comfort of your own home.
- Telehealth services: Telehealth services offer a convenient way to access healthcare professionals who specialize in brain health, including psychiatrists, psychologists, and neurologists. These services allow individuals to receive support and guidance on brain health from anywhere with an internet connection.

3.3 *Improved Multitasking Skills*

The internet and digital era have provided many opportunities for individuals to improve their multitasking skills. Here are some ways that the internet and digital tools have improved multitasking skills:

- Multiple windows and tabs: Modern web browsers allow users to open multiple windows and tabs simultaneously, enabling them to switch between different tasks quickly and easily.
- Mobile devices: Smartphones and tablets allow users to access multiple apps simultaneously, making it easier to multitask while on the go.
- Productivity apps: There are many productivity apps available that offer features such as task management, note-taking, and calendar organization. These apps can help individuals keep track of multiple tasks and stay organized.
- Collaboration tools: Collaboration tools such as Google Docs and Slack allow individuals to work together on projects in real time, enabling them to multitask and work more efficiently.
- Online learning: Online courses and tutorials allow individuals to learn new skills while multitasking. For example, someone could watch a video tutorial on how to use a new software program while also working on a different task.

Overall, the internet and digital tools have provided many opportunities for individuals to improve their multitasking skills. However, it is important to note that multitasking can also have negative effects on productivity and mental health. It is important to find a balance between multitasking and focusing on one task at a time. Additionally, it is important to prioritize tasks and set realistic goals to avoid feeling overwhelmed or burnt out.

3.4 *Working Memory and Fluid Intelligence*

The internet and digital era have provided many opportunities for individuals to improve their working memory and fluid intelligence. Here are some ways that the internet and digital tools have improved working memory and fluid intelligence:

- Brain training games and apps: There are many brain training games and apps available that have been designed to improve working memory and fluid intelligence. These games and apps may include tasks such as memory games, attention exercises, and problem-solving tasks.
- Online courses and tutorials: Online courses and tutorials can help individuals improve their working memory and fluid intelligence by teaching them new skills and knowledge. These courses and tutorials may include topics such as coding, language learning, and critical thinking.
- Social media and online communities: Social media and online communities can also improve working memory and fluid intelligence by providing opportunities

for social interaction, debate, and discussion. These activities can help individuals develop their critical thinking and problem-solving skills.

- Online research and information retrieval: The internet provides a vast amount of information on almost any topic, and individuals who are skilled in finding, organizing, and retaining this information are likely to have strong working memory and fluid intelligence.
- Online collaboration and teamwork: The internet has made it easier than ever to collaborate with others on projects and tasks. Working with others online can help individuals develop their teamwork skills, problem-solving abilities, and communication skills.

3.5 Visual Attention Reaction Time

The internet and digital era have also provided opportunities for individuals to improve their visual attention reaction time. Here are some ways that the internet and digital tools have improved visual attention reaction time:

- Video games: Video games can improve visual attention reaction time by requiring the player to quickly respond to visual cues on the screen. Games such as first-person shooters or racing games can improve reaction times and visual attention.
- Online sports and fitness training: Online sports and fitness training can also improve visual attention reaction time by requiring the user to react quickly to visual stimuli. Training programs such as agility drills or reaction time exercises can improve visual attention and reaction time.
- Virtual and augmented reality: Virtual and augmented reality technologies can provide immersive environments that require the user to react quickly to visual stimuli. These technologies can improve visual attention and reaction time by simulating real-world scenarios that require quick reactions.

3.6 Telemedicine

Telemedicine, which involves the use of digital technology to provide remote medical care, has the potential to improve brain health in the digital era in several ways:

- Improved access to healthcare: Telemedicine allows individuals to receive medical care and support for brain health challenges from the comfort of their homes, regardless of their location. This can improve access to care for individuals who live in remote areas or have mobility challenges that make it difficult to access traditional healthcare services.

- Increased convenience: Telemedicine offers the convenience of receiving care without the need to travel to a healthcare facility, which can be especially beneficial for individuals with busy schedules or mobility challenges.
- Enhanced monitoring and management: Telemedicine technology can be used to remotely monitor and manage brain health conditions, such as dementia or Parkinson's disease. This allows for early detection of changes in symptoms and timely adjustments to treatment plans.
- Access to specialists: Telemedicine technology can provide access to specialists in the field of brain health, even if they are located in a different city or country. This can improve the quality of care for individuals with complex brain health conditions who require specialized expertise.
- Increased patient engagement: Telemedicine can increase patient engagement in their own healthcare by providing access to digital tools that support brain health, such as cognitive training apps or online therapy platforms.

Overall, telemedicine can be a valuable tool for improving brain health in the digital era by increasing access to care, enhancing convenience, and improving patient engagement and outcomes.

4 Discussions

In this chapter, the impact of digital media on the human brain was examined. While it was discovered that digital technologies and media can have both negative and positive effects, excessive use can be harmful and potentially damage the brain. However, if used in moderation, there can be benefits as well. The increasing use of digital media in the modern era has raised concerns about its impact on the human brain. This chapter highlights that while there are some benefits associated with the use of digital media, the negative consequences of excessive use cannot be ignored. Research has shown that excessive use of digital media can lead to addiction, depression, anxiety, decreased attention span, and decreased cognitive abilities. However, it is important to note that the impact of digital media on the brain is not entirely negative. In some cases, it can have positive effects, such as improving cognitive abilities and increasing access to information. For example, digital media can be used to promote brain health through the use of cognitive training apps, online therapy platforms, and telemedicine.

In order to improve the brain health, there are certain recommendations which may be taken into consideration depending upon the age-group, as listed in Table 2.

Following are some of the technical and standard recommendations to improve brain health in the digital era:

- Use technology responsibly: To minimize the negative effects of digital technology on brain health, it is important to use it responsibly. This includes setting limits on screen time, taking regular breaks, and using tools such as blue light filters to reduce the impact of digital devices on sleep.

Table 2 Recommendations for reducing effects of digital technologies [10]

Sr. No.	Age-group	Recommendations
1	Younger than 18 months	Should avoid screen time other than video calling
2	1824 months	Spend time in other high-quality programs
3	2–5 years	1 h/day supervised high quality programming
4	6 years and above	Place consistency in limits of using media

- Follow ergonomic guidelines: To reduce physical strain and injury associated with computer use, follow ergonomic guidelines such as positioning your computer screen at eye level, using an ergonomic keyboard and mouse, and taking regular breaks to stretch and move.
- Use assistive technology: If you have a condition that affects your ability to use digital devices, such as a visual impairment or a mobility impairment, consider using assistive technology such as screen readers or voice-activated assistants.
- Follow security best practices: To protect your brain health and personal information online, follow security best practices such as using strong passwords, avoiding public Wi-Fi networks, and being cautious about clicking on links or downloading attachments from unknown sources.
- Use evidence-based digital tools: When choosing digital tools to support brain health, look for evidence-based tools that have been scientifically validated to improve brain function, such as cognitive training apps or virtual reality therapy.
- Seek professional support: If you are experiencing mental health challenges or cognitive impairment, seek professional support from a qualified healthcare provider. Online therapy platforms and telehealth services can provide access to mental health support and cognitive assessments from the comfort of your home.

By following these technical and standard recommendations, you can help improve brain health in the digital era while minimizing the negative impacts of digital technology on your well-being. To reap the benefits of the digital era while minimizing the negative consequences, it is important to use digital media in moderation. The chapter provides age group-wise recommendations to promote responsible use of digital media. For children and teenagers, it is recommended to limit screen time, prioritize physical activity and social interaction, and promote healthy sleep habits. For adults, it is recommended to limit screen time before bed, take breaks from digital media, and engage in activities that promote brain health, such as exercise, reading, and meditation.

5 Conclusions

In conclusion, the impact of digital media on brain health is complex and multifaceted. While it can have both positive and negative consequences, responsible use and moderation are key to promoting brain health in the digital era. The recommendations provided in this chapter can serve as a guide for individuals to make informed decisions about their use of digital media and promote healthy brain function.Conflicts of InterestNo author has any potential conflicts of interest.

References

1. American Academy of Pediatrics. Committee on public education, "American Academy of Pediatrics: children, adolescents, and television,". Pediatrics. 2001;107:423–6.
2. Inergency. Determinants of mental health among youths and adolescents in the digital era: Roles of cyber and traditional bullying, violence, loneliness, and environment factors. https://inergency.com/determinants-of-mental-health-among-youths-and-adolescents-in-the-digital-era-roles-of-cyber-and-traditional-bullying-violence-loneliness-and-environment-factors/.
3. Cheng C, Li AY. Internet addiction prevalence and quality of (real) life: a meta-analysis of 31 nations across seven world regions. Cyberpsychol Behav Soc Netw. 2014;17(12):755–60.
4. Kirsh SJ, Mounts JWR. Violent video game play impacts facial emotion recognition. Aggress Behav. 2007;33(4):353–8.
5. OECD. Childhood in digital age. 2019. http://www.oecd-ilibrary.org/sites/2d4352c2-en/index.html?itemId=/content/component/2d4352c2-en#Figureure-d1e494. Accessed 15 Jan 2023.
6. Negative Effects of Technology. Mobicip Blog. https://www.mobicip.com/blog/negative-effects-of-technology. Accessed 12 Jan 2023.
7. Nicholson NR. A review of social isolation: an important but underassessed condition in older adults. J Prim Prev. 2012;33(2–3):137–52.
8. Dong G, Li H, Potenza MN. Short-term internet-search training is associated with increased fractional anisotropy in the superior longitudinal fasciculus in the parietal lobe. Front Neurosci. 2017;11:372. https://doi.org/10.3389/fnins.2017.00372.
9. These are the best apps to keep your brain active. Healthline, 2022. https://www.healthline.com/health/mental-health/apps-to-keep-brain-busy#fa-qs. Accessed 14 Jan 2023.
10. Singh P, Das J, Das ZJ. Effect of digital technology on our brain health. IJAR. 2022;8(2):380–4.

Brain Health in the Digital Era

Syed Sarosh Mahdi, Shilpa Gunjal, Muneer Gohar Babar, Sakina Syeda, and Niekla Survia Andiesta

Abstract *Introduction:* Digital technologies have completely transformed the way humans work, communicate, and socialize over the last three decades. Human beings are now completely dependent on their digital devices to interact with the world. That transformation has not come without challenges. Digital technologies have impacted the mental well-being of humans like no other technology before it has done.

Methodology: The book chapter examined the complex relationship between the digital world and how it is impacting the mental well-being of individuals. The preceding chapters present both pros and cons of the digital era with regard to brain health as well as policy recommendations.

Conclusion: Digital technologies have the potential to provide solutions to the most pressing questions humanity is facing today. The perfect balance will require moderation and oversight when interacting with the digital world.

Keywords Brain health · Digital era · Mental health · Social media · Technology · Internet · Digital hygiene

1 Introduction

The human brain is complex and acts as the control center to the entire nervous system which allows the entire body to function effectively at different levels. These functions range from control of body movements to maintenance of cognitive, mental, and emotional functions which are responsible for our normal social well-being

S. S. Mahdi (✉) · S. Gunjal · M. G. Babar · N. S. Andiesta
Division of Clinical Oral Health Sciences, School of Dentistry, International Medical University, Kuala Lumpur, Malaysia
e-mail: syedsarosh.mahdi@unicam.it

S. Syeda
Department of Sociology, University of North Texas, Denton, TX, USA

G. Battineni et al. (eds.), *Computational Methods in Psychiatry*,
https://doi.org/10.1007/978-981-99-6637-0_7

[1]. The American Heart Association/American Stroke Association (AHA/ASA) defines brain health as the "average performance levels among all people at that age who are free of known brain or other organ system diseases in terms of decline from function levels, or as adequacy to perform all activities that the individual wishes to undertake" [2].

Maintaining sound health of the brain is key for a sound well-being. However, modern lifestyle comes with a lot of significant and persistent cognitive demands. This somehow leads to increased mental illness and less well-being. The human prefrontal cortex manages these demands, usually without difficulty. When the demands become chronic and stressful, the prefrontal cortex struggles and may fail. The result is a broadened vulnerability to mental disorders for all citizens of modernity [3]. Numerous factors that affect the health of our brain are reduced attention, impaired emotional and social intelligence, technology addiction, social isolation, sleep disturbance, and adverse impact on cognitive and brain development [4]. Physical damage to the brain through trauma, tumors, and inflammatory conditions can cause certain neurological disorders. Functional impairments can be the features associated with neurodegenerative diseases (Parkinson's disease, Alzheimer's disease, and dementia) or the mental disorders (schizophrenia, alcoholism, or drug abuse). The latest factor, but not the least, that is now considered to play a key role in the maintenance of mental health is the association of the present generation with digital technology.

Digital technology has transformed the way people live for the past two to three decades. Digital technology has influenced people of all ages. Majority of adults use the internet daily with one in four adults being online all the time [5]. This has resulted in a great impact on the way humanity functions, especially the way they communicate, form relationships, and obtain the information they need. All age group people have now able to access vast online information available and are able to connect with others. This technology helps us to generate, store, and process enormous amounts of information and interact with each other rapidly and efficiently [4].

Digital technologies are believed to have many good factors and can affect mental health in a better way. The common digital tasks studied online are internet browsing, searching, gaming and educational apps. Online searching may play a role in neural exercise as it brings about stimulating exercise to the brain and may bring about myelination of the brain tissue. Such neural training associated with sound health exercises can depict lower pre-cortical metabolism, which can be interpreted as greater cognitive ability [4]. At the same time, studies have shown that it may bring about cognitive training to the brain and aids in overall development, multitasking skills, enhanced memory, and improved motor skill [6]. However, specific programs, videogames, and other online tools may provide mental exercises that activate neural circuitry, improve cognitive functioning, reduce anxiety, increase restful sleep, and offer other brain-health benefits. Future research needs to elucidate underlying mechanisms and causal relationships between technology use and brain health, with a focus on both the positive and negative impact of digital technology use.

However, today's adolescents have grown up in the digital era. More than any generation before, their life has been shaped by the constant availability of online contents and services, the 24/7 possibility to reach and be reached by others, and the easy access to gratifying and personalized contents and functionalities on screen-based devices. Concerns have been raised in the adolescent population about the extensive dissemination of screen-based devices which includes smartphones, laptops, tablets on the clinical and psychological effects of overuse of screen time [7]. Numerous research has studied the negative effects of the utilization of technology. Screen time has shown to have some relation with the reduced attention and are linked with disorders like attention deficit hyperactivity disorders (ADHD). This may also lead to less face-to-face communication with impaired intelligence and differed cognitive development. This may also bring about changes like social isolation and impaired sleep disorders [6].

Numerous reports have clearly identified the extensive uses of social media like Facebook, Twitter, Snapchat, and Instagram by the young population. The association between the usage of social media and social isolation is being established in few studies [8, 9]. The increased screen time has also been closely associated with the impaired cognitive development like poorer language development, especially in children [10]. So, the World Health Organization (WHO) have issued a concern, recommending that children younger than 5 years old should spend no more than 1 h in front of a screen on any day [11]. A systematic review has reported relationship between media use and ADHD-related behaviors in children and adolescents [12]. Adolescents with more screen time were associated with overt improper and disturbed sleep [13]. Due to these findings, neuroscientists have started focusing their attention on how digital technology may be changing our brains and behavior.

The information age as they call it has been extremely exciting and beneficial for mankind. Ever since the internet came into existence humanity has seen almost every aspect of life being influenced by the technologies associated with information technology and the internet [14]. Like with all previous technologies, there have been both benefits and harms associated with digital technologies and the internet. While the benefits mostly outweigh the harmful effects, the digital age hasn't been without its cons and vices. Throughout this century, we have seen the proliferation of digital technologies with a relentless speed. The creation of the smartphone and its ubiquitous presence has massively exposed people of all ages to digital technologies like never before in the history of humanity [15]. It is almost impossible not to feel the impact of digital technologies and they are present in almost household.

Technological advances usually outpace our understanding of how they affect humanity both at the physical and mental level, that is also true for all technologies associated with the digital era. Universal access to the internet through smartphones has also led to the rise of social media giants like Facebook, Snapchat, Twitter, Instagram, and many others. What began as a way communicate with friends, family, and acquaintances virtually and keep humans connected has led to the rise of criminal activity, cyber stalking, harassment, impersonations, financial fraud, suicides, and a plethora of complex problems for people of all ages but particularly for vulnerable populations like women and children [16]. The mental health crisis is exacerbated by the 24/7 presence of social media in our lives and the societal pressure it creates on ordinary and gullible humans. Influencer culture has resulted in extremely fake personas being marketed as "achievable" by ordinary people. This is putting pressure, especially on immature minds like teenagers.

The coming years will present even greater challenges for mental health due to the rapid advancements in the field of artificial intelligence and machine learning. Social media platforms will get better at understanding human minds and target aspects of our personalities that trigger a favorable response for the platform (like spending more time on a specific platform, buying products, and engaging in news articles), etc. All this will be achieved more effectively as the algorithm becomes stronger through AI, predictive modeling, and machine learning [17]. Their understanding of each of us will be more complete as we spend more and more time on digital platforms. The "FOMO" fear of missing out will get even more frenzied, particularly for teenager and younger adults. This will lead to a complex web of social, economic, and mental health issues. The tech giants have shown that they have the money, power, and political connections to control the narrative on digital technologies and also thwart or misdirect regulations and legislation. The next chapters will highlight how digital technologies are impacting various facets of human lives and their possible solutions. The preceding chapters will discuss the implication on digital era on various segments of society.

2 Digital Era and Mental Health of Children

Children are most vulnerable to the vagaries and complexities of the digital age. The child's mind is not developed enough to understand the dangers and hazards of social media [18]. Children are generally forbidden by social media apps from joining but there is a very simple way around this issue. They can simply certify that they were over 18 and no more questions are asked. Digital technologies also impact children, as children also spend a lot of time online. Excessive use of digital technologies can negatively impact a children mental health. It can lead to sleep disturbances, low attention span, and poor quality of sleep. Some studies suggest excessive team can also lead to myopia. Children who spend excessive time online do so at the expense of physical activities which can lead to obesity as well as poor communication skills due to lack of traditional face-to-face interactions [19].

2.1 *Digital Era and Issues Related to Security, Privacy, and Mental Health of Teenagers*

Teenagers represent perhaps the most avid users of social media platform. A significant proportion of teenage population worldwide is hooked to various social media platforms and spends a considerable amount of time on online platforms. Teenagers primarily use social media platforms to communicate and socialize. Teenage brain like the brains of children, but not to that extent, is still evolving and growing, teenagers suffer from depression, anxiety, and issues related to negative self-image more than the adult population [20]. Social media amplifies and promotes the seeking of social status, unrealistic goals, shortcuts, hedonistic lifestyle, and detachment from reality. The constant social media stream puts the teenage mind in a state of neurosis and hence detrimental to mental health. Teenagers are also prone to blackmailing, revenge porn, grooming, and other forms of abuse online. Monitoring of teenager's social media use by parents and caregivers is highly recommended [21].

Excessive use of social media can also have a detrimental effect on the development of the brain as it changes the brain's reward system, which in turn can make it difficult for teenage girls and boys to regulate and control their impulses. Excessive use can also result in low self-esteem, addiction, cyberbullying, and poor emotional control. Social media use can also hamper the development of communication skills as it doesn't involve face-to-face communication, hence impeding the development of communication skills and empathy [22].

2.2 *Cyberstalking and Female Mental Health*

Cyberstalking, the practice of continually harassing, threatening, or monitoring someone else online or through social media, can have detrimental repercussions on a person's mental and physical health, especially in women. Cyberstalking, according to research, can result in emotions such as dread, worry, and depression as well as a loss of privacy and control over one's personal information. This may result in the victim having trouble sleeping, having their appetites shift, and feeling uneasy all around. Additionally, the ongoing surveillance and harassment might cause emotions of helplessness and loneliness [23].

Cyberstalking can have detrimental effects on one's physical health. Cyberstalking victims' immune systems may become compromised because of the ongoing stress and anxiety it causes, making them more vulnerable to sickness. High blood pressure, palpitations, and headaches are additional effects of stress. Additionally, PTSD (post-traumatic stress disorder) symptoms like flashbacks, nightmares, and avoidance behaviors can develop as a result of cyberstalking. This may negatively affect one's mental health over time and make it challenging to manage daily life [24].

It's vital to remember that cyberstalking is illegal, and victims should contact the police as well as their friends, family, and mental health experts for support. The effects of cyberstalking can be managed and victims' sense of control over their life can be regained with the aid of support groups and counseling. Online harassment can cause significant harm to mental and emotional health of the victim and anonymity accorded by the internet empowers the abusers who feels he has the license to harm the victim.

It is important to understand that digital technologies are still evolving and there is a need to monitor their effect on the mental well-being of humanity. Moderation and supervision are the key when it comes to use of these technologies. States should also come up with legislation protecting the health and well-being of their citizens. The well-being of humans should be above all considerations including the interest of large tech firms and social media giants.

2.3 Revenge Porn and Brain Health

Revenge porn, or the release of sexually explicit photographs or material of someone without their knowledge, can have severe psychological and emotional repercussions, including post-traumatic stress disorder (PTSD), anxiety, sadness for the distressed individual (PTSD) [25, 26]. It can also lead to social isolation and the inability to build or maintain connections. There is no research on the direct effects of revenge porn on brain health, but it is plausible that the psychological and emotional pain induced by revenge porn can indirectly impair brain function.

3 Impact of Videogames on Brain Health

The effects of video games on cognitive function are still being investigated, and so far, the results have been contradictory. Cognitive abilities like focus, memory, and the ability to solve problems may all benefit from time spent playing video games, according to some research. Other research has shown that playing video games for long periods of time can have detrimental impacts on the brain, including addiction, diminished social connections, and a loss of gray matter in key regions of the brain [27].

It's worth noting that different themed games, differing amounts of time spent playing, different personality types of different age-groups, and with different health histories might all have varying effects on the brain. Furthermore, studies have shown that moderate amount of gaming can have positive impacts on the brain, including elevating mood, decreasing stress and anxiety, and fostering creativity [28]. Although there is still a lack of a complete understanding about the effects of video games on brain health and research is still ongoing, it is generally accepted that moderation is the key and that excessive video game play should be avoided.

3.1 *Virtual Reality and Brain Health*

Virtual reality (VR) is yet another ancillary of the myriad of digital technologies that have mushroomed in the recent past, through VR, users interact with a simulated three-dimensional environment by wearing a headset that has a display and several sensors. Many studies have been published to examine the effects of virtual reality on the human brain, but the results have been inconclusive, thus far [29].

Research has shown that virtual reality can help with things like memory retention and focus, as well as conditions like anxiety, PTSD, and phobias. People with mental health issues or physical ailments like pain have benefited from VR treatment, which has been used to alter their reactions to various stimuli and alleviate symptoms like phantom limb discomfort [30].

Headaches, eye strain, and motion sickness have all been linked to too much time spent in virtual space, according to other research. As VR technology is in such a nascent stage, more research over extended periods of time is required to fully understand the potential negative/positive effects of VR on long-term brain health. Like other digital technologies, the impact of VR on different people is expected to be variable. Variables such as age, gender, personality types, and cultural ethos will all likely impact how VR impacts a particular individual.

It's important to remember that VR is still in its infancy, so more research is required before humanity can completely grasp the effects it has on brain health and determine how best to apply the technology therapeutically.

3.2 *Use of Digital Technologies for Augmenting and Supporting Mental Health*

Digital technologies like all technologies can play a very constructive role in brain health, diagnosis of mental health, treatment modalities, and as an auxiliary to other treatments. Many neurodegenerative diseases lead to lifetime debilitation for those inflicted by these diseases. Digital technologies can aid these patients in improving their quality of life [31].

Brain–computer interface (BCI) technology can assist those suffering from any form of paralysis like (locked in syndrome, spinal cord injury, brainstem stroke, muscular dystrophy, and amyotrophic lateral sclerosis). Patients suffering from these conditions usually lack ability to walk, talk, write, and communicate due to loss of fine motor function but their thinking capabilities are usually fully intact. Brain interface technology has shown promise in making lives of such patients better, as it could potentially allow such patients to communicate with the outside world, surf the web, send email, and communicate their thoughts to their loved ones through these technologies [32, 33].

BCI technology focuses on enhancing the quality of life for people with severe motor disabilities through the development of gadgets that aid in daily activities.

This comprises instruments for communication through direct brain-device connections, as well as rehabilitation aids and the control of prosthetics, computers, and other gadgets. Moreover, BCIs exhibit promise in gaming, teaching, and training.

3.3 Telemedicine Based Technologies to Improve Mental Health-

We have seen a proliferation of telemedicine-based technologies in recent years, particularly after the COVID-19 pandemic. Telemedicine is the use of information technology to improve health outcomes across all healthcare domains. The technology uses information technology and internet-based technology transfer mediums to transmit information from the physician's side from the comfort of his home. It is used in situations where the medical personnel are not readily available, such as remote locations like ships in international waters, remote and rural areas, and also in situations where the patient has very limited mobility [33].

Over the years, telemedicine-based services have been used to improve the mental health outcomes of patients. Telemedicine-based interventions were key to addressing mental health needs to patient during the COVID-19 pandemic. COVID-19 pandemic caused a lot of anxiety and fear among people worldwide, and we saw an increase of general anxiety and PTSD due to fear of the unknown and contagion during the acute phase of the pandemic [34].

Telemedicine-based technologies can be very useful to help vulnerable segments of the population to get mental health even when they are not in the presence of a trained mental health professional or a psychologist. Telemedicine is now ubiquitous technology that can reach anywhere in the globe, no matter how remote the location is, the only prerequisite is the presence of an internet connection on both ends. Telemedicine can also help people with mental health issues, addictions, and those facing abuse of any sort to seek professional help from the comfort of their own house. Telemedicine combines the use case of traditional medicine with latest advancements in information technology to provide tailor made solutions for all forms of health services. It can be used to provide one-on-one counseling to those seeking advice and consultation for various mental health issues [35].

Millions of people around the world are suffering from addictions of various forms including addition from hardcore drugs like cocaine, heroin, and other forms of highly dangerous psychoactive drugs. Many of these drug addicts don't seek medical attention due to stigma, financial issues, and other societal constraints. Telemedicine-based services could provide the perfect platform for those afflicted by addictions to remain anonymous, in the comfort of their homes and seek medical advice and counseling. Telemedicine could offer out of the box solutions in terms of drug rehabilitation and integration of former drug addicts back in the society. Similarly, women and men suffering violence, bullying or domestic violence of any form can also use telemedicine-based digital services to talk to a trained mental health professional who can council them and provide best possible solutions to their mental health needs.

Telemedicine-based technologies can also supplement mental health needs to children who have suffered child abuse, bullying or any other form of abuse resulting in depression, anxiety, and PTSD. Children are also often very averse to seeking help, particularly after getting abused. Telemedicine provides the opportunity for such children to receive face-to-face therapy albeit digitally from the comfort of their homes. This could be used to build trust with the mental health professional providing therapy and counseling, setting the stage for one-to-one traditional therapy sessions later [36].

People suffering from learning disorders like autism and other autism spectrum disorders can also benefit from the use of digital technologies and learning aids. The COVID-19 pandemic hit people with disabilities differently than most other groups. People suffering from learning disorders were already living a very secluded life and the pandemic only exacerbated the problem .

4 Screen Time and Mental Health

The ubiquitous presence of smart phones has upended almost every aspect of human society. Excessive screen time can cause problems related to attention deficit disorder and sleep disorder. Children aged 2–5 should ideally be allowed no more than 1 h per day, 6 years, and older 2 h per day. It is important that parents should control screen time and not allow children unfiltered screen time. Excessive screen time can also lead to communication problem in growing age children. Attention deficit syndrome can lead to learning disabilities that can cause problems even in adulthood. Children with attention deficit disorder will have problems later in life in academics, work life, and personal life. That is why it is important to create a balanced relationship with technology. Parents should encourage digital hygiene and open discussion regarding the use of digital technologies with children. Parents should monitor the content their children are consuming online and try to avoid their exposure to extreme and harmful content. Parents should also develop a trusting relationship with their children where children are willing to discuss their problems with ease [37]. Parents should also create rules in consultation with their children about screen time and what content they are allowed to consume. Increased screen times is linked depression and anxiety in both children and adults. The internet also has great potential for children as there is very good content available online which fosters growth, creativity, and self-expression. Digital technologies for children should be always used with caution and under parental guidance [38].

4.1 *Suicide and Digital Technologies*

There is evidence to suggest that internet and related digital technologies have led to increase in suicides due to cyber bullying, harassment, and low self-esteem. The pressure to present the ideal image forces young adults into going to extremes to present that ideal (which doesn't exist in the real world), when those ideals are shattered it can put the individual at risk of suicide, depression, and suicidal thoughts [39]. Negative feedback on the internet can lead to low self-esteem, feelings of helplessness, and sense of hopelessness, which in turn can turn into a cocktail of negative emotions triggering suicidal thoughts. Individuals should seek support when feeling these emotions. Organizations and Governments have a responsibility of preventing suicides through support networks and legislations [40].

4.2 *Radicalization in the Digital Era*

Internet is an unregulated space hence it can encourage negative and harmful behaviors such as extremist propaganda, criminal behavior, anti-social activities, and radicalization [41]. Extremist propaganda has the potential to turn young minds into radicalized bots willing to do bidding of any extremist outfit based on false or misguided ideals. Extremist propaganda can be racist, political, or religious. Conspiracy theories have been extremely disruptive and polarized societies [42].The COVID-19 pandemic was also turned into a fertile ground by conspiracy theorist who tried to cash on a natural calamity and turned uncertainty into a profitable business by churning out conspiracies about the origins of COVID-19 and even created doubts about the vaccine. The pandemic saw the world divided once again due to ridiculous conspiracy theories which resulted in confusion, fear, and paranoia. Exposure to conspiracy theories also resulted in many declining the COVID-19 vaccine resulting in increased mortality and morbidity. The recent past we have seen how the Islamic state of Iraq and Syria exploited the internet to recruit young people into their violent organization by radicalization vulnerable teenagers and youngsters into an ideal that only leads to death and destruction. The ISIS devised a very methodological online campaign which helped it recruit thousands of vulnerable and disgruntled individuals to its violent platform [43]. It is important to regulate the internet and what viewers can watch online. Political and religious extremist propaganda can result in negative health outcomes. Propaganda can only result in polarization,paranoia, and loneliness. People indoctrinated online who hold extreme political and religious views can feel isolated and falsely believe that their views are misunderstood. Government and private organization must enable an environment that encourages open debates but not conspiracy theories. Material that is openly false/fake should be labeled as such, or better removed entirely from the internet. Religious and political indoctrination can have real life consequences like the rise of the Nazi party and the ISIS. These are sensitive issues and the world .

4.3 Family Functioning and Digital Era

Digital era has also had an impact on the personal lives of all individuals. Social media and the internet have led to new challenges with regard to privacy, trust, and communication. The widespread presence of 24/7 communication has led to increase in illicit affairs leading to marital issues and even divorces. The easy availability, deniability, and urge to engage in online affairs can erode trust and boding in relationships [38].

However, there are also positive interpersonal effects of digital technologies. The elderly can be in touch with their offspring's even when they are not in the vicinity. Communication software with video calling capabilities can create a sense of proximity even when families are apart due to various reasons. Social media has also facilitated long-distance relationships which can often transform into lifelong bonds of friends and partnerships [44]. People with shy demeanor who tend avoid real-life encounters with people of the opposite sex can also benefit greatly from the detachment and obscurity offered by the internet in seeking partnerships, friendship, and romance. Online dating has several pros for those trying to seek lifelong healthy relationships without putting themselves out there in the real world for judgment. People suffering from low self-esteem and confidence can also benefit from online dating as it gives them an opportunity to present themselves in a positive light [37].

5 Impact of Remote Working During COVID-19 on Mental Health

COVID-19 pandemic has changed the way we work. The terms remote working and work from home became common place during the pandemic as the world reimagined work during the pandemic. The traditional workplace was disrupted as it was no longer possible for a large group of people to work together in a confined space. That helped foster a new culture of remote working through applications like Zoom and Microsoft teams. On the positive side, work from home can offer flexibility, work-life balance, and can reduce commute time, which in turn help improve mental well-being, but on the contrary, it can also cause feelings of isolation, lack of boundaries between work and personal life, and decrease opportunities for face-to-face interactions and connections with others,which can especially effect those who struggle with such interactive workspaces [45]. It is important for individuals and companies to create boundaries while working from home and creating a routine. Work-life balance should be prioritized even while working from home [46].

6 Conclusion

Digital age has been very challenging for the mental health of individuals across the world. The pandemic has only exacerbated these concerns. Digital technologies have been made all aspects of life easier and more accessible but it also come with certain caveats. The need to strike balance between digital life and mental health has never been greater as these technologies are ubiquitous. Moderation remains the key and oversight is required when these technologies are being used by minors. Government legislation is also required to protect the digital rights of citizens.

References

1. Wang Y, Pan Y, Li H. What is brain health and why is it important? BMJ. 2020;9(371):m3683.
2. Gorelick PB, Furie KL, Iadecola C, Smith EE, Waddy SP, Lloyd-Jones DM, Bae HJ, Bauman MA, Dichgans M, Duncan PW, Girgus M, Howard VJ, Lazar RM, Seshadri S, Testai FD, van Gaal S, Yaffe K, Wasiak H, Zerna C; American Heart Association/American Stroke Association. Defining optimal brain health in adults: a presidential advisory from the American Heart Association/American Stroke Association. Stroke 2017 ;48(10): e284-e303.
3. https://www.psychologytoday.com/us/blog/modern-world-modern-mind/202205/how-the-brain-handles-modern-life.
4. Small GW, Lee J, Kaufman A, Jalil J, Siddarth P, Gaddipati H, Moody TD, Bookheimer SY. Brain health consequences of digital technology use. Dialogues Clin Neurosci. 2020;22(2):179–87.
5. Firth J, Torous J, Stubbs B, Firth JA, Steiner GZ, Smith L, Alvarez-Jimenez M, Gleeson J, Vancampfort D, Armitage CJ, Sarris J. The "online brain": how the Internet may be changing our cognition. World Psychiatry 2019 ;18(2):119–129.
6. Singh P, Das J, Das ZJ. Effect of digital technology on our brain health. Int J Appl Res. 2022;8(2):380–4.
7. Domingues-Montanari S. Clinical and psychological effects of excessive screen time on children. J Paediatr Child Health. 2017;53:333–8.
8. Nicholson NR. A review of social isolation: an important but underassessed condition in older adults. J Prim Prev. 2012;33(2–3):137–52.
9. Primack BA, Shensa A, Sidani JE, et al. Social media use and perceived social isolation among young adults in the U.S. Am J Prev Med. 2017;53(1):1–8.
10. Horowitz-Kraus T, Hutton JS. Brain connectivity in children is increased by the time they spend reading books and decreased by the length of exposure to screen-based media. Acta Paediatr. 2018;107(4):685–93.
11. https://www.medicalnewstoday.com/articles/325461. Accessed 19 Jan 2023.
12. Nikkelen SW, Valkenburg PM, Huizinga M, Bushman BJ. Media use and ADHD-related behaviors in children and adolescents: a meta-analysis. Dev Psychol. 2014;50(9):2228–41.
13. Christensen MA, Bettencourt L, Kaye L, et al. Direct measurements of smartphone screen-time: relationships with demographics and sleep. PLoS One. 2016;11(11):e0165331.
14. Nemec PB, Chan S. Behavioral health workforce development challenges in the digital health era. Psychiatr Rehabil J. 2017;40:339–41.
15. Brand M, Young KS, Laier C. Prefrontal control and internet addiction: a theoretical model and review of neuropsychological and neuroimaging findings. Front Hum Neurosci. 2014;8:375.
16. Crone EA, Konijn EA. Media use and brain development during adolescence. Nat Commun. 2018;9:588. https://doi.org/10.1038/s41467-018-03126-x.

17. Harris B, Regan T, Schueler J, Fields SA. Problematic mobile phone and smartphone use scales: a systematic review. Front Psychol. 2020;11:672. https://doi.org/10.3389/fpsyg.2020.0067.
18. Livingstone S, et al. Children's online risks and opportunities: comparative findings from EU kids online and net children go Mobile. London School of Economics; 2014.
19. Koo C, et al. Internet-addicted kids and south Korean government efforts: boot-camp case. Cyberpsychol Behav Soc Netw. 2011;14(6):391–4. https://doi.org/10.1089/cyber.2009.0331.
20. Caballero A, Granberg R, Tseng KY. Mechanisms contributing to prefrontal cortex maturation during adolescence. Neurosci Biobehav Rev. 2016;70:4–12. https://doi.org/10.1016/j.neubiorev.2016.05.013.
21. Casey BJ, Caudle K. The teenage brain: self control. Curr Dir Psychol Sci. 2013;22:82–7. https://doi.org/10.1177/0963721413480170.
22. Burnett S, Sebastian C, Cohen KK, Blakemore S-J. The social brain in adolescence: evidence from functional magnetic resonance imaging and behavioural studies. Neurosci Biobehav Rev. 2011;35:1654–64.
23. Bottino S, et al. Cyberbullying and adolescent mental health: systematic review. Cadernos de Saúde Pública. 2015;31:463–75.
24. Camerini A-L, Marciano L, Carrara A, Schulz PJ. Cyberbullying perpetration and victimization among children and adolescents: a systematic review of longitudinal studies. Telematics Inform. 2020b;49:101362.
25. Takahashi K, Huang Y, Feng Y, Lee J, Yao L. The influence of exposure to online revenge porn on mental health: a cross-sectional study. J Affect Disord. 2021;279:31–7.
26. Thompson ML, Stough C, Singh MK. The impact of revenge porn on mental health and Well-being: a review. Trauma Violence Abuse. 2019;20(4):447–57.
27. Ferguson CJ. The good, the bad, and the ugly: a meta-analytic review of positive and negative effects of violent video games. Psychol Bull. 2007;133(4):551–73.
28. Kuss DJ, Griffiths MD. Internet gaming addiction: a systematic review of epidemiological research for the last decade. Curr Pharm Des. 2012;18(32):52438–52.
29. Slater M, Sanchez-Vives MV. Enhancing our lives with immersive virtual reality. Front Neurosci. 2016;10:191.
30. Rizzo AA, Kim GJ, Lafleur MF, Difede J. A review of virtual reality exposure therapy for post-traumatic stress disorder. Depress Anxiety. 2014;31(12):970–82.
31. Lu CB, Hughes JN, Fan YY, Liang KY, Luo JL, Zhang XH, Li C, Fang X, Sun X, Ma Y. Digital interventions for mental health care. Lancet Psychiatry. 2017;4(10):765–74.
32. Christensen H, Baumeister H, Ritterband LM, Andrews G. Internet-based interventions for depression. Cochrane Database Syst Rev. 2010;7:CD008096.
33. Cuijpers P, Cristea IA, Karyotaki E, Reijnders M, Huibers MJ. The effects of guided self-help for depression and anxiety disorders: a meta-analysis. Behav Res Ther. 2016;86:17–26.
34. Knaevelsrud C, Maercker A. Internet-based treatment for PTSD: a systematic review. Depress Anxiety. 2007;24(3):169–80.
35. Oladeji BD, Ola BA, Adebayo ET, Adejumo PO, Adekeye OA. Telepsychiatry for mental health care delivery in low- and middle-income countries: a scoping review. BMC Psychiatry. 2019;19(1):278.
36. Hickie IB, Naismith SL, Scott EM, Guastella AJ, Sherring N, Hermens DF. A review of the impact of telepsychiatry on the quality and access of mental health care services. Aust N Z J Psychiatry. 2015;49(12):1069–79.
37. Twenge JM, Campbell WK. Increases in depressive symptoms, sleep disruption, and substance use among U.S. adolescents after 2012 and links to screen time during the COVID-19 pandemic. JAMA Netw Open. 2020;3(11):e2025756.
38. Rosen LD, Carrier LM, Cheever NA. Does the internet increase, decrease, or supplement social capital? Social networks, participation, and community commitment. Am Behav Sci. 2013;57(10):1369–91.
39. Price M, Bailey A, Batterham P, Niehaus M, Weare K. Understanding the role of social media in suicide prevention: a qualitative investigation. J Med Internet Res. 2015;17(12):e289.

40. Christofides N, Goldner EM, Deans D, Darlington G. Social media and suicide: a critical review of the literature. J Med Internet Res. 2016;18(10):e263.
41. Brossard D, Scheufele DA. Science, new media, and the public. Science. 2013;340(6128):40–1.
42. López-Rodríguez C, Boix A. The use of online media in political campaigns: a review of the literature. Int J Electron Gov Res. 2015;11(2):1–22.
43. Naji SA, Zaidi Z, Bibi Y. Understanding religious extremism and terrorism: a review of the literature. J Relig Health. 2021;60(2):487–500.
44. Lin YC, Shih TC. Family conflict and family cohesion: the impact of family Members' internet use and dependence. J Child Adolesc Behav. 2014;2(5)
45. Glaser J, Dolan P, Huang R, Toussaint J, Backonja M, Covinsky K. Remote work during the COVID-19 pandemic: mental health effects. Lancet Psychiatry. 2021;8(2):159–60.
46. Haase A, Eckardt J, Göritz AS. The impact of the COVID-19 pandemic on mental health and Well-being: a rapid systematic review. Int J Environ Res Public Health. 2020;17(22)

Work from Home and its Impact on Lifestyle of Humanoid in the Context of COVID-19

Y. Sarada Devi, A. Vijayasankar, and D. Venkatarao

Abstract The COVID-19 epidemic has shaped the major disturbance of all living in the history, disturbing billions, in more than 200 countries. Staying home because of lockdown were put into practice as the desirable act to reduce the affect and have a control over the spread of the disease. The COVID-19 epidemic brought the concept of working from home (WFH), the novel method of work for personnel. Many had to shift, abruptly, for the first time to distant work and without any groundwork. Accepting this flexibility in work was a deliberate option that needed time, groundwork, and getting adapted to efficiently support output for ensuring balance in life and work. COVID-19, though, the outburst has considerably required most administrations to accept this style of work. Few studies described pros and cons of remote work. The effects of WFH were sightseen. Other side of coin speaks the necessity to inspect how work from home, as a "innovative method" has exaggerated the sustainability and and efficiency of staff by stating precise circumstances in work during the COVID-19. The purpose of this work is to explore the impact of WFH from the survey done considering stress, adaptability to work environment, work satisfaction, time management, health, well-being, and anxiety with data collected from different individuals under different age groups both male and female. The results examined the work from home experience among the individuals had both positive and negative influence, respectively, on workflow.

Keywords COVID-19 · Work from home · Work efficiency · Work-life balance

Y. S. Devi (✉) · A. Vijayasankar · D. Venkatarao
V R Siddhartha Engineering College, Vijayawada, Andhra Pradesh, India
e-mail: vijayasankar.anumala@vrsiddhartha.ac.in

G. Battineni et al. (eds.), *Computational Methods in Psychiatry*,
https://doi.org/10.1007/978-981-99-6637-0_8

1 Introduction

The current quick universal spread of a new COVID-19 virus contamination introduced an economic recession globally. A total lockdown was instructed by the government announcing to the complete shutdown of all activities that are not essential which crested inconvenience to many working atmospheres. Serious challenges arouse in traditional working atmospheres. Long-term sequences also started similar to crisis in 2008 which had a great impact on the global economy. Education and health-care were the areas which were impacted pronouncedly along with industries. A flexible working atmosphere was adopted by few companies and industries to decrease the spread of virus taking into consideration the health of people. Throughout the COVID-19 disaster, people used online as well as digital businesses and work from home (WFH). This crisis also changed the patterns of work and the concept of working from home changed rapidly. The corresponding side-effects also arouse along with the start of WFH as explained by authors in [1].

WFH required people to practise novel online skills with practical skills in communication work. Along with this, working at home also has a need for confidentiality of data which raises a necessity to get adapted to a different environment. Secondly, person from home, will have a shortage of direct contact with contemporaries, and when difficulties rise at workplace, it was problematic to resolve rapidly online. Psychological pressure and nervousness were increased in spite of online system communication. In count, work from home leads to the livelihood of space of family members. Care of the children, tasks of the family, household work were few of the difficulties faced by the people who work from home which created a struggle amid work and family. The inequity amid family and work created a negative impact on job efficiency that should be seriously considered by the HR experts to compensate the effect.

Even, the culture of the firm might be overlooked by the employees when the work style of office is once changed. Meanwhile employed from household only can connect and toil virtually, individuals may incline towards ignoring the part of office culture. The training detected that WFH had both pros and cons affecting various throughout pandemic, like struggles in personal, being unable to accustom to communicate, and absence of care from colleagues. Special office skills are to be learnt by the employees who worked from home. WFH made individuals sense remote and lead to emotional pressure. Throughout the pandemic, employees repeatedly faced struggle amid taking care for their relations and work. Hence, this study consolidates the impact of work from home based on the above aspects considered.

2 Literature Survey

2.1 Work from Home

WFH has always been deliberated during pandemic for the reason that of distorting limits of not being absent at work about personal, work and non-work, and social significances, the hazards and aids of flexible hours of work. According to Kniffin et al., [2] there were few rewards of work from home, like, planning for time, to take attention on family, the choice to effort for the most imaginative time, and opportunity to work from home in situation of illness. Experiential trainings create numerous consequences of WFH, like performance of job, satisfaction in job, smaller income intents, and condensed levels of pressure as said by Moretti et al. [3]. Work from home was accepted out by numerous public and private parts to work without harm by adjusting the concepts of WFH.

According to Milasi et al. [4] and Hunter et al. [5], WFH is a two-edged weapon that has a varied result on well-being, work-lifetime equilibrium and fulfilment. Home-based work increases job satisfaction. Numerous academics have discussed how working remotely or from home might affect work-life balance both positively and adversely. As said by Ervasti, J.; Aalto, V.; Pentti, J.; Oksanen, T.; Kivimäki, M.; Vahtera, J [6] when working from home, stress levels are typically greater & if one has a flexible schedule, stress levels are lower. Recent research of 40 knowledge workers by [7] 2021 who were required to work from home during COVID discovered some productivity benefits of WFH but also raised some questions about the practice's long-term efficacy, creative potential, and individual resiliency.

Evidence from a sizable sample of email and meeting metadata reveals sharp increases in virtual meetings and emails following government-enacted lockdowns during COVID (which in effect forced WFH on sizable samples of employees), perhaps to make up for the loss of in-person connections. This project made several contributions to the WFH literature as explained by authors in [8]. First, most studies on WFH have traditionally concentrated on employees who perform standardised tasks or who were in highly certain disciplines. By exploring the effects of WHF as narrated by authors in [9] arrangements on a wider range of workers and industries and by presenting fresh data on the distinctions between independent workers and managers, we add to the body of literature on this subject.

Additionally interesting is the quantity of detail that was gathered regarding the workers' WFH-related time consumption. These data allow us to look at changes in the actual time (not than aggregate memory) spent on personal and professional activities (such as meetings for work, reading/writing reports, and personal time) across time and for a large sample of people. A comprehensive investigation on the impact of WFH during COVID-19 on collaboration in a sample of Microsoft US employees was carried out by Yang et al. (2020).

According to their findings, the impact of WFH is mitigated by a person's remote collaboration experience. They also found that the preferred method of collaboration has changed: instant messages were utilised more frequently than scheduled meetings.

However, the analysis suggests that the observed changes are primarily due to factors related to the COVID-19 pandemic and that WFH under normal circumstances is likely to decrease collaboration and increase focus time. The findings also show more total collaboration hours, more meeting hours, and fewer focus hours. A switch to WFH, the authors wrote in their conclusion, "may be good for individuals participating in concentrated work that demands big blocks of free time but may be negative for those engaging in work that is more collaborative in character". This assertion emphasises the necessity for research into the varied effects of COVID-19 WFH on various categories of knowledge workers.

2.2 Level of Living

A person's mental health and psychological welfare may be significantly and profoundly impacted by pandemic breakouts and other upsetting life experiences. Stress, anxiety, mental confusion, social isolation, and depression are some of the mental or psychological issues that may develop. Additionally, those who are quarantined due to COVID-19 infection frequently experience anxiety, dread, and dissatisfaction. Moreover, significant schedule changes have been linked to COVID-19 unpredictability, which could result in an increase in stress, hopelessness, and anxiety. The COVID-19 outbreak and individual well-being have also been the subject of a review of the literature by authors in [10]. An element that is believed to have an effect on a person's quality of life is anxiety.

One of the most prevalent mental health conditions affecting people of all ages globally is anxiety [11]. Because they are unable to handle the stress, at least 11% of people worldwide experience anxiety each year (Craske and Stein, 2016). This also dealt with anxiety. Due to uncertain situations and survival resources that are considered to be life threatening, various groups within the global society have experienced symptoms of anxiety.

One of the first mental health conditions to get attention is anxiety due to COVID-19. Certain academics' interest as they perform an exploratory study into assessment techniques and additional psychological impacts or remedies brought on by the epidemic.

Two key aspects that explain how stress is produced were the main focus of research on stress at work. The first topic that has been covered over the years is the normal stress factors associated with employment. The studies looked at how demanding psychosocial aspects of the workplace, like growing workloads, role ambiguity, a lack of control, and a lack of social support, may lead to workplace stress and impair work performance. The second topic covered is environmental factors, including assessing how an employee's talents and their physical surroundings affect their performance and how an environment misfit would have negative psychological as well as physiological repercussions.

However, uncertainty and possibly hazardous conditions at work are also a key element that might raise stress levels among employees. As a result, elements of the external environment interfere with employees' ability to perform or place unwarranted demands on them, which hinders job performance by elevating stress levels [12].

Assumption 1 *(H1): Work ability and psychological and physical stress symptoms are negatively impacted by the percentage of time spent working from home (Factor 1).*

2.2.1 Job Satisfaction of Staff in Home Offices

Job satisfaction among employees and mental health are directly related as suggested by authors in [13, 14]. The level of an employee's fulfilment with their work can be referred to as job satisfaction. It is also the joyful emotional condition brought on by the professional experience. Working remotely for a while can improve organisational dedication, the calibre of relationships with leaders, and reduce conflict at the office. Therefore, the unplanned and transient transition to WFH caused by COVID-19 may enhance job satisfaction. Previous research on the effect of WFH on job satisfaction, however, has shown mixed results, such as a decline in the quality of relationships with co-workers.

Job satisfaction is substantially influenced by social contacts at work. Consequently, social isolation may have a negative effect on job satisfaction as a result of the laws against social distance and WFH during the COVID-19 epidemic. Social isolation was found to have a detrimental impact on distant job satisfaction in a study by Toscano and Zappalá [15]. However, Bouziri and colleagues point out that numerous businesses entirely moved to remote work, allowing all staff to work from home, to curb the COVID-19 pandemic. As a result, these businesses exclusively use digital technologies for communication. According to Bouziri and colleagues, the risk of social isolation in this situation is lower than it was for teleworkers in times before to the epidemic. While some of their co-workers engaged in face-to-face conversations, the latter worked from home.

Assumption 2 *(H2): Job satisfaction is positively impacted by Factor 1, which is the percentage of time spent working from home.*

The current study's innovative focus is on investigating particular WFH features. The technological equipment at home (Factor 2), the availability of a company requirement for WFH (Factor 3), and the flexibility provided by the employer for one's job (Factor 4) were the four different aspects of WFH that we looked at. Furthermore, as a subjective quality of the home office, we concentrated on the impression of greater autonomy (Factor 5). The effects of each of the four traits on an employee's job happiness, work capacity, and symptoms of psychological and physical stress are examined.

Employees that work in WFH are reliant on information and communication technologies (ICT), which might comprise a variety of technical tools. In response to the COVID-19 pandemic's inception, spread, and containment efforts, many workers and businesses swiftly shifted to WFH and other types of mobile working.

As a result, a sizable share of workers with disabilities brought on by technology would be working from home. However, there are no laws governing the furnishings that should be used in home offices. We assume that certain employees do not have access to enough technical equipment at the home office because it is not required by law and because the COVID-19-related move to WFH was unplanned and rapid. We therefore assume that numerous health indices, as well as employee job satisfaction, are influenced by the efficacy of technologies for working from home.

Assumption 3 *(H3): The presence of a corporate policy allowing for remote work has a favourable impact on factors, work ability, physical and mental stress symptoms, and job satisfaction.*

WFH is under a lot of pressure during the COVID-19 pandemic. The right resources are necessary for employees to handle them in a healthy manner. We presume that the ability to be flexible in one's own work, enabled by the employer, is a crucial tool for coping with the ambiguous and ever-changing needs of the workplace as also suggested by researchers in [16]. The participants were specifically questioned if they could plan their working hours while WFH on their own or if arrangements with superiors were required. WFH can be linked to more flexibility in terms of working hours, breaks, and job sequencing, allowing workers to exercise more autonomy. According to studies, the core characteristics of WFH such as greater individual responsibility, greater flexibility, and freedom have an impact on job satisfaction. Employees can combine professional and personal duties, giving them more freedom in their work-life balance, which is one benefit of the greater flexibility. Numerous studies have revealed that WFH contains some elements that are health-promoting, such as more flexible working hours. These may result in improved performance, motivation, and satisfaction.

3 Methods

3.1 Techniques: Sample

Professionals who began working from home after the pandemic's breakout were given the questionnaire designed to gather data. The convenience sampling method was employed for the respondents. Participants were primarily IT professionals because telework adoption rates were shown to be higher in knowledge-based service bvusinesses. It was made clear to participants that their participation was optional and anonymous. Participants' age, demographic data, including sex were requested in the questionnaires to give a more complete picture of the sample.

3.1.1 Data Gathering

The data was gathered using the survey method, with an internet questionnaire serving as an instrument. By describing the purpose of the questionnaire to the respondents, data were gathered by email using a google form. Out of the 675 surveys that were first sent through email, the process resulted in 472, for a response rate of 69.9%. Different scales were included in the questionnaire with various hypotheses: stress, adaptability to work environment, work satisfaction, time management, health, well-being, and anxiety.

3.1.2 Questionnaire

Based on the below survey, its stated that COVID-19 work from home had noteworthy influence on responsibilities, both adaptive and relative.

Did the concept of work from home affect

- The efficiency of work
- Timings of work
- Family space
- Work satisfaction
- Time management
- Health
- Workflow
- Stress levels
- Adaptability to work environment
- Well-being
- Anxiety levels

3.1.3 Demographic Data

A total of 472 surveys as listed in Table 1 were collected on 5-point scale considering different domains.

5 points indicating accepting the effect and its impact extremely.

0 points stating no impact of WFH on the parameter.

The results of WFH can be divided into two categories: results for the "job domain" and "life domain". Studies have shown that WFH improves work domain outcomes like productivity, job satisfaction, flexibility, and engagement. A self-explanatory analysis of WFH's assets, drawbacks, prospects, and pressures was conducted with a particular focus on the IT industry.

Table 1 Demographic data representing the count of surveys in different domains

Gender	Count	%	Age (Years)	Count	%	Work experience in years	Count	%	Education	Count	%
Male	298	63	22–30	386	82	1–5	386	82	UG	378	80
Female	174	37	31–40	47	10	10–15	47	10	PG	94	20
			41–50	32	7	20–25	32	7			
			51–55	7	1	>25	7	1			
Total	472	100		472	100		472	100		472	100

4 Discussion

With the rise of multiple family workforces, COVID-19 allowed everyone the chance to experience WFH, which had long been a sought employment alternative for many. The problem of caring for elderly parents and/or young children while working in a demanding setting has been raised.

4.1 Did the Concept of Work from Home Affect the Efficiency of Work?

The survey collected from different individuals working in IT sector stated that around 62% of individuals state that there is no impact of working from home on their efficiency of work as shown in Fig. 1. The opinion of the people is crucial to take into account, along with the efficacy of the WFH procedures. An overwhelming majority of the feedback the practise received was positive.

WFH is influenced by both organisational and "individual and family factors", with "self-control, self-motivation, ability to work self-reliantly, determination, self-organization, self-confidence, time managing skills, computer knowledge" being some of the factors that need to be addressed.

4.2 Did the Concept of Work from Home Affect Timings of Work?

The poll estimated that productivity has decreased significantly, by as much as 20%, because the goals had not changed but working hours had. According to the poll, "these results are consistent with employees becoming less productive during WFH

Fig. 1 Effect of work efficiency in IT sector

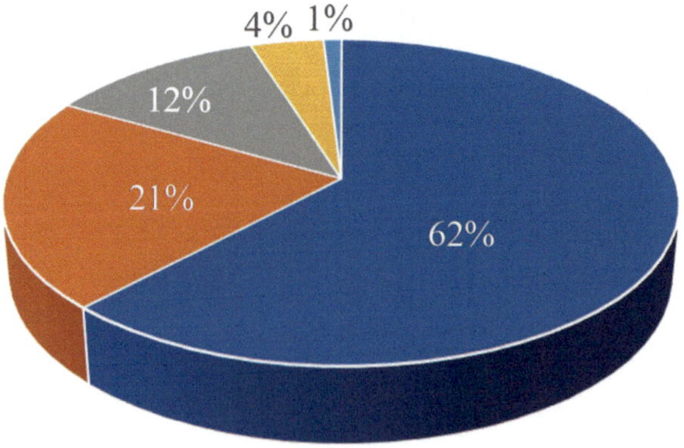

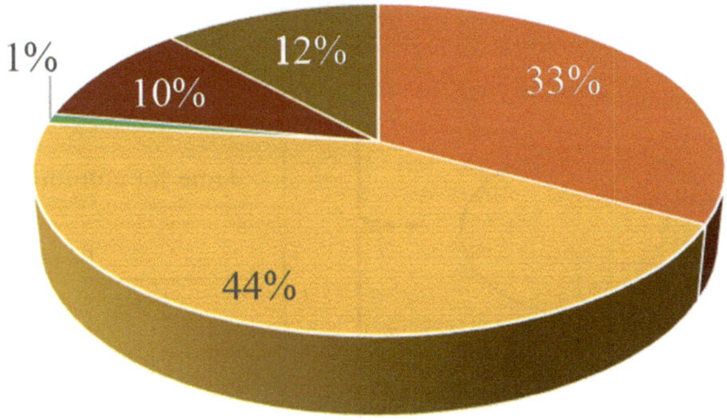

Fig. 2 WFH effect on timings of work

and working longer hours to make up for it". The study determined that around 44% of employees spent more time participating in various sorts of formal and informal meetings during WFH, especially video conferences, as the cause of this reduction in productivity is shown in Fig. 2. Another factor was that they worked for significantly less time uninterrupted. They also spent less time receiving coaching or having one-on-one meetings with managers, as well as networking both inside the company and with clients.

Employees who had children at home extended their working hours considerably more than those who did not, which led to a higher decline in productivity. The study stated that businesses should not undervalue the value of networking and uninterrupted work time on employee productivity. "Among other considerations, these and previous data imply that communication, coordination, and collaboration are inhibited under WFH", it said.

4.3 *Did the Concept of Work from Home Affect Family Space?*

Family dynamics significantly affects work and life satisfaction, which is related to the harmony of work and life. Individuals' adaptation mechanisms are also influenced by the quality of family relationships. Quality of family relationships and adaptive mechanisms are inversely correlated. Overall, the current study's findings largely confirmed the conceptual model that was suggested regarding the relationships between WFH, demographic variations, adaptive processes, and family connection quality. The perceived amount of time spent with family members was favourably correlated with WFH, which in turn positively correlated with the quality of the family relationships. Among 472 responses collected, 389 mentioned that due to continuous and non-timely online meetings, family time was disturbed. Family connection happiness increased as a result of better work-life balance, but family relationship satisfaction itself was a poor predictor of work-life balance.

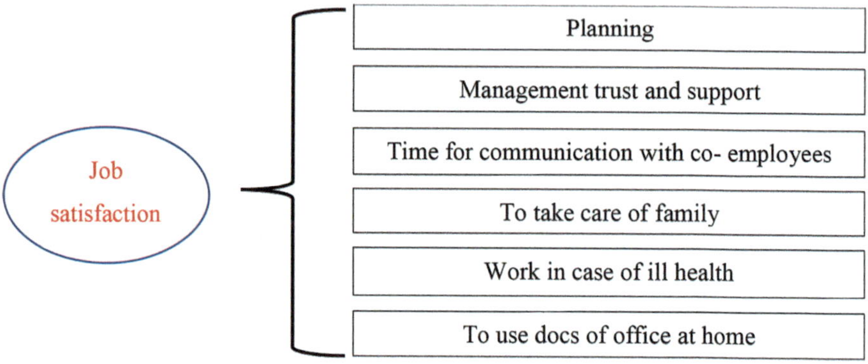

Fig. 3 Parameters illustrating the job satisfaction

Fig. 4 WFH effect on work satisfaction

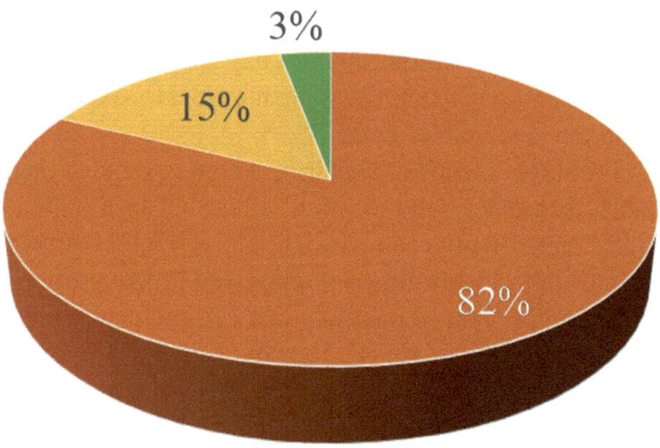

4.4 Did the Concept of Work from Home Affect Work Satisfaction?

A key element influencing the work from home arrangement is satisfaction or the capacity to schedule time to complete activities before due dates when working from home. Different parameters that show impact on job satisfaction are as listed in Fig. 3. When working from home, employees could alter or choose their daily timetable or routine. Good time management skills are viewed as a valuable resource when working independently from home, and the freedom to set one's own schedule is considered a benefit of remote work. Flexible scheduling is possible while working from home, and it gives you the freedom to work late into the night, schedule personal appointments during working hours, and finish chores in the evenings or on days off. Figure 4 illustrates around 82% predominantly accepted that there is job satisfaction even worked from home.

4.5 *Did the Concept of Work from Home Affect Time Management?*

One of the biggest time wasters whenever it comes to managing the workday is immediately eliminated while working from home. It's crucial to understand how to take advantage of these new timetables, though.

4.5.1 Improved Timeliness

Anyone can be more prone to complete work and duties on time, indicating that one is skilful at meeting deadlines. The more on-time projects finished, the less pressure there will be to worry about losing a client or failing your boss.

4.5.2 Improved Job Standards

Utilising the most precious hours to concentrate on the most difficult activities is part of successful time management. A greater quality of work may result from learning what to do with the bulk of brainpower.

4.5.3 Greater Output

By managing time, more time can be spent getting things done and less time deciding what to do next. One can find rushing toward goals at even a greater rate while using smart goals as a guide.

4.5.4 Decreased Stress and Anxiety

It can cause a lot of worry and anxiety to feel that one is constantly falling behind at work. As a result, productivity suffers, and general life quality and health suffer. Work from home affects on health, workflow, stress levels, adaptability to work environment, well-being, and anxiety levels.

A worker with good time management abilities will frequently have exposure to more boss-approved opportunities for interesting new assignments and may even find new opportunities for promotions. Additionally, it has been demonstrated that people can prosper in a real world.

Just as effective time management has a wealth of advantages, poor time management has several drawbacks. Without a plan for your day, you'll find yourself fumbling between one task to the next without ever receiving the proper level of focus. Even though remote working environments can be beneficial, they can also result in stress, procrastination, and low productivity if they are not well managed. Delay, the most obvious outcome of bad time management, occurs when there is uncertain about what ought to be done at any time. When there is no clear strategy

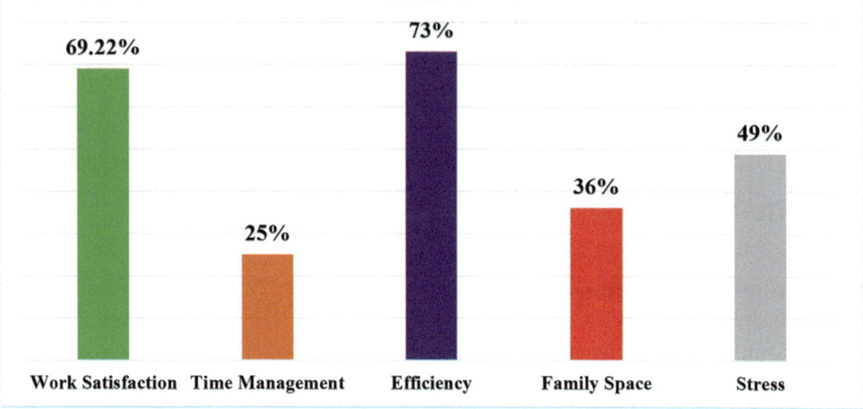

Fig. 5 Overall statistics of the data collected

in place, it's simple to start with simple activities and postpone more tough ones. Utilising effective time management techniques enables to work efficiently.

It might be difficult to get moving when there is an enormous amount of work before. Learning time management skills will help feel more at ease during every workday. As a result, one can get more motivated and can use energy in the best way possible. When one doesn't know how to efficiently manage time, it frequently takes longer to complete some tasks. This could mean that longer hours should be spent to complete important jobs. There exists a sign of burning out which raises exposure to illness.

From Fig. 5 the survey states that:

- 69.22% of the qualitative responses showed support for WFH and showed satisfaction towards WFH. The elimination of commuting times and the ensuing decrease in stress were factors in the enhanced quality of work.
- Some participants confirmed the WFH had badly impacted their productivity, or that their output had decreased. The respondents believed that working 24 hours a day was a new demand by supervisors who did not honour personal time, and that there were distractions at home as a result of the WFH's longer working hours, absence of a formal lunchtime, tea/snack break, and even dinner time. Only 25% felt that they could effectively manage time between work and family.
- Many participants expressed the opinion that the family atmosphere was encouraging and boosted productivity. It also true to responders who had past knowledge of WFH, although for smaller lengths of time.
- Other answers from women included being completely numb because of the COVID and WFH's various duties, including being a spouse, mother, and parents-in-law at home in addition to being a team manager at work, and occasionally overwhelmed since there is no time restriction for women. Especially its clear from the statistics that almost 49% of the total survey felt that WFH created stress and the data was mostly from women.

5 Conclusion

The once-desired, highly desirable WFH has not consistently shown to be one of the better solutions for the majority, according to research. WFH still has interest, but not in the way it does right now. To effectively regulate and make WFH practicable, the government needs implement better rules and regulations. The provision of advice on how to adjust to distant online work is one area of policy where preparation and implementation are essential. Without any instructions, the decision to halt in-person meetings and work was quickly put into effect. Workers lack the tools necessary for this transition, such as software, access to formal papers, and a suitable workspace, and many are unclear of what WFH implies.

References

1. Bouziri H, Smith DRM, Descatha A, Dab W, Jean K. Working from home in the time of COVID-19: how to best preserve occupational health? Occup Environ Med. 2020;77(7):509–10. https://doi.org/10.1136/oemed-2020-106599.
2. Kniffin KM, Narayanan J, Anseel F, Antonakis J, Ashford SP, Bakker AB, Bamberger P, Bapuji H, Bhave DP, Choi VK. COVID-19 and the workplace: implications, issues, and insights for future research and action. Am Psychol. 2021;76:63.
3. Moretti A, Menna F, Aulicino M, Paoletta M, Liguori S, Iolascon G. Characterization of home working population during COVID-19 emergency: A cross-sectional analysis. Int. J. Environ. Res. Public Health. 2020;17:6284.
4. Milasi S, Fernandez-Macias E, Gonzalez-Vasques I. Telework in the EU before and after the COVID-19: where we were, where we head to. Eur. Union 2020, 2020, 1–8.OCED. Teleworking in the COVID-19 pandemic: trends and prospects. Paris, France: OECD; 2021.
5. Hunter JR, Meiring RM, Cripps A, Suppiah HT, Vicendese D, Kingsley MI, Gordon BA. Relationships between physical activity, work ability, absenteeism and Presenteeism in Australian and New Zealand adults during COVID-19. Int J EnvironRes Public Health. 2021;18:12563. [PubMed]
6. Ervasti J, Aalto V, Pentti J, Oksanen T, Kivimäki M, Vahtera J. Association of changes in work due to COVID-19 pandemic with psychosocial work environment and employee health: a cohort study of 24 299 Finnish public sector employees, vol. 79. Occup. Environ Med; 2021. p. 233.
7. Meyer B, Zill A, Dilba D, Gerlach R, Schumann S. Employee psychological Well-being during the COVID-19 pandemic in Germany: a longitudinal study of demands, resources, and exhaustion. Int J Psychol. 2021;56:532.
8. Bullinska-Stangrecka H, Bagienska A. The role of employee relations in shaping job satisfaction as an element promoting positive mental health at work in the era of COVID-19. Int J Environ Res Public Health. 2021;18:1903.
9. Ebener M, Hasselhorn HM. Validation of short measures of work ability for research and employee surveys. Int. J. Environ.Res. Public Health. 2019;16:3386.
10. Lu Y, Liu Q, Yan H, Gao S, Liu T. Job burnout and its impact on work ability in biosafety laboratory staff during the COVID-19 epidemic in Xinjiang. BMC Psychiatry. 2021;21:543.
11. Siqueira LTD, Dos Santos AP, RLF S, PAM M, da Silva Vitor J, Ribeiro VV. Vocal self-perception of home office workers during the COVID-19 pandemic. J Voice. 2020;37(1):144.e15–22.
12. McDowell CP, Herring MP, Lansing J, Brower C, Meyer JD. Working from home and job loss due to the COVID-19 pandemic are associated with greater time in sedentary behaviours. Front Public Health. 2020;8:750.

13. Stickley A, Koyanagi A. Loneliness, common mental disorders and suicidal behaviour: findings from a general population survey. J Affect Disord. 2016;197:81–7.
14. Killgore WD, Cloonan SA, Taylor EC, Dailey NS. Loneliness: a signature mental health concern in the era of COVID-19. Psychiatry Res. 2020;290:113117.
15. Toscano F, Zappalà S. Social isolation and stress as predictors of productivity perception and remote work satisfaction during the COVID-19 pandemic: the role of concern about the virus in a moderated double mediation. Sustainability. 2020;12:9804.
16. Kröll C, Nüesch S. The effects of flexible work practices on employee attitudes: evidence from a large-scale panel study in Germany. Int J Hum Resour Manag. 2019;30:1505–25.

Deep Feedforward Neural Networks for Prediction of Mental Health

Ramasamy Mariappan and Gopi Battineni

Abstract Mental health disorders or psychiatric issues such as Alzheimer's disease (AD), cognitive impairments, and depression have an impact on physical health. The early detection of patients who are at risk of a mental health crisis is of paramount importance to reduce burdens and costs that can result from. However, the high prevalence of mental health issues makes it impractical to manually review complicated patient health records to make proactive psychiatric health care decisions. Artificial intelligence (AI) techniques have recently been developed to aid mental health professionals, such as psychiatrists and psychologists, in making clinical decisions. Recently, deep learning approaches find great attention among biomedical researchers due to their unmatchable ability to use very large size datasets to predict medical results. One such tremendous application is the use of deep learning for the prediction of psychiatric disorders. However, typical deep learning (DL) approaches suffer from limitations due to their significant presumptions, which make this not suitable for medical imaging. This book chapter reviews the literature on DL algorithm applications in predictive research on psychiatric health. In particular, it gives a succinct overview of contemporary DL techniques in psychiatric health research. This chapter proposed a novel deep learning method using deep feedforward neural networks coupled with psychiatric tools, which could hasten a new way for integration into prognostic research in digital psychiatry and eventually lead to its use in clinical results. In our final section, it examined the major difficulties in applying DL algorithms and psychiatric tools to enhance the prognosis and prediction of mental health disorders and leveraging several interesting applications for DL algorithms along with physician's intelligence for enhancing mental health treatment.

Keywords Mental health · Psychiatric tools · EEG · DL · Neural networks

R. Mariappan (✉)
School of Computer Science and Engineering, VIT University, Vellore, Tamil Nadu, India

G. Battineni
Clinical Research Center, School of Medicinal and Health Products Sciences, University of Camerino, Camerino, Italy
e-mail: gopi.battineni@unicam.it

G. Battineni et al. (eds.), *Computational Methods in Psychiatry*,
https://doi.org/10.1007/978-981-99-6637-0_9

1 Introduction

The digital mental health sector has experienced rapid growth over the past decade due to the proliferation of digital tools and technical advancements, increasing consumer preferences for digital health, and the impacts of COVID-19 and natural disasters on the user's ability to access face-to-face services [1]. However, despite the rapid growth of the digital mental health sector, supply and demand barriers continue to exist, impeding the effective operation of the sector [1–3]. Consumers can experience issues accessing services due to poor health or digital literacy, digital infrastructure, or pre-existing social inequalities. Some may also be hesitant to use digital mental health services due to mistrust in their efficacy or concerns about the use of their data. Poor awareness and distrust are also experienced by health professionals, in part due to an underdeveloped evidence base for how digital mental health services could be best used [4]. In particular, there is limited evidence to understand the suitability of digital interventions for low prevalence and complex mental health issues, and vulnerable or at-risk population cohorts. While health professionals understand the need to cater to the unique needs and preferences of consumers, they can find it overly complex to navigate the digital mental health ecosystem and match consumers to the right services.

Cognitive challenges are suggestive highlights of all psychological messes. High paces of mental indications, prominently tension, sorrow, self-destructive conduct, and posttraumatic stress disorder have been accounted for in the all-inclusive community following past nCoV scourges, independent of irresistible status. An investigation of 90 COVID-19 cases with a 97% reaction rate also demonstrated undeniable degrees of mental trouble with 59% determined to have mental problems furthermore [5]. The modest quantity of data accessible from creature examines and past respiratory scourges recommend not just that novel coronavirus may influence the cerebrum, but that the subsequent impact on cognitive operations might persevere for a significant stretch after recuperation. While new cases of very much described neurological problems resulting from the current pestilence might be moderately simple to distinguish, enduring sub-clinical problems, for example, mild cognitive decline, focal memory and speech loss, or intensification of previous degenerative neuropathology like vascular dementia, and Alzheimer's illness, may effectively go undetected or then again be ascribed to mental responses and social change produced by the pandemic.

The current longitudinal studies of neurological disorders should be expanded to collect data on COVID-19 openness and immune response status in addition to the psychological functioning, brain imaging, and disease biomarker data that are now collected [3]. The development of new COVID-19 mice models, which will enable the assessment of the interaction between viral pathology and neurodegeneration and contribute to the advancement of new therapies, will encourage preclinical studies aimed at determining the robotic relationship between COVID contamination and neurological illness [6]. The common barriers to cognitive assessment are listed below:

- Poor coordination of psychological evaluations with EMR frameworks makes a significant clerical work burden to archive the yield of a cognitive performance assessment.
- Moreover, the absence of an appropriate combination with the EMR framework additionally restricts the capacity to follow a person's cognitive/psychological insight over the long run.
- In certain conditions, testing apparatuses are ineffectively planned and additionally unintuitive for clients.
- Also, numerous cognitive tests have exhibited restricted worth when sent to a heterogeneous patient populace. This constraint arises due to the initial development and testing being inhomogeneous.
- Early identification of MCI is challenging because of constraints related to cognitive diseases. Symptoms or signs identified with the underlying beginning of MCI can change altogether between people, contingent upon etiology, intellectual hold, and variable requests of everyday living, among different elements.
- Alzheimer's association encourages parental care to be aware of the main indication of the presence of COVID-19 disease in people with dementia or AD.

By aiming at the above-mentioned factors, the current chapter proposes to examine the wide scope of mental health issues, neuropsychiatric ramifications, neurological issues, psychiatry issues, and neuropsychiatric issues like disarray and cognizance. Even though extreme neuropsychiatric consequences are relatively rare, a sizable number of people would be impacted globally. Since previous flu pandemics were linked to long-lasting neuropsychiatric effects, it is plausible that new viral contaminations with a wide range could also generate persistent mental gloom.

The majority of psychiatric studies, which have used machine learning, have been on categorization or diagnosis. However, researchers have pointed out that the existing methods underperform due to a lack of understanding of the constraints of the various machine learning techniques or psychiatric issues and their associated procedures and highlighting the challenge in developing and validating such models. Previous studies have shown that the analysis of neuroimages using deep learning (DL) techniques can offer evidence of mental health issues, which can be applied in clinical settings and aid in the identification of mental illnesses [7]. However, to accomplish this goal, numerous issues must be resolved.

- Because the DL architectures often need large data samples to train the models, the analysis of neuroimaging data may be difficult due to the absence of such data.
- The imaging data typically occupy a high-dimensional space; for instance, a 64 2D neuroimage can yield 4096 characteristics [8]. As a result, there is a chance that the DL models will overfit.
- One potential solution to this problem is to use feature engineering to make the data less dimensional before supplying it to the DL models.

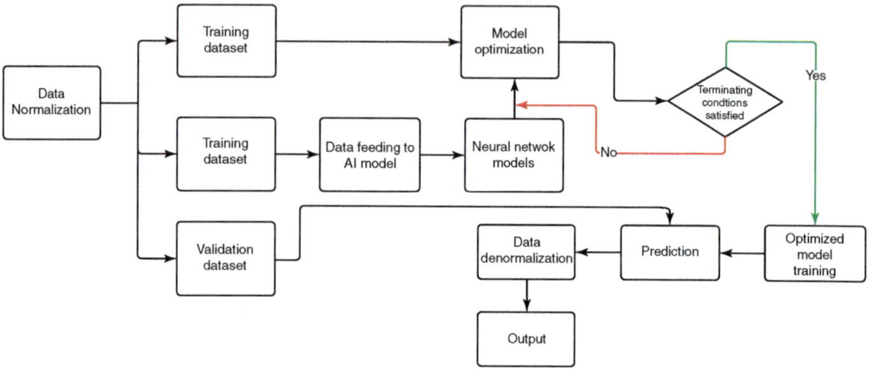

Fig. 1 Deep learning architecture

The DL models have been proven to perform better than the conventional ML models in the prediction of several disorders, including depression, and schizophrenia [9, 10]. These models can profit from feature engineering techniques. However, because these techniques extract features based on past knowledge, they might leave out some details that are important for mental outcome study. Using convolutional neural networks (CNN) to automatically extract information from the raw data is an alternate method [11, 12]. Figure 1 presents the architecture of DL model, and it is indicated that neural networks are effective in processing unprocessed neuroimage data.

One of the simplest and most often used neurological symptom diagnostics in the literature is electroencephalography (EEG) [13, 14]. The EEG data are typically categorized as high-density, continuous streaming data. There are several difficulties despite the early success of using DL algorithms to evaluate EEG data for researching various mental health issues.

- One significant issue is the amount of inaccurate, noisy, and redundant information present in raw EEG data obtained from sensors due to depleted batteries, errors in sensor readings, and sporadic communication failure in wireless sensor networks.
- The raw EEG signal must first undergo several preprocessing stages (such as data denoising, data interpolation, data transformation, and data segmentation) before being fed to the DL models.
- The analysis of the EEG streaming data is computationally due to the dense properties of the raw EEG data, which presents a challenge for the model architecture choice. One solution is to use a dimensionality reduction technique using feature engineering.
- On the one hand, using feature selection/extraction techniques, several types of features can be gleaned from the raw data.
- The ability of DL to learn relevant features from "all" available data is one of its intuitive qualities, hence feature selection procedures are less frequently used in DL application scenarios.

- One option is to pre-train a deep neural network using a sizable source dataset using Google Inception v3 model is fully connected layers on top of the network, and then use traditional backpropagation to fine-tune the network using the small target dataset.

Some of the major mental health issues are addressed and listed below:

- Schizophrenia is a severe mental illness that causes aberrant reality interpretation.
- An extreme mental health disease called bipolar disorder, also known as manic depression, generates emotional highs (mania or hypomania) and lows (depression).
- Attention Deficit Hyperactivity Disorder (ADHD): A brain disorder that impairs your ability to focus, remain still, and maintain behavioral control (common in children) [15].
- Anxiety is a state of unease, anxiety, or dread. Extreme mood swings, such as emotional highs and lows, are a sign of bipolar disorder.
- Depression is a common and serious medical disorder that negatively affects a person's feelings, thoughts, and behavior.
- After experiencing a traumatic, frightening, or hazardous event, some people develop.
- Post Traumatic Stress Disorder (PTSD): A disorder, which affects people who suffered from a traumatic, frightening, or dangerous incident.

The methods and classification modes presented in Table 1 majorly highlighted and used in the current literature to predict and classify psychiatric issues.

A new method for the proactive prediction of mental health or psychiatric issues using digital psychiatric tools and a feedforward deep convolution neural network (FFDCNN) was discussed in this work. The rest of the manuscript is organized as

Table 1 List of classification and prediction models

Prediction models	Classification
Bayesian network model	Gaussian classification
Naive Bayes algorithm	Logistic regression algorithm
Logistic regression algorithm	Neural networks model
Multilayer perceptron model	Random forest algorithm
Sequential minimal optimization	Support vector machine
K-star model	XGBoost algorithm
Random subspace model	K-nearest neighbors model
J48 algorithm	
Random forest algorithm	
Random tree	
LASSO model	
Linear regression algorithm	
SVM classifier	
CatBoost algorithm	
XGBoost algorithm	
KNN classifier	

follows. Section 2 explores the psychiatric tools and their biomarkers. Section 3 provides brief introduction on FFDNN, followed by a discussion, and a few future challenges ahead in Sect. 4. Section 5 concludes the chapter with possible future works ahead for further work.

2 Psychiatry Tools

There are numerous neurological complications, psychological complications, and mental health complications. The following neuropsychological complications are observed among psychiatric patients, as shown in Table 2. In the current literature, there are numerous analog psychiatry tools such as anxiety scales, anxiety inventory, PTSD inventory, depression inventory, cardiac anxiety questionnaires, ICD questionnaires, etc.

2.1 *Electroencephalogram (EEG)*

EEG is one of the easiest and most important neurological analytical tests that can alter clinical decisions. Determining whether a patient has neurological entanglements is beneficial. Scientists found that around 33% of COVID patients who were given an EEG had unusual neuroimaging restricted in the frontal flap of the mind [16]. A portion of the EEG adjustments found in COVID-19 patients may show harm to the brain that probably won't have the option to be fixed in the wake of recuperating from the sickness. EEG stays vital in the assessment of the patient with impeded cognizance, especially with the end goal of barring non-convulsive seizures and status epilepticus. It may not generally be the infection acting straightforwardly on the cerebrum causing the strange EEG readings, it is very well may be the

Table 2 Neurological/psychological/mental health complications

Neurological complications	Psychological complications	Mental health complications
• Developmental dyslexia • Encephalopathy • Encephalitis • Epilepsy • Hereditary ataxia • Huntington's disease • Juvenile myoclonic epilepsy • Myelitis • Parkinson's disease • Progressive supranuclear palsy • Stroke	• Attention deficit hyperactivity disorder (ADHD) • Anorexia nervosa • Autism • Anxiety • Asperger syndrome • Addiction • Bipolar affective disorder • Depression • Obsessive-compulsive disorder (OCD) • Panic disorder • Post traumatic stress	• Dementia in Alzheimer's disease • Dementia in Parkinson's • Frontotemporal dementia • Cognitive decline • Mild cognitive decline (MCD) • Memory loss

oxygen admission, heart issues identified with COVID-19, or another kind of result, which is the reason he says that exhaustive patient consideration ought to incorporate more imaging of the cerebrum or EEG testing as important. Specifically, EEG can be utilized to survey encephalopathy, epileptogenicity, also, any central anomalies in patients with COVID-19 [17]. Previous studies have proven that the EEG is a vital tool that shows the neurological complications, mental health issues, etc. associated with various diseases. Hence, this research paper proposes to investigate mental health issues and psychiatric issues, especially those affected with neurocognitive impairments.

Measurement of EEG to diagnose psychiatric disorders using a novel methodology was proposed. It will also investigate the effect of COVID on mental health and psychological complications including stress, depression, cognitive deficits, motor palsies, sensory deficits, cranial nerve deficits, and cerebella affection such as ataxia or nystagmus, etc. by monitoring brain waves through brain–computer interface (BCI) [18]. In this work, it can be evaluating the EEG parameters of patients encountering shifting levels of encephalopathy concerning an essential COVID-19 ailment. This will help us to get sufficient details on variations in mental health and neuropsychiatric parameters due to the COVID attack. A multi-channel brain wave EEG equipment will be used to record the brain waves of the COVID patient who is affected or who has recovered. Theta waves are obtained during the COVID attack by filtering the brain waves acquired by the BCI mind-wave kit. Theta wave power levels are then compared before and after the COVID-19 attack using the BCI Graphical User Interface (GUI) software tool. The following neuropsychological complications will be analyzed. At the patient's bedside, an experienced neurophysiologist will record the patient's EEG. The EEG data will be recorded using a minimum of 9 silver/silver chloride recording electrodes, arranged according to the 10–20 international standard, with the extra ground and reference electrodes. The EEGs will be acquired during a 20–30-min period by a BCI-based EEG system (Refer to Fig. 2). Filters with low and high frequencies of 0.53 Hz and 70 Hz, respectively, were applied to the EEG channels at a 3 dB level. A single-channel ECG was concurrently recorded. The variations in frequency bands across a range of psychiatric diseases are described in Table 3 in the resting state condition.

The brain waves alpha, beta, and theta can be visualized using an EEG device and its associated eSense meter, as shown in Fig. 3. The EEG Lab brainwave visualizer uses a signal processing method using MATLAB, applying FIR filter and wavelet transform to extract the brain wave frequencies, respectively, alpha 1, alpha 2, and delta signals.

2.2 QEEG

The Quantitative Electro Encephalo Gram (QEEG), more commonly known as a brain map, is a very powerful tool, which is used to get very important objective information about the brain [19]. The computerized EEG spectral analysis of a

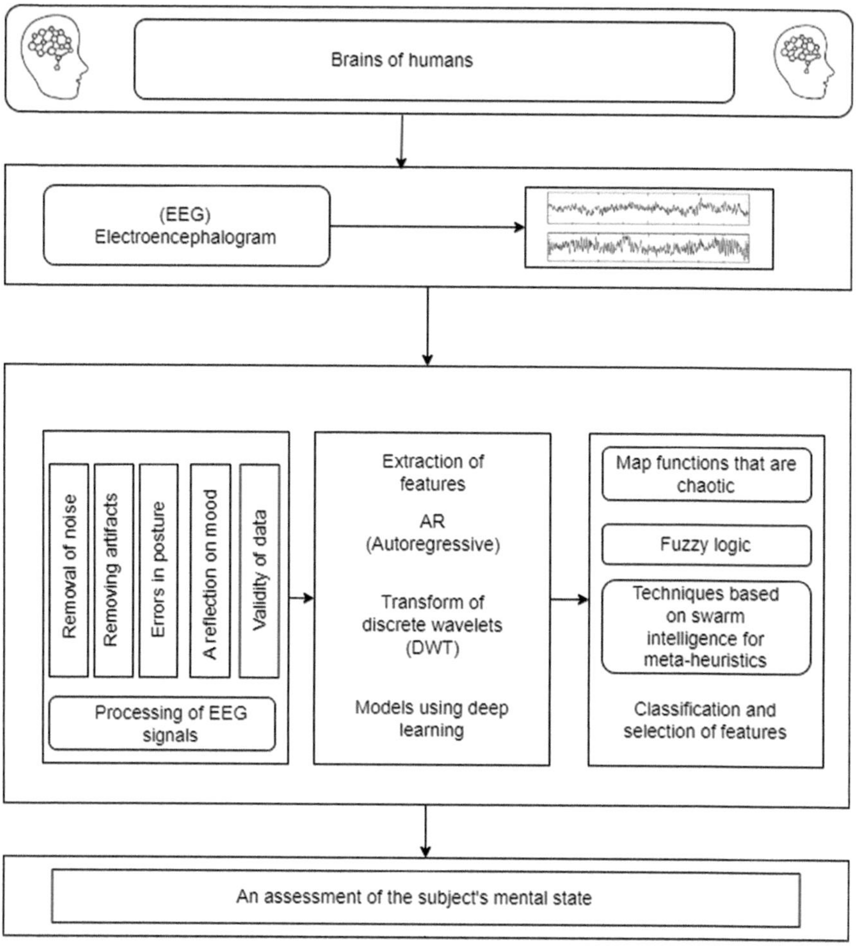

Fig. 2 EEG based on neuropsychological/mental health monitoring

Table 3 Features of EEG and qEEG

EEG features	qEEG features
Linear features: • Low-frequency power • Decay from lower to higher frequencies • Alpha -power, frequency, dispersion • A baseline of the entire frequency spectrum *Non-linear features:* • Sample-Entropy, Approx Entropy (ApEn) • Correlation dimension (CD) • Lyapunov exponent (LLE), Hurst exp (H)	• Power in $\alpha1$,$\alpha2$,$\beta1$,$\beta2$, δ ,θ • Relative strength in the specified frequency spectrum • Relative strength in the specified frequency spectrum • Relative strength in the band of frequencies 1 • Relative strength in the band of frequencies 1 • Relative strength in the band of frequencies 2 • Relative strength in the specified frequency spectrum • The EEG power spectrum's overall strength • Beta Ratio, Theta (TBR) • Alpha to Theta ratio (TAR)

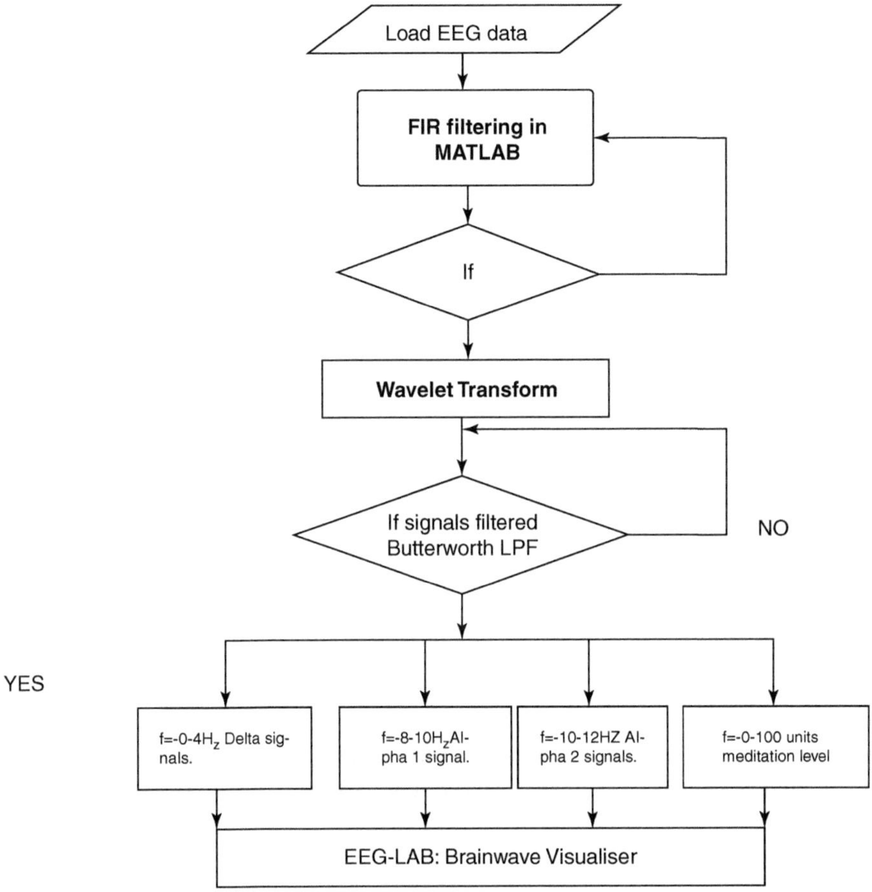

Fig. 3 Visualizing brain waves with eSense meter

neuro-cognitive impaired person provides more quantitative data than visual analysis of EEG.

- qEEG provides absolute and relative power of brain waves
- Z-transform of qEEG indicates deviation from the mean value
- Z-scores were summed to yield an accordance value for each electrode in each frequency band.

All the more explicitly, qEEG estimates profoundly coordinated large-scale level neurophysiological marvels in the cerebrum, which catch the activities of enormous scope cortical organizations of neuronal gatherings and which are astoundingly related to perception, and psychological well-being. The salient spectral features of EEG as well as qEEG are listed in Table 3.

The main cognitive and psychological factors that influence COVID's effect will be quantified by the qEEG experiment. COVID generates a qEEG profile that depicts

Table 4 Biomarkers for qEEG

Spatial biomarkers	Temporal biomarkers	Spectral biomarkers
Spearman correlations of the amplitude Envelope across channels	Analysis of detrended fluctuations Widest multifractal spectrum Duration of oscillation bursts Duration of stable phase bursts Stable frequency; standard deviation Inter-quartile range of the central frequency, maximum wavelet frequency, and phase values Oscillations per window number Kurtosis, skewness, inter-quartile range, median, range, and variance are amplitude envelope metrics	Power, both absolute and relative middle frequency Central frequency power spectral edge and bandwidth Activity, complexity, and mobility of Hjorth Strength, global frequency, and spatial complexity of the Wackerman Global Field Amplitude, frequency, and spectral purity of Barlow Peak frequency and width for alpha The baseline for alpha peak power corrected for 1/f peak frequency and width for beta Beta peak power with baseline correction for 1/f

the patient's physiological condition. An accessible technique to comprehend quantitative parameters for otherwise complex neuro-physiological entities is provided by the qEEG metrics and associated scales. The z-score will then be determined and compared to the normative individual. The difference between the value of the COVID-attacked person and the mean of the population divided by the population's standard deviation (SD) is known as the *Z*-score, which is a great statistic to use.

$$Z = \frac{x_i - \overline{X}}{SD}$$

where the *z*-score indicates how much variation of the measured value from the standard optimal value. The qEEG experimental profile reveals the following biomarkers as shown in Table 4.

Neuro-feedback is the "blueprint" for changing the electrical activity of the central nervous system using feedback from the brain. It can be done using a brain–computer interface such as a mind-wave kit/sensors/electrodes placed on the scalp and ears. The BCI is then connected to the specialized neuro-feedback computer, where the software tool detects, measures, and stores brain activities. Before applying the neuro-feedback approach, QEEG is used to objectively analyze the physiological state and brain activity as shown in Fig. 4.

The psychiatric data is analyzed using psychiatric tools and the DL model. The acquired EEG data is fed into data normalization, followed by segmentation and optimal allocation of samples for getting feature selection. Then, the data size is reduced to the optimal one by using dimensionality reduction techniques with linear discriminant analysis (LDA), followed by the least square support vector (LS-SVM)

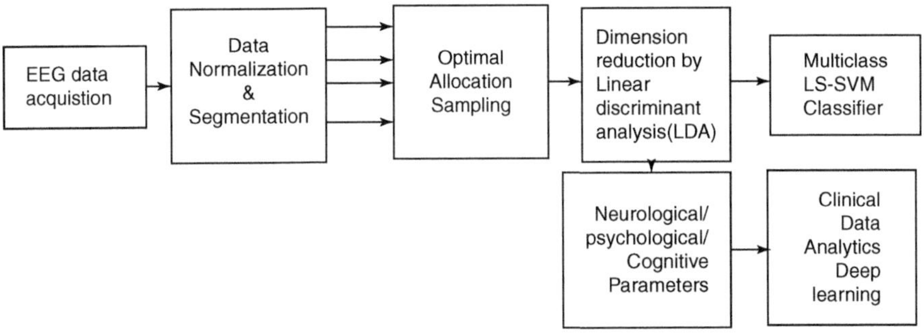

Fig. 4 Neuropsychiatric data analytics using deep learning

based classifier [20]. From the LDA analysis, the neurological/psychological parameters are finally passed into clinical data analytics using the DL model.

The multi-channel BCI kit interfaced with the EEG lab tool and Montreal Cognitive Assessment (MOCA) tool for evaluating the EEG and cognitive parameters including cognitive index (CI) is as follows.

- Encephalopathy: Glasgow Coma Scale (GCS)
- Level and the grade of hepatic encephalopathy (HE): "p" or class of liver cirrhosis
- EEG parameters: Alpha, Beta, Gamma, and theta
- Cognition parameters: Cognitive Index (CI), Cognitive Symptom Index (CSI), Emotional Symptom Index (ESI), MOCA score, etc.
- Mild cognitive decline (MCI) with Glasgow Coma Scale <13 or "severe Cognitive decline (SGD)" (GCS > 13) and reduced consciousness were only noted when patients were off sedation
- Performance Parameters: Classification accuracy, correlation coefficient, and Confidence Interval (CI).

where cross-correlation *(rxy) = Cov (X,Y)/SDx, SDy*

Generalized configuration score (GCS) = classification accuracy + correlation coefficient

Classification accuracy = No. of cases correctly classified/Total no. of cases

3 Feedforward Neural Networks

With the help of past and current data, predictive modeling is a statistical technique that uses machine learning and data mining to anticipate and forecast likely future outcomes. It functions by looking at both recent and historical data, then applying what it discovers to a model created to predict future outcomes. Nowadays, DL models are used to acquire or predict specific types of information. Data science, which also encompasses statistics and predictive modeling, contains deep learning as a key component. The artificial neural network (ANN) is working based on the

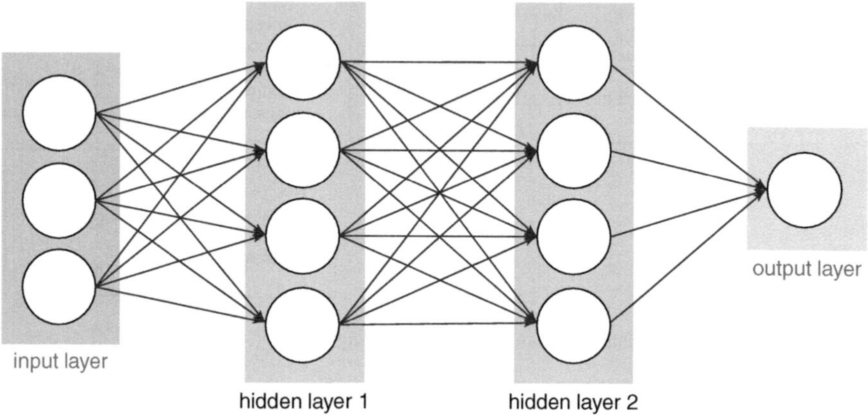

Fig. 5 Feedforward DNN with multiple hidden layers [22]

neuron relations between input and output functions through certain weights [21]. The weights and input/output functions assigned to the unit determine how the ANN will behave. For the output of each unit in this case, we will utilize the Sigmoid function. Linear and threshold are some additional functions. In comparison to the threshold and linear functions, the sigmoid function is more closely related to real neurons. We must carefully select the connections and appropriately weigh the connections for a neural network to learn.

As shown in Fig. 5, in the feedforward neural network, each connection has a weight ϴ j. There are three hidden layers, namely hidden layers 2, 3, and 4. The jth layer is connected to the j + 1th layer through the weighted connection. Weight (θ) and activation value together find the activation value of the next layer. Data fed into the network is represented by input layer activity. The weights between the layers and the activity of the preceding levels define the activity of each buried layer. The weight between the previous layer's activity and that of the output layer determines the activity of the latter.

In the above network, we have two layers. Given input vectors are

$X = [x_0, x_1, x_2]$ where $x_0 = 1$ and $a_0 = 1$ are biased terms

We calculate $z_j^l = \sum_i a_i^l \theta_{ij}^l$ $where\, a_j^l = g(z) = \frac{1}{1+e^{-z}}$; g is the sigmoid function,

where a_i^l is the activity of ith unit in the l–1th layer and θ_{ij}^l is the weight of the connection between the ith and jth unit.

The back propagation neural network algorithm is also known as backpropagation of errors since it transfers faults from output nodes to input nodes. A popular algorithm for training feedforward neural networks is backpropagation [23]. It calculates the loss function's gradient about the network weights. It is far more effective than simply computing the gradient for each weight directly. Gradient methods, including variations like gradient descent or stochastic gradient descent, are frequently used to train multilayer networks and update weights to reduce loss due to this efficiency. Using the chain rule and computing the gradient layer by layer, the backpropagation method calculates the gradient of the loss function concerning each weight. The back propagation neural network algorithm is defined in Algorithm 1.

Algorithm 1 Backpropagation Neural Network Algorithm

Step 1: Inputs X, arrives through the pre-connected path.

Step 2: The input is modeled using true weights W. Weights are usually chosen randomly.

Step 3: Calculate the output of each neuron from the input layer to the hidden layer to the output layer.

Step 4: Calculate the error in the outputs

Backpropagation Error = Actual Output – Desired Output

Step 5: From the output layer, go back to the hidden layer to adjust the weights to reduce the error.

Step 6: Repeat the process until the desired output is achieved.

4 Discussion

This book chapter has reviewed the existing literature on the prediction of psychiatric disorders with the application of internet and communication technologies (ICT) tools such as ML and DL algorithms. The prediction of psychiatric issues such as multiple conditions like depression, schizophrenia, and ADHD is analyzed with the help of EEG as a psychiatric tool, applied with a feedforward deep learning neural network. However, there are future challenges ahead to investigate the following issues.

Table 5 presents the different psychological issues combined with biomarkers. Cognitive, emotional, and behavioral impairments can be caused by mental illnesses. Psychiatric disorders can interfere with children's learning abilities. Mental illness can also cause inconvenience for adults, especially in their families, workplaces, and communities. Schizophrenia, depression, bipolar disorder, and anxiety are just some of the mental illnesses that exist.

People suffering from mental illness undoubtedly experience emotional problems, cognitive difficulties, and social difficulties. In light of these issues, it can be concluded that mental illness has serious consequences for societies across the world. In addition, new strategies are necessary to prevent and treat it. For these goals to be achieved, it is crucial to detect mental illness early. Predictive analytics will revolutionize healthcare. Self-reports of mental illness, which include questionnaires that analyze patterns of feelings and social interactions, are used to diagnose mental illness. When the right treatment and care are provided, many people can recover from mental illness or emotional disorders.

Table 5 Psychiatric disorders and associated biomarkers

Psychiatric disorders	Psychiatric tools	Psychiatric biomarkers
AD	Brain imaging	Complete brain atrophy
		Increased CSF level
Bipolar disorder	Brain imaging	Reduction in hippocampus
		Brain-derived neurotrophic factor and pro-inflammatory biomarkers
		Brain proteins
		Retinal binding protein-4
		Growth differentiation factor-15
		Hemopexin, hepsin, matrix metalloproteinase- 7
	Neurotrophic method	Decreased serum BDNF level
Depression	PHQ-9 Electrophysiological	Determination of MDD score Variation in EEG frequencies at rest EEG—α and θ waves Variation in O and P activity of EEG PTEN gene C-reactive protein, interleukin-6, tumor necrosis factor-a
ADHD	SNAP25 gene	SNAP-25 gene Ddel and Mull-polymorphisms
Major psychiatric disorders	Inflammatory	Pro-inflammatory biomarkers
	Gut microbiota	Bacterial translocation via chronic stress, leaky gut
Major depressive disorder		Long non-coding RNAs (lncRNAs)
		a-1 anti-trypsin, brain-derived neurotrophic factor, Epo-lipo-protein C3, epidermal growth factor, cortisol, resistin, prolactin, myeloperoxidase, tumor necrosis factor-a receptor type-II
Schizophrenia	Inflammatory	Increased CRP
		Up-regulation of mRNA
	Neurotransmitter	Increased synaptic dopamine concentration
		Decreased plasma level of GABA
		DISC1-gene
		Protein phosphorylation patterns

It is now possible to model mental health and understand health outcomes using social media. A variety of psychological disorders are now being predicted quantitatively, including depression, anxiety, and suicidality. Using this research can help monitor mental health statuses, diagnose problems, and design interventions for these conditions. The research and methodology used in these studies are not standardized, so it is impossible to evaluate their validity. Data collected during regular medical examinations, such as wearable data, blood samples, and urine samples, can also be used as biomarkers. Researchers have found that tryptophan concentration is particularly useful for classifying people with depression based on multiple blood metabolites [24].

In addition to providing relevant data to complement clinical care, computational approaches to mental health could also identify risky behaviors, provide timely interventions, or reach populations that traditional clinical approaches are unable to reach. Because this field is still nascent, identifying trends in research modes and practices is vital for identifying gaps before they emerge systemically. In addition to reflecting scholarly research quality, these issues also demonstrate the impact clinical care and social media predictions can have on the mental health of individuals.

Machine learning is believed to have originated from machine learning. As an example, supervised learning and unsupervised learning are two of the most commonly used machine learning approaches. An approach called supervised learning predicts outcomes based on labeled input data. Classification and regression problems are excellent candidates for supervised learning. Data is being analyzed to specific measurements to make sense of the data. Unlike supervised learning, unsupervised learning aims to make sense of data on its own. Measurements and guidelines are not present in unsupervised learning. As well as being a strategy to solve a particular problem, ensemble learning strategically combines multiple classifiers. In ensemble learning, models are improved, or a reduced chance of selecting poorly performing models is reduced.

To make mental healthcare more effective and tailored, it seems essential to predict the outcomes of individual participants. Machine learning-based predictions have, however, received surprisingly little attention in digital mental health interventions. In machine learning, advanced statistical and probabilistic techniques are applied to construct systems that can learn from experience and improve over time. Mental health prediction can be greatly enhanced by using this tool. Research can be acquired from the data, personalized experiences can be provided, and intelligent algorithms can be developed. Support vector machines, random forests, and artificial neural networks are widely used algorithms in the field of machine learning for predicting and categorizing future events.

The opportunities with machine learning involve the extent of neurological conditions connected to COVID-19 and its intellectual symptoms. The fundamental connection between the pathophysiology of infection and the dissemination of viruses and their associated pro-inflammatory modifications can be studied. The challenges involve the duration and intensity of neurological and psychosocial alterations that occur after an acute viral illness. Short-term and long-term memory capacity can be affected by viral illness severity and psychological effects.

The possible future research contributions are developing suitable deep learning algorithms, which can handle high-dimensional data space with the aid of feature engineering. More research work is needed to extract appropriate psychiatric biomarkers, which are fed as input to the DL-based training model. Moreover, the development of web applications or mobile applications equipped with digital psychiatric tools as well as DL models can be easily accessible by psychiatric patients to know about the impact of psychiatric issues on their mental health.

5 Conclusions

This book chapter reviews the literature on deep learning techniques and their applications in predictive research on psychiatric health. This chapter proposed a novel deep learning method using deep feedforward neural networks coupled with psychiatric tools, which could hasten a new way for the integration into prognostic research in digital psychiatry and eventually lead to its use in clinical results. Our final section explores the challenges ahead for the prediction of mental health disorders and leveraging some interesting applications for DL algorithms along with physicians' intelligence for enhancing mental health treatment.

Conflicts of Interest No author has any conflicts of interest.

References

1. Hossain MM, et al. Epidemiology of mental health problems in COVID-19: a review. F1000Res. 2020;9:636. https://doi.org/10.12688/f1000research.24457.1.
2. Pandey K, et al. Mental health issues during and after COVID-19 vaccine era. Brain Res Bull. 2021;176:161–73. https://doi.org/10.1016/j.brainresbull.2021.08.012.
3. Jones EAK, Mitra AK, Bhuiyan AR. Impact of covid-19 on mental health in adolescents: a systematic review. Int J Environ Res Public Health. 2021;18(5):1–9. https://doi.org/10.3390/ijerph18052470.
4. The Lancet Psychiatry. COVID-19 and mental health. Lancet Psychiatry. 2021;8(2):87. https://doi.org/10.1016/S2215-0366(21)00005-5.
5. Talevi D, et al. Mental health outcomes of the CoViD-19 pandemic. Riv Psichiatr. 2020;55(3):137–44. https://doi.org/10.1708/3382.33569.
6. Park JG, Pino PA, Akhter A, Alvarez X, Torrelles JB, Martinez-Sobrido L. Animal models of COVID-19: transgenic mouse model. Methods Mol Biol. 2022;2452:259–89. https://doi.org/10.1007/978-1-0716-2111-0_16.
7. Lin E, Lin CH, Lane HY. Deep learning with neuroimaging and genomics in Alzheimer's disease. Int J Mol Sci. 2021;22(15):7911. https://doi.org/10.3390/IJMS22157911.
8. Awate SP, Yushkevich PA, Song Z, Licht DJ, Gee JC. Cerebral cortical folding analysis with multivariate modeling and testing: studies on gender differences and neonatal development. Neuroimage. 2010;53(2):450–9. https://doi.org/10.1016/J.NEUROIMAGE.2010.06.072.
9. Richards BA, et al. A deep learning framework for neuroscience. Nat Neurosci. 2019;22(11):1761–70. https://doi.org/10.1038/S41593-019-0520-2.
10. Zaharchuk G, Gong E, Wintermark M, Rubin D, Langlotz CP. Deep learning in neuroradiology. Am J Neuroradiol. 2018;39(10):1776–84. https://doi.org/10.3174/AJNR.A5543.
11. Gong Y, Liu L, Yang M, Bourdev L. Compressing deep convolutional networks using vector quantization. 2014.
12. Gu J, et al. Recent advances in convolutional neural networks. Pattern Recogn. 2018;77:354–77. https://doi.org/10.1016/J.PATCOG.2017.10.013.
13. Romagnoli S, Franchi F, Ricci Z. Processed EEG monitoring for anesthesia and intensive care practice. Minerva Anestesiol. 2019;85(11):1219–30. https://doi.org/10.23736/S0375-9393.19.13478-5.
14. Fung FW, Abend NS. EEG monitoring after convulsive status epilepticus. J Clin Neurophysiol. 2020;37(5):406–10. https://doi.org/10.1097/WNP.0000000000000664.

15. ThaparA,CooperM.Attentiondeficithyperactivitydisorder.Lancet.2016;387(10024):1240–50. https://doi.org/10.1016/S0140-6736(15)00238-X.
16. Cecchetti G, et al. Cognitive, EEG, and MRI features of COVID-19 survivors: a 10-month study. J Neurol. 2022;269(7):3400–12. https://doi.org/10.1007/S00415-022-11047-5.
17. Kubota T, Gajera PK, Kuroda N. Meta-analysis of EEG findings in patients with COVID-19. Epilepsy Behav. 2021;115:107682. https://doi.org/10.1016/j.yebeh.2020.107682.
18. Nijboer F, et al. An auditory brain–computer interface (BCI). J Neurosci Methods. 2008;167(1):43–50. https://doi.org/10.1016/J.JNEUMETH.2007.02.009.
19. Duffy FH, Hughes JR, Miranda F, Bernad P, Cook P. Status of quantitative EEG (QEEG) in clinical practice. Clin EEG Neurosci. 1994;25(4):vi–xxii. https://doi.org/10.1177/155005949402500403/ASSET/155005949402500403.FP.PNG_V03.
20. Pham QB, Yang TC, Kuo CM, Tseng HW, Yu PS. Combing random forest and least square support vector regression for improving extreme rainfall downscaling. Water. 2019;11(3):451. https://doi.org/10.3390/W11030451.
21. Jain AK, Mao J, Mohiuddin KM. Artificial neural networks: a tutorial. Computer (Long Beach). 1996;29(3):31–44. https://doi.org/10.1109/2.485891.
22. Brunel N, Hakim V, Richardson MJE. Single neuron dynamics and computation. Curr Opin Neurobiol. 2014;25:149–55. https://doi.org/10.1016/j.conb.2014.01.005.
23. Rajput N, Verma SK. Back propagation feed forward neural network approach for speech recognition. In: Proc. 2014 3rd Int. Conf. Reliab. Infocom Technol. Optim. Trends Futur. Dir. ICRITO 2014, 2015. https://doi.org/10.1109/ICRITO.2014.7014712.
24. Setoyama D, et al. Plasma metabolites predict severity of depression and suicidal ideation in psychiatric patients-a multicenter pilot analysis. PLoS One. 2016;11(12):e0165267. https://doi.org/10.1371/JOURNAL.PONE.0165267.

The Challenge of Self-diagnosis on Mental Health Through Social Media: A Qualitative Study

Seda Yıldırım

Abstract People usually get some health information or read similar health cases from internet and other digital media channels to self-diagnose. The COVID-19 pandemic has spurred self-diagnosis, and people motivated to be self-diagnosis by finding health information on social media. In this context, this study aims to explore how social media influences self-diagnosis behavior and mental health. Firstly, this study will review prior studies and reports to give a holistic approach for the link between self-diagnosis, mental health, and social media. Then, recent news and reports will be analyzed to give qualitative evidence for the significant link between self-diagnosis and mental health and social media based on Turkish cases. As a result, it is planned to compare the positive and negative sides of self-diagnosis when considering its effect on mental health and to give an original model examining the link between social media and self-diagnosis.

Keywords Self-diagnosis · Mental health · Cyberchondria · Social media · Fake medicine · Fake news · COVID-19 pandemic

1 Introduction

The twenty-first century refers to a digital age in the literature, and it is seen that the internet meets the basic information needs of society during this period [1]. Especially, it can be said that digital transformation leads everyone in society to digital areas as a result of the development of mobile technologies and internet infrastructures [1–3]. Algorithms and machine learning (ML) enable people to do many tasks in their daily lives more easily. With the introduction of this technology into our lives, digital adaptation also increases people's interest in this technology [4]. In this respect, it is seen that the number of people seeking for information on

---

S. Yıldırım (✉)
Faculty of Economics and Administrative Sciences, Department of Business Administration, Tekirdag Namık Kemal University, Tekirdag, Turkey

G. Battineni et al. (eds.), *Computational Methods in Psychiatry*,
https://doi.org/10.1007/978-981-99-6637-0_10

disease and health through digital systems has increased, recently [5]. Some patients prefer to use digital tools such as chatbots and other portals with AI (Artificial Intelligence) drivers, and some of them prefer to seek health information on the internet and social media. For example, Ayonrinde and Michaelson (1998) determined that patients receive assistance from electronic resources and allow digital resources to guide them when making health-focused decisions [6]. Fan et al. (2021) investigated employing self-diagnosis by health chatbots in China, and they emphasized that health chatbots should be designed based on patient (consumer) expectations and needs [7]. Ćirković (2020) pointed out that patients can benefit from self-diagnosis applications based on AI systems. He investigated alternative digital applications for self-diagnosis as "Ada (Berlin-based app), Babylon (London-based app), Buoy Health (Harvard Medical School based) and Your.MD (Oslo and London)." However, he determined that healthcare professionals should be careful about the outcomes and threats of using AI application for medical consultant and self-diagnosis in long term [4].

You and Gui (2021) investigated how users perceived chatbot-based symptom checker (CSC) apps based on AI. The chatbot is a computer program that can chat (interactively communicate) with people. CSC applications used for medical diagnostics can evaluate users' medical symptoms. People get a diagnosis according to their symptoms by talking with the CSC application. Of course, there are expected threats in these applications as well. In cases where users have high-risk diseases, these applications may cause people's health to be worsened [8].

Nundy and Patel (2020) said that self-diagnosis can be useful implication during unusual conditions such as COVID-19 pandemic. During the COVID-19 pandemic, the "car service test" practices used in the United States have also found their place in other countries. It is thought that the increase in self-testing practices for COVID-19 has allowed physicians and other healthcare professionals to concentrate on more serious cases [9]. Essentially, the use of self-diagnosis during pandemics is a pre-COVID-19 practice. Self-diagnosis is considered as the primary step for disease control and management during pandemic and epidemic periods. In this case, leaflets were distributed to patients during the 2009 pandemic, and the symptoms of the disease were explained. Although pre-diagnosis has an auxiliary effect on epidemic control, there should be a control mechanism within self-diagnosis practices [10]. It is a fact that self-diagnosis is an effective implication during the pandemic such as COVID-19 pandemic when there is a complex management procedure for healthcare services. However, free usage of self-diagnosis so frequently can be harmful for individuals' health [11]. Lewis (2016) investigated the experience of self-diagnosis of autism spectrum among adults. He determined that most of participations employed self-diagnosis before having a formal medical diagnosis. Individuals used the internet and digital channels to get information and self-diagnosis when waiting for an official diagnosis [12].

The expected benefit and ease of use in the adoption of technology affect the adaptation. It can be difficult to evaluate the effectiveness of technologies used in medical services such as medical diagnosis and to determine how effective this technology is for the consumer. As it is known, consumers seem to be inclined to adapt and use digital services that are easy to use and fast accessible [13]. At this point, excessive use of self-diagnosis practices and the complete abandonment of consulting physicians may result in risky results.

This study focuses on explaining the impact of social media on self-diagnosis and mental health. The main contribution of this study is expected to give a brief view of the link between social media and self-diagnosis. In addition, investigating recent selected cases, there will be useful practical implications. As it is purposed, this study has four main parts as "introduction, literature review, descriptive study and conclusion." The importance of the related issue, aim, research design, and contribution of the study are all explained in the first part. In literature review, the links between social media usage, self-diagnosis, and mental health problems are explained. Then, the third part explains selected sample cases and includes descriptive findings. In the conclusion part, descriptive findings are discussed by giving some future recommendations.

This study employs qualitative research methodology and uses descriptive content analysis to find answers for the below questions:

- RQ1: What is the link between self-diagnosis and mental health problems?
- RQ2: How do social media influence self-diagnosis?
- RQ3: What does self-diagnosis cause?

2 Self-diagnosis, Mental Health, and Social Media

Historically, medical consultation was a process between patient and doctor during clinical encounters. The basic element required for medical consultation is that the doctor and the patient meet under appropriate conditions. However, in some circumstances, the clinical environment may not be very conducive to the medical consultation process. Long waiting times, difficulties in getting an appointment and other physical restrictions create significant barriers to medical consultation. Digital opportunities, on the other hand, provide an important support in overcoming physical restrictions and obstacles [7].

It can be said that there is a close relationship between self-diagnosis and digital applications. Increasing usage of social media sources and social media makes individuals more awareness of some mental health problems and makes people concern about their health when looking some disease symptoms on social media. In this part, this study explains the link between self-diagnosis, mental health problems, and social media usage.

Social media and internet usage encourage self-diagnosis and consumption of vitamins and dietary supplement. For example, many patients with mental disorders take nutritional supplements, but it is very difficult to establish a precise understanding of the way these patients use nutritional supplements. In the study, it was observed that Twitter users who self-diagnosed with a mental disorder stated that they actively took nutritional supplements on Twitter. In addition, these people were found to have more negative emotions than those who did not mention their dietary supplement intake [14]. Sadagheyani and Tatari (2021) stated in their study that social media can have negative and positive effects on mental health. In the study, it was seen that as a result of social media use, mental problems such as anxiety, depression, loneliness, bad sleep, self-harm, and suicide may occur. On the other hand, it has been stated that accessing other people's health experiences and expert health information may be beneficial in terms of managing depression more effectively [15].

Increasing self-diagnosis by taking advantage of social media may cause people to attribute simple disease symptoms to larger and more serious diseases. For example, many people who review social media for headaches may self-interpret a diagnosis of brain cancer. Most people suffer from anxiety, stress, and other mental illnesses because they see every illness they see on social media appropriate for themselves. The use of digital tools such as social media mostly by young people may cause young people to be more exposed to self-diagnosis and mental health problems. On the other hand, on social media platforms such as Instagram and TikTok, untrained professionals transfer information to people in the form of life coaching and wellness coaching in increasing numbers. The rise of talk about self-care and health is leading people to more self-diagnosis behavior [16]. As a result of the searches people do on their mental health in the Google search engine, they push many people into the habit of self-diagnosis. Experts state that people who engage in self-diagnosis behavior become vulnerable to some dangers. At this point, according to Micheline Maalouf (A Licensed mental health counselor), many people on social media are asking if they have a mental health problem. A client said she thought she might have obsessive-compulsive disorder (OCD), and she saw that the client diagnosed her by looking at the symptoms in the TikTok video. According to Lindsay Fleming (licensed professional counselor–LPC), people need mental health answers more. According to Kaileen McMickle (licensed professional counselor–LPC), the higher a person's anxiety, the more likely they are to seek information about their experience. Therefore, Google and social media tools are also suitable tools for these people [17]. While it is certain that social media is the most used tool for self-diagnosis and identifying mental health problems, experts have a great job here. In cases where it comes to self-diagnosis, it may be difficult to reveal the true diagnosis of people. People may begin to follow the wrong treatment methods because they attribute the wrong diseases to themselves. Unfortunately, there are videos about various mental health problems in many places on social media such as TikTok, and such videos become more relevant. On popular social media platforms such as TikTok and YouTube, young people exhibit self-diagnosis behavior according to the media content they see. There is a growing influx of people who have been diagnosed with many personality disorders and are seeking treatment. On the positive side, while young people are more aware of the importance of mental health, people are more likely to have depression, anxiety, and suicidal thoughts due to misdiagnosis and treatments [18]. With increasing social media usage, self-diagnosis can worsen an individual's existing mental disorders and complicate the right treatment. In other words, social media can worsen undiagnosed mental health disorders and worsen self-esteem and lead people to engage in self-harming behaviors such as suicidal thoughts [19]. As seen in Fig. 1, various mental illnesses can be increased as a result of excessive usage of social media.

The heaps of advertisements and phenomenon content that present health conditions in a simpler way on social media support the self-diagnosis craze. Users face a great danger. Upon the complaints received, some advertising content on TikTok and Instagram was removed from the broadcast because it provided harmful medical information. However, these practices do not prevent false health referrals. TikTok has stated that it "removes ads that promote self-diagnosis or are intended to discourage you from seeking appropriate medical advice from a healthcare professional." But there are still many gaps in the control of applications. In addition, as a result of the increased search for health information due to the COVID-19 crisis, social media has been filled with health content. In particular, there seems to be a lot of mental health content. In the last 2 years, the number of phenomena that produce content by focusing on conditions such as OCD, dissociative identity disorder, and autism has increased tremendously. For example, on TikTok, the ADHD hashtag 10.6 billion, anxiety 13.1 billion, neurodivergent has about 3 billion views. While the danger of self-diagnosis mostly covers young people, the tendency of young people to follow peer groups also supports this type of behavior [20].

Table 1 presents views from experts on self-diagnosis. When considering literature and experts' opinion, it is seen that self-diagnosis is a threat to young people with mental illness. Social media make is more accessible for people who seek for

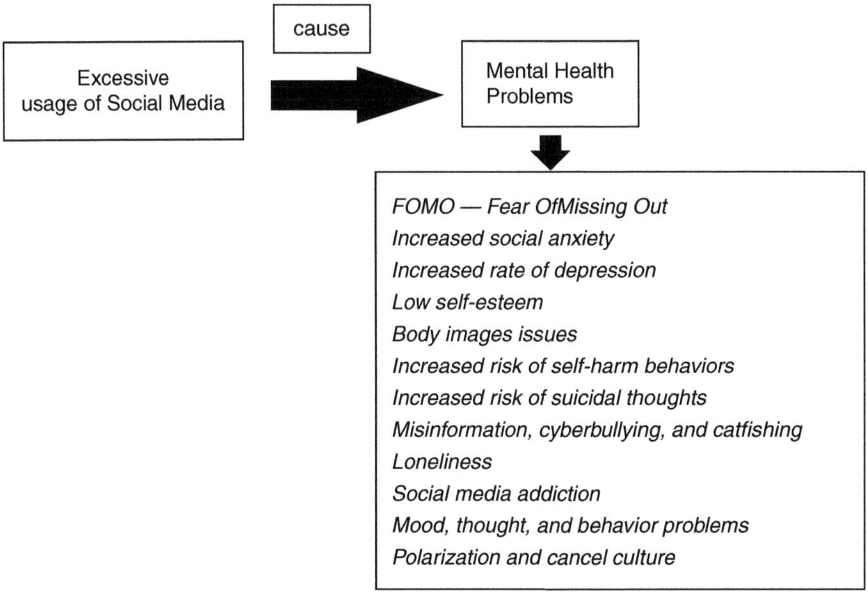

Fig. 1 Social media and mental illness (Source: based on [19] and created by author)

Table 1 Some findings: expert opinions based on self-diagnosis, mental illness, and social media association

Elements	What experts say	Key findings
Demographics	Most experts said that young adults had a higher potential to self-diagnose through social media or internet	Teenagers and young adults appear to be more open to self-diagnosis and are more prone to self-diagnosis because of greater peer influence
Health status	Most experts determined that people who have already some mental illness, are more open to self-diagnose rather than healthy people in general	It can be said that patients with mental disorders such as depression or anxiety disorder search more for disease information on the internet. Therefore, they are closer to seeking treatment with self-diagnosis
Social media	Social media content offers a wide variety of disease and treatment information, but their accuracy is unknown	The rise of social media usage makes it easier to self-diagnose for people who search for health and illness info
Health concern	Self-diagnosis can increase health concerns for people	People who self-diagnose have more health concerns in the long run
Information search	Internet and social media present much info about health, treatment, and illness. Access information is so easy through social media contents	As a result of the selection and registration of social media content according to the interests of the people, people who are in search of illness and treatment are unwittingly exposed to more health and treatment content
Advertisements through social media	A large number of social media content makes it very difficult to audit. Pharmaceutical companies can also encourage people to use the wrong drug by publishing their advertisements on social media	Drug advertisements published on social media may cause people who self-diagnose to use these drugs more
Mental illness	The symptoms of some mental illnesses are similar and social media people share these symptoms without being an expert	Even though a person has no mental health problems, most people think they have some illness due to self-diagnosis

health and treatment info to self-diagnose. In addition, the more people self-diagnose, the more anxious they become in long term.

3 Descriptive Study

This part explains the link between self-diagnosis, social media, and mental health problems by exploring sample cases from Türkiye. As employing qualitative research methodology, this study collected some sample cases through internet sources and then cases were analyzed by descriptive content analysis. This study employed purposive sampling methodology to select specific cases from Türkiye.

According to prior literature, it is mostly seen that self-diagnosis also cause over-consumption of drugs or vitamins without any physician control and internet usage encourages self-diagnosis. The following criteria were adopted in the purposive sampling method. The study included cases related to self-diagnosis, mental health, and social media and its outcomes in Türkiye. This study selected the below cases:

- **Case 1:** The most common situation in the counterfeit drug market is the introduction of substandard or counterfeit versions of drugs. Products that do not contain the active substance of the original drug or contain other substances are sold. In addition, illegally bringing original drugs to the country, changing the barcode and data matrix information on them and selling them are among the methods frequently used. On the other hand, since there is a high demand for weight loss pills and pills that are claimed to increase sexual power (erection support, aphrodisiac supplements), various supplements are also among the favorites of scammers. According to Prof. Mustafa Cetiner (Acıbadem Hospital, Internal Diseases, Hematology), "the number of buyers of supplements that are claimed to contain aphrodisiacs, increase sexual power and help with erection problems is substantial. This demand can be attributed to the fact that individuals avoid talking about their problems due to the fact that sexuality is seen as a 'taboo' in Turkish society." People who cannot open to a specialist doctor hope to benefit from such drugs [21].
- **Case 2:** Gangs that produce counterfeit drugs open websites with the names of pharmacies and sell on the internet and social media. Food supplements, herbal medicines, vitamins, burn creams, muscle relaxants, eye drops stand out among the most sold products. Products that are forbidden to enter Türkiye from abroad are also offered for sale on these sites, as well as counterfeit products of world-famous drug brands. The vast majority of people who use counterfeit drugs consult a doctor as a result of serious reactions. In the complaints, it is stated that there are side effects such as dizziness, vomiting, high fever, itching, and swelling [22].
- **Case 3:** Pharmacist Şeker Pınar Özcan (Member of the Board of the Istanbul Chamber of Pharmacists) stated that there has been a serious increase in demand for vitamins with the pandemic. This increase is a physical but uncontrolled increase. Some patients order from the internet or buy products from the market or gas station other than the pharmacy, see the side effects of this and get sick or do not see any benefit. Unfortunately, it appears to be a very unconscious use. It is necessary not to be fooled by various images from the internet. Sometimes real product images are used, but a completely different product is delivered to people. The patient who uses it can sometimes be a blood pressure patient. For example, a person thinks that he only bought a simple vitamin or something with herbal ingredients from the internet, but this may have triggered his blood pressure. Some drugs can cause bleeding when used together. Pharmacist Özcan determined that many patients suffered from problems due to the unconscious usage of drugs [23].

- **Case 4:** Exp. Bio. Çiğdem Üregen stated that vitamin intake was mostly provided by self-diagnosis detection of individuals from pharmacies and digital channels. This situation was extremely dangerous. People did not know by themselves whether there was a vitamin deficiency in their body. A single vitamin cannot make up for the deficiency of another vitamin. Therefore, before taking vitamins, it is necessary to consult a specialist and doctor and use it under his direction. Doctors can recommend the right vitamin to people in the right amounts. Hypervitaminosis occurs when unnecessary vitamins are taken. It is known that vitamins taken from natural foods as much as daily needs do not cause any problems. On the other hand, the need for additional vitamins should be planned according to the doctor's advice [24].
- **Case 5:** Prof. Vefik Arıca (Dean of Yalova University Faculty of Medicine) stated that it has been observed that families take vitamins for their children without consulting the physician. For the use of vitamins, the child must first undergo a medical examination. The use of vitamins should be started after the necessary examinations are made and which vitamin deficiency is determined. Therefore, vitamins should not be taken by self-diagnosis without consulting the physician and pharmacist. Prof. Arıca stated that during the epidemic period, the vitamins that were taken outside the control of the doctor and without consulting the pharmacist, under the counter and whose effectiveness has not been proven cause some problems. The main problem in unconscious vitamin consumption is seen in children. In unconscious use, vitamin syrup whose effectiveness has not been proven may not have completed the missing vitamin in our body. If the child has iron deficiency, learning difficulties, autism, and retardation in IQ may occur in the future. According to Prof. Arıca, the internet threats individuals' health by selling fake and dangerous medicines, vitamins, etc. [25].
- **Case 6:** Exp. Dr. Filiz Arabacı stated that due to the Coronavirus, people prefer vitamins D and C to protect their body resistance. The unconscious use of vitamins has increased during the epidemic period. However, people have chronic diseases, and unconscious use of vitamins can cause serious systemic problems. For example, unnecessary and irrespective use of vitamin D causes very serious consequences. Before using vitamin D, the blood level should be checked and if the blood level is low, vitamin D should be taken. This should be with the recommendation of the doctor. With self-diagnosis, people go directly to the pharmacy and buy vitamin D. Long-term use of vitamin D and high levels of vitamin D in the blood lead to kidney diseases, kidney stone disorders, and high blood pressure in long term [26].
- **Case 7:** Dr. Aslı Karadeniz (Maltepe University Faculty of Medicine, Infectious Diseases and Clinical Microbiology) stated that if antibiotics and other drugs are not used in the right dose and time, the body may be harmed, unexpected diseases and side effects may occur. For example, allergic reactions may occur, liver and kidney failures may occur, different drug interactions and side effects may occur. In order to prevent the negative effects of excessive, unnecessary and wrong drug use, it is necessary to use drugs at the right time and in the right way,

with the advice of a doctor. Even if there are side effects, the patient will be under control. Physicians have an important responsibility in rational drug use. Unconscious drug use may complicate the control of the disease. Stating that the treatment of cold and flu can mostly be done with rest, plenty of fluids, and simple medicines at home, Dr. Karadeniz stated that unconscious drug use can make it difficult to control the disease. Dr. Karadeniz pointed out that the drugs given in influenza infections should not be used uncontrolled and warned that vitamins should not be taken without a doctor's advice. In some cases, it is seen that patients stop taking the drug on their own [27].

- **Case 8:** The Ministry of Health announced some data on antidepressant drug use in Türkiye on February 2, 2015. Accordingly, 1 out of every 10 people in Türkiye uses antidepressants. These high rates show that there are prescriptions issued by physicians who are not in the field of mental health, drugs recommended by pharmacy staff, drugs used with "neighbor advice," and unconscious use. People may start to use drugs incorrectly, not be able to cope with drug side effects, worry, and withdraw from treatment. During the treatment process related to mental health, people cannot be patient enough and go to frequent doctor changes and frequent drug changes and can cause them to enter a vicious circle again. Sometimes, relapse or chronicity of symptoms and unresponsiveness to treatment can be seen because people stop taking the drug early without consulting their doctor as soon as their symptoms improve [28].
- **Case 9:** Prof. Abdurrahman Altındag (Gaziantep University Faculty of Medicine, Department of Psychiatry), the increase in the pace of life and competition and the weakening of social bonds have isolated people and increased the risk of depression. Psychiatric diseases have a prevalence of 10% in women and 5% in men. When they get depressed, people look for various solutions and start trying other people's drugs. Non-prescription drugs can be easily purchased from pharmacies. Unconscious use of antidepressants can lead to the worsening of the person's mental state or to the emergence of different disorders. The side effects of some drugs are not suitable for the use of the patient. Antidepressants should be used under the supervision of a doctor, in doses that he deems appropriate [29].
- **Case 10:** According to Prof. Karaduman, help should not be sought from people who are not experts in the treatment processes of the low back, neck, and joint pains. Commonly in the community, people talk about their experiences and offer mutual advice for solving illness or pain. The recommended exercises can make people physically sicker. Unconscious sports exercises can worsen the health of patients [30].
- **Case 11:** Evaluating the results of the research in the news of M. Günay from Milliyet newspaper, there is an interview with Dr. Aylin Tutgun Ünal about cyberchondria. According to Dr. Ünal, with the increase in the time spent at home during the epidemic, internet use has also increased. It has brought a new problem in the field of health to the agenda in the new media era. The prevalence of moderate cyberchondria in all generations between the ages of 18 and 75 also revealed the extent of the danger. Twenty-two percent of them stated that they

constantly searched for a disease on the internet, thinking that they had an undiagnosed disease. Unfortunately, when Gen Z realizes something about their body that they can't explain, they search for it online many times. He takes the information he obtains from the internet seriously rather than the opinion of his family doctor or specialist doctor. While researching the symptoms of the disease on the internet, he also visits forum sites where the medical conditions, symptoms, and experiences of people with the disease are discussed. In the study, it was also seen that the generations who applied to the family health center searched more diseases on the internet and were highly cyberchondria [31].

- **Case 12:** The concepts of health and disease are among the most talked about and discussed topics in the digital environment today. According to Dr. Alptekin Çetin, "Shares, comments, different treatment options and results of these treatment options have become easily accessible on the internet." However, inferences and diagnoses for serious diseases can emerge from simple symptoms. For example, a person who takes over the internet search engines for heartburn may be in a position to diagnose him with stomach cancer at the end of the day. People with symptoms of cyberchondria also have higher levels of health anxiety. People who do not receive professional help for a disease they think they have, or who do not prefer to receive it, believe that they have different health problems based on non-scientific comments on the internet based only on personal experiences [32].
- **Case 13:** Cyberchondriac disorder is a variant of hypochondriasis under the somatoform disorders. Cyberchondria disease is the state of "*trying to diagnose or treat him by searching information, documents and treatment methods on the internet about the diseases he thinks he has.*" Cyberchondriacs do not trust doctors very much. They think that the procedures are insufficient, even though they go to the hospitals many times because of their complaints. Although the physicians exhibit a compelling attitude in the examination and analysis procedures, all the examinations are normal. This situation may make them more ambitious and continue their research on the internet for self-diagnosis. They can browse forums, blogs, or even start researching foreign articles. Worst of all, the cyberchondriac person doesn't deal with just one complaint. They investigate the slightest disruption or discomfort in their bodies, often with exaggerated conclusions. However, it is natural treatments that attract the most attention of cyberchondriac patients. Because they don't trust drugs too much. They do not find it very reassuring because they always read the package inserts of the drugs. For this reason, they can also access expert-level knowledge about medicinal plants over time [33].
- **Case 14:** Çiftçi (2022) interviewed with Clinical Psychologist Cemre Ece Gökpınar about self-diagnosis. According to Gökpınar, cyberchondria increased health concerns, and people try to feel relax when searching health info on the internet without going to any expert or medical doctor. Unfortunately, digital media present many health info and some of them are very dangerous for the health of society. For example, websites that offer some natural and herbal mix-

tures cause people to try these mixtures regardless of whether they are allergic or not, and people's health is worsened [34].

- **Case 15:** Dr. Rıdvan Üney (Psychiatrist/Psychotherapist) has identified some situations related to the behavior of searching for illness on the internet. Health sites on the internet are attracting a lot of attention. When people notice a symptom of a disease in them, they first research on the internet. Some people call this behavior Google doctors. The state of being overly worried about their health is called Health Anxiety (Health Anxiety). This anxiety ranges from simple curiosity to sickness. As the health concern increases, so do searches for the disease on the internet. Now, at the slightest indication, a person spends a lot of time on the internet. This condition is called "Illustration Searching on the Internet" or "Cyberchondria." Searching for a disease on the internet can cause the following types of damage according to Dr. Üney [35]:

  (a) The person can find dozens of diseases as the cause of the slightest symptom.
  (b) While searching for illness on the internet, a person may first feel relief and then be exposed to negative information.
  (c) As people find illness, their health concerns increase.
  (d) People can access wrong disease information from their symptoms.
  (e) Although people have a simple symptom, they may have a fear that it may be fatal.
  (f) Due to the information pollution on the internet, in order to cope with his illness, he receives treatment information from sites that have no scientific basis.
  (g) Due to self-diagnosis, people apply too many vitamins or use nonsensical herbal medicines.
  (h) They shop from completely commercial sites that are not remotely related to health. They endanger their own health.

This study provides some descriptive findings based on selected cases from Turkey as below:

3.1 Descriptive Evidence

This study selected some cases related to self-diagnosis, mental health, and social media from Türkiye. Based on selected cases, some descriptive findings can be presented as below:

Table 2 presents main themes related to self-diagnosis, mental health, and social media based on Turkish cases. It can be said that experts mostly determine the link between social media and self-diagnosis by terms of "Cyberchondria, Health concern and anxiety, Internet and Social Media, Fake Treatment, Fake Medicine and Counterfeit Drug, Overdose of Vitamins and food supplement in Türkiye." Self-diagnosis is mostly related to the level of health concern and anxiety, then

Table 2 Findings about the link between self-diagnosis, mental illness, and social media from Turkish cases

Main titles	Key points
Cyberchondria	As the health concern increases, the addiction behavior of searching illness through internet increases too Cyberchondria mostly depends on health concern, and self-diagnosis is also related with cyberchondria
Health concern and anxiety	Health concerns and anxiety encourage people to search for illness or treatment through internet and social media
Internet and social media	Internet and social media make it easier to access health info for households
Fake treatment	Self-diagnosis can cause fake treatment for people
Fake medicine and counterfeit drug	The industry of fake medicine and counterfeit drug increases through self-diagnosis
Overdose of vitamins and food supplement	During the COVID-19 pandemic, people become to consume vitamins and food supplement more

Table 3 Risks of self-diagnosis through social media

Variables	Key points	The level during the COVID-19 pandemic
Fake treatment and fake diagnosis	People search some sign of a medical problem by social media and then they self-diagnose. Unfortunately, nobody knows what kinds of treatment or diagnosis will be occurred	Increase
Fake experts	During the COVID-19 pandemic, social media included higher numbers of health contents and many fake experts suggest some health recommendation for households	Increase
Fake news	Fake news increased by social media and people who mostly self-diagnosed, believed this news much more	Increase
Fake medicine consumption	Fake medicine consumption increases due to self-diagnosis, and digital media provides a huge marketplace for the fake medicine industry	Increase
Mental illness	Self-diagnosis causes mental illness such as depression or addictive	Increase
Allergies and health hazard	The consumption of overdose of vitamins and food supplements will make allergies and health hazard	Increase

cyberchondria increases based on health concerns. The vicious circle between self-diagnosis and health concern is dangerous for society's health in long term.

Table 3 shows how self-diagnosis can threaten human health in long term. Unfortunately, social media channels give many fake news and info about health issues. For example, influencers or some fake experts suggest some vitamins or organic mixture for people and people tend to believe them as they self-diagnose through social media. The COVID-19 pandemic made people more anxious about their health and self-diagnosis and cyberchondria increased.

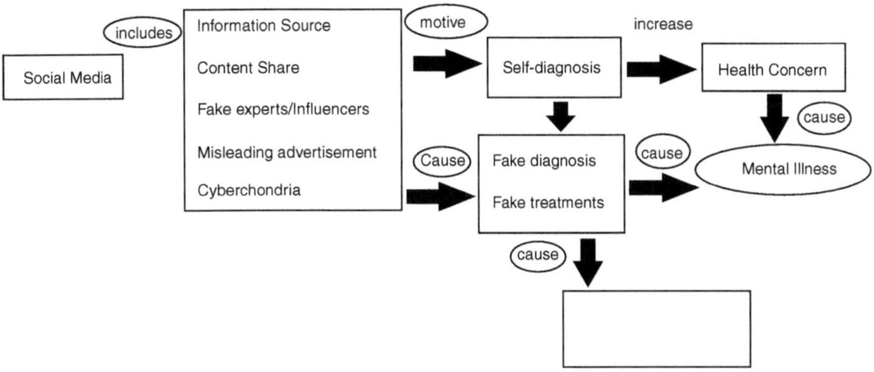

Fig. 2 A conceptual model (Source: created by author)

3.2 A Model: The Link Between Social Media Usage, Self-diagnosis, and Mental Health

As determined by the literature review and selected Turkish cases, some key points can guide for the link between social media, self-diagnosis, and mental illness. Figure 2 shows an alternative model as below:

4 Conclusion and Discussion

The COVID-19 pandemic has changed the lifestyles of people globally and almost forever when considering its effect on the rapid digital transformation. In other words, the COVID-19 pandemic has accelerated digital adaptation from younger to older. However, it has been expected that digitalized world would be the new universe for people since the beginning of twenty-first century [36, 37]. As accessing information in an easy and fast way through digital media, people challenge with over-information, too. The main trouble is finding or accessing real information from digital media channels. Unfortunately, there are lots of digital media channels and information in the digital world. In this point, self-diagnosis is another problem related to rising digitalization in recent days. In this context, this study aims to explore how the internet influences self-diagnosis by analyzing its impact on mental health. Accessible applications for physicians and specialists can deliver efficient results in healthcare. On the other hand, self-diagnosis practices used by people who are not healthcare professionals can have dangerous consequences. Therefore, it is necessary to pay attention to the use of AI-based digital health applications [4]. The internet can cause wrong diagnosis and misunderstanding by decreasing the belief in healthcare professionals [12]. Self-diagnosis can provide some benefits but digitalization has caused individuals to overuse the internet and social media channels, and accessing false information through digital channels has brought serious health problems. In particular, people can make themselves sick as a result of unconscious consumption of vitamins and supplements through self-diagnosis. Exp. Bio. Cigdem Üregen stated that when fat-soluble vitamins (vitamins A, D, E, K) are taken in excess, they cause accumulation in the body. Due to the uncontrolled usage, it causes an excess of vitamins called "hypervitaminosis" [25]. Hypervitaminosis can occur acutely and chronically. Acute hypervitaminosis occurs as a result of the use of one or more vitamins, depending on the high dose. Chronic hypervitaminosis occurs when clinical symptoms occur with a latent course. The toxicity of water-soluble and fat-soluble vitamins causes poisoning syndrome [38].

When considering the link between self-diagnosis and social media usage, it is seen that using fake drugs or overconsumption of vitamins are critical threats for sustainability of society's health in long term. The counterfeit drug market which is exceeding 300 billion dollars worldwide continues to grow day by day due to the development of social media channels. According to the 2021 data of the World Health Organization, 10–15% of the pharmaceutical market is in the hands of the counterfeit medicine market and more than one million people die every year due to counterfeit medicine [21]. During the COVID-19 pandemic, it has been seen that many people turn to vitamins and food supplements to strengthen their immune systems. Citizens started to buy vitamins through websites, not pharmacies, as they met many of their needs by shopping online due to the epidemic. However, when talking about clothes, shoes, and electronic materials, now fake vitamins are offered for sale on e-commerce platforms. Recently, the number of people complaining in consultation with their pharmacist that the vitamin they buy online is different from the ones they bought before has increased [23].

While using the internet for reliable information about mental health problems, the following may be recommended [18]:

- Information can be obtained from sites ending with the ".gov" suffix because they are supported by the federal government.
- Sites ending in ".edu" may be more reliable because they are managed by medical schools or universities.
- Information on health sites ending with ".org" may be more reliable because they are maintained by non-profit organizations.
- Articles from scientific journals or medical journals can be read.
- Diagnoses themselves can be complex. Therefore, mental health problems should not be solved by self-diagnosis alone without professional help.
- Many people who are not licensed and educated on social media present themselves as experts and give health advice. Therefore, it is important to check whether the people from whom health advice will be sought are truly experts.

While social media channels support the counterfeit drug market [1], self-diagnosis has also become a driving force for the vitamin market and other supplement markets. Economically, self-diagnosis has become a profit tool for digital platforms, but it is a threat to the sustainability of public health. As it is known, the COVID-19 pandemic has increased health concern and people tend to self-diagnose much more than ever. When considering digital transformation in health industry

[39], digitalized tools and digital media channels will be core source in the future. In this point, people should be aware of fake news [40, 41] fake medicines, fake experts [1], and fake treatments to save their health.

This study has some limitations such as data selection, case selection, sample, and methodology. Future studies can explore the impact of self-diagnosis on mental health for different countries by using different methodologies. However, this study is thought to guide future studies by giving some descriptive evidence for the link between self-diagnosis, social media, and mental health as a result of investigating Turkish cases.

Acknowledgments This study used available open access data and secondary data. Turkish references are translated into English.

References

1. Yıldırım S. The rising aesthetic concern with digitalization: qualitative evidences from Turkey. In: Mittal M, Goyal LM, editors. Predictive analytics of psychological disorders in healthcare, Lecture notes on data engineering and communications technologies, vol. 128. Singapore: Springer; 2022.
2. Öncü MA, Yıldırım S, Bostancı S, Erdoğan F. The effect of COVID-19 pandemic on health management and health services: a case of Turkey. Duzce Med J. 2021;23:61–70.
3. Yıldırım S, Bostancı SH. The efficiency of e-government portal management from a citizen perspective: evidences from Turkey. World J Sci Technol Sustain Dev. 2021;18(3):259–73.
4. Ćirković A. Evaluation of four artificial intelligence–assisted self-diagnosis apps on three diagnoses: two-year follow-up study. J Med Internet Res. 2020;22(12):e18097.
5. Bostancı S, Yıldırım S, Erdoğan F. A review on e-government portal's services within hospital information system during Covid-19 pandemic. Konuralp Med J. 2022;14:271.
6. Ayonrinde O, Michaelson S. Self-diagnosis and attitude change through the information super highway. Psychiatr Bull. 1998;22:581–3.
7. Fan X, Chao D, Zhang Z, Wang D, Li X, Tian F. Utilization of self-diagnosis health chatbots in real-world settings: case study. J Med Internet Res. 2021;23(1):e19928. https://doi.org/10.2196/19928.
8. You Y, Gui X. Self-diagnosis through AI-enabled Chatbot-based symptom checkers: user experiences and design considerations. AMIA Annu Symp Proc. 2021;2020:1354–63.
9. Nundy S, Patel KK. Self-service diagnosis of COVID-19—ready for prime time? JAMA Health Forum. 2020;1(3):e200333. https://doi.org/10.1001/jamahealthforum.2020.0333.
10. Jutel A, Baker MG, Stanley J, Huang QS, Bandaranayake D. Self-diagnosis of influenza during a pandemic: a cross-sectional survey. BMJ Open. 2011;1:e000234.
11. Mouliou DS, Pantazopoulos I, Gourgoulianis KI. Societal criticism towards COVID-19: assessing the theory of self-diagnosis contrasted to medical diagnosis. Diagnostics. 2021;11:1777.
12. Lewis LF. Exploring the experience of self-diagnosis of autism spectrum disorder in adults. Arch Psychiatr Nurs. 2016;30(2016):575–80.
13. Lanseng EJ, Andreassen TW. Electronic healthcare: a study of people's readiness and attitude toward performing self-diagnosis. Int J Serv Ind Manag. 2007;18(4):394–417.
14. Wang Y, Zhao Y, Zhang J, Bian J, Zhang R. Detecting associations between dietary supplement intake and sentiments within mental disorder tweets. Health Informatics J. 2020;26(2):803–15.
15. Sadagheyanı HE, Tatari F. Investigating the role of social media on mental health. Ment Health Soc Incl. 2021;25(1):41–51.

16. ViewPoint Center. (t.y.). The harm of self-diagnosis on social media. https://www.viewpoint-center.com/the-harm-of-self-diagnosis-on-social-media/#:~:text=Self%2Ddiagnosing%20on%20social%20media,health%20issues%2C%20like%20anxiety%20disorders.
17. Phillips L. Self-diagnosis in a digital world, counseling today, cover stories. 2022. https://ct.counseling.org/2022/03/self-diagnosis-in-a-digital-world/.
18. Warner M. A challenge with social media: self-diagnosing mental health. 2021. https://med.uth.edu/psychiatry/2021/03/26/a-challenge-with-social-media-self-diagnosing-mental-health/.
19. Fuller K. The dangers of using social media to self-diagnose a mental health disorder. 2022. https://www.akuamindbody.com/the-dangers-of-using-social-media-to-self-diagnose-a-mental-health-disorder/.
20. Murphy H. Self-diagnosis ads on TikTok blur mental health fears with reality. Financial times. 2022. https://www.ft.com/content/dd63fb93-fa81-4a29-918e-93fa06fb8c4c.
21. Elmacıoglu L. Milyarlarca dolarlık sahte ilaç pazarı dolandırıcıların iştahını kabartıyor (The billion-dollar counterfeit drug market is whetting the appetite of fraudsters). 2022. https://www.indyturk.com/node/466491/sa%C4%9Flik/milyarlarca-dolarl%C4%B1k-sahte-ila%C3%A7-pazar%C4%B1-doland%C4%B1r%C4%B1c%C4%B1lar%C4%B1n-i%C5%9Ftah%C4%B1n%C4%B1-kabart%C4%B1yor.
22. Erdemir F. İnternetten ölümüne ticaret: Sahte ilaç satışı patladı (Online trading to the death: Counterfeit drug sales explode). 2021. https://www.tgrthaber.com.tr/gundem/internetten-olumune-ticaret-sahte-ilac-satisi-patladi-2800360.
23. DHA. Uzmanlar uyarıyor… İnternetten alınan vitamin ve gıda takviyeleri sahte olabilir. (Experts warn… Vitamin and food supplements bought online can be fake). 2021. https://www.cnnturk.com/saglik/uzmanlar-uyariyor-internetten-alinan-vitamin-ve-gida-takviyeleri-sahte-olabilir?page=1.
24. CNN. Türk.com. Fazla vitamin kullanımı ne gibi sorunlara yol açıyor? (What kind of problems does excessive vitamin use cause?). 2022. https://www.cnnturk.com/saglik/fazla-vitamin-kullanimi-ne-gibi-sorunlara-yol-aciyor?page=1.
25. Küçük E. Çocuklara bilinçsiz vitamin kullandırılmamalı (Children should not be given unconscious vitamins). 2021. https://www.aa.com.tr/tr/saglik/cocuklara-bilincsiz-vitamin-kullandirilmamali/2411525#:~:text=%22Bilin%C3%A7siz%20kullan%C4%B1mda%2C%20etkinli%C4%9Fi%20kan%C4%B1tlanmam%C4%B1%C5%9F%20bir,geli%C5%9Fiminde%20s%C4%B1k%C4%B1nt%C4%B1%20varsa%20onlar%20geli%C5%9Fmeyecek.
26. İHA. Bilinçsiz kullanılan vitaminler çok ciddi sağlık sorunlarına yol açabilir (Unconsciously used vitamins can cause very serious health problems). 2020. https://www.hurriyet.com.tr/aile/bilincsiz-kullanilan-vitaminler-cok-ciddi-saglik-sorunlarina-yol-acabilir-41671525.
27. Kara K. Bilinçsiz ilaç kullanımı daha çok hasta ediyor (Unconscious drug use makes more patients sick). 2019. https://www.aa.com.tr/tr/saglik/bilincsiz-ilac-kullanimi-daha-cok-hasta-ediyor/1687431#:~:text=olumsuzluklar%C4%B1%20%C5%9F%C3%B6yle%20anlatt%C4%B1%3A-,%22Fazla%20ve%20gereksiz%20ila%C3%A7%20kullan%C4%B1m%C4%B1n%C4%B1n%20istenmeyen%20etkileri%20olabilir.,ila%C3%A7%20etkile%C5%9Fimleri%2C%20yan%20etkileri%20olabilir.
28. https://arzuerkan.com/depresyon-sikligindaki-artis-nedenleri-yetersiz-uygunsuz-ilac-kullanimi/.
29. Haber 7. Bilinçsiz antidepresan kullanmayın (Do not use unconscious antidepressants). 2012. https://www.haber7.com/saglik/haber/839359-bilincsiz-antidepresan-kullanmayin.
30. Zobar G. Bilinçsiz tedavi ve egzersizler büyük sağlık sorunlarına yol açıyor (Unconscious treatment and exercises cause major health problems). 2017. https://www.aa.com.tr/tr/saglik/bilincsiz-tedavi-ve-egzersizler-buyuk-saglik-sorunlarina-yol-aciyor/821586.
31. Ntv.com.tr. İnternetten hastalık arama hastalığı: Siberkondri (En çok Z kuşağı başvuruyor). (The disease of searching for a disease on the Internet: Cyberchondria (The Z generation is mostly applying)). 2020. https://www.ntv.com.tr/teknoloji/internetten-hastalik-arama-hastaligi-siberkondri-en-cok-z-kusagi-basvuruyor,yYGx6QJpNk6F_A_dfhPgwA.

32. Milliyet.com. İnternetten hastalık araştırıp kendine tanı koyma: Siberkondri (Searching for a disease on the Internet and self-diagnosing: Cyberchondria). n.d. https://www.milliyet.com.tr/pembenar/internetten-hastalik-arastirip-kendine-tani-koyma-siberkondri-6541584.
33. Yavuz M. İnternet hastalık hastalığı, siberhondrik bozukluk (Internet sickness sickness, cyberchondric disorder). 2021. https://www.haberler.com/yazarlar/dr-mehmet-yavuz/internet-hastalik-hastaligi-siberhondrik-bozukluk-617/.
34. Çiftçi MY. İnternette hastalık teşhisi hasta ediyor (Internet diagnosis is sickening). 2022. https://www.trthaber.com/haber/saglik/internette-hastalik-teshisi-hasta-ediyor-689863.html.
35. Hürriyet. Yaşadığınız sağlık sorunlarına internetten bakıp teşhis koymayın (Do not diagnose your health problems by looking at the internet). 2020. https://www.hurriyet.com.tr/aile/yasadiginiz-saglik-sorunlarina-internetten-bakip-teshis-koymayin-429926.
36. Yildirim S, Demirtas I, Yildirim DC. A review of alternative economic approaches to achieve sustainable development: the rising digitalization and degrowth post COVID-19. In: Castanho R, editor. Handbook of research on sustainable development goals, climate change, and digitalization. Hershey: IGI Global; 2022. p. 288–307.
37. Yıldırım S, Bostancı S. A qualitative approach to developments in the digital economy during the impact of Covid-19 crisis. J Emerg Econ Policy. 2022;7(1):32–44.
38. Roop JK. Hypervitaminosis—an emerging pathological condition. Int J Health Sci Res. 2018;8(10):280–8.
39. Mittal M, Kaur I, Pandey SC, Verma A, Goyal LM. Opinion mining for the tweets in healthcare sector using fuzzy association rule. EAI Endorsed Trans Pervasive Health Technol. 2019;4(16):e2.
40. Agarwal A, Mittal M, Pathak P, Goyal LM. Fake news detection using a blend of neural networks: an application of deep learning. SN Comput Sci. 2020;1:143.
41. Aggarwal A, Chauhan A, Kumar D, Mittal M, Verma S. Classification of fake news by fine-tuning deep bidirectional transformers based language model. EAI Endorsed Trans Scalable Inform Syst. 2020;7(27):e10.

Relationship Between Mortality and Mental Health Disorders

Aarti K. Thakre, Nitin G. Dumore, and Monali N. Dumore

Abstract Background: The potential value of comprehending extra mortality among individuals with mental illnesses. It is unknown how professionally determined mental illnesses affect mortality. The major causes of impairment worldwide are severe mental diseases. With ageing, their prevalence decreases, probably as a result of early mortality. However, it is unknown whether those with serious mental problems who live longer still have shorter life expectancies than their peers and whether their causes of death are different.

Aim: To investigate the relationship between mental illnesses and cause-specific mortality.

Method: Data sources—Our search method includes terms for mortality, particular diagnoses (such as schizophrenia, depression, anxiety, and bipolar disorder), and mental disorders. In order to find articles that cited acceptable articles, we also used Google Scholar. We observed the several mortality rate (SMR) on Tamil Nadu in 2011–2015. The total number of several mental disorders (SMD) patients, their sociodemographic characteristics, their alive/dead status, and the reason of death were recorded. For the calculation of SMR, which is determined by the formula, observed deaths/expected deaths, we utilized the crude death rates (CDR) for rural Tamil Nadu from 2011 to 2015 as a reference.

Result: The figures are astounding. In low-income countries, there are at least a billion people suffering from mental illness, of whom roughly 75% go untreated. Every year, 3–4 billion people die as a result of drug abuse. One suicide happens every 40 s. The SMR of SMD patients in Tamil Nadu was 3.33, 2.76, 2.11, 1.91, and 1.89 between 2011 and 2015. Out of the 74 deaths that occurred overall over these 5 years, 62 (83.7%) were caused by natural causes, and 12.2% were suicides. Age, education, and marital status between SMD patients who were living and died

---

A. K. Thakre (✉) · N. G. Dumore
Dadasaheb Balpande College of Diploma in Pharmacy, Nagpur, Maharashtra, India
e-mail: dbcdip.office@gmail.com

M. N. Dumore
Dadasaheb Balpande College of Pharmacy, Nagpur, Maharashtra, India

G. Battineni et al. (eds.), *Computational Methods in Psychiatry*,
https://doi.org/10.1007/978-981-99-6637-0_11

differed statistically significantly. The aggregated relative risk of mortality among people with mental illnesses for all causes of death was 2.22.

Conclusion: According to these data, mental disorders affect mortality. The significance of mental illnesses in avoidable death has to be better taken into account in efforts to assess and manage the global burden of sickness. An enhanced risk of mortality is linked to mental illnesses including schizophrenia and depression and patients with SMD showed nearly two times higher the mortality, according to our findings.

Keywords Schizophrenia · Suicide · Depression · Several mortality rate (SMR) · Several mental disorders (SMD) · Crude death rates (CDR)

Abbreviations

CDR	Crude death rate
CI	Confidential interval
PANSS	Positive and negative syndrome scale
SHR	Sub-hazard ratio
SMD	Several mental disorders
SMR	Several mortality rate

1 Introduction

Researchers have consistently found that as compared to the general population, those with mental problems had higher mortality rates. In New York, the death rate among psychiatric inpatients was higher than the average [1]. Since then, additional research and evaluations on the mortality risks of people with a range of mental disorders 2–6 and particular diagnoses have been done [1] (e.g., schizophrenia [2], depression [3, 4], and bipolar disorder [5]). Mortality risk is higher in psychiatric patient. The danger of passing away too soon is increased by psychiatric diagnoses in and of itself [6]. Alcohol-related disorders are more prevalent in men [7]. Excessive mortality is linked to anxiety or panic disorder [7, 8]. An increased risk of dying from cardiovascular disease is associated with neurotic depression [9]. Establishing the importance of mental problems as indicators of disease-specific mortality was our goal.

Mentally ill persons typically pass away earlier than those who are not. A study on the Danish population revealed that people with mental illnesses pass away 7 and 10 years earlier than people who are otherwise of similar age and sex. People who have various mental problems (such as mood disorders, schizophrenia, etc.) are more likely to die young and have shorter life spans overall [10, 11].

Globally, men, women, and children are all affected by mental diseases. Early-onset intellectual disability and diseases of the autistic spectrum increase the chance of mental illnesses, which also persists into old ages with schizophrenia, depressive disorders, and anxiety disorders [12]. According to recent research from study on the global burden of disease, mental and addiction illnesses contributed to 7% of the total global burden of disease as assessed by disability [13]. Disability was present for 19% of all years lived and adjusted life-years.

Given that a number of biological, psychological, and social elements appear to be involved, the relationship between mortality and several mental disorders SMD is complex. Because of the handicap they cause rather than the mortality, mental disorders are one of the leading causes of the global burden of diseases [14, 15]. Mortality in SMD is more to 2–3.5 than the general population, according to the majority of systematic reviews [16, 17]. Furthermore, recent data suggests that this difference is widening. The majority of deaths are caused by physical health conditions, particularly cancer, respiratory and cardiovascular diseases [18]. One of the main non-natural causes of mortality for those with serious mental illness is suicide. Other elements like drug use, disregard for medication instructions, ignorance of the need for medical attention, and discrimination may also be important [19]. The risk factors for excess mortality among SMD were divided by the World Health Organization with three categories: personal characteristics, health system issues, and social determinants of health. Few researches have looked at death as an outcome, despite the fact that several studies from India have looked at the long-term clinical and functional outcomes [14, 15] of people with SMD. Even current research on SMDs like bipolar disease and depression with psychotic symptoms is limited to schizophrenia [20].

Around the world, mental and drug use problems are the main factors contributing to years spent disabled [21]. Furthermore, there is proof that those with severe mental illnesses have life expectancies lower than those of the general population [9], primarily as a result of the high rate of cardiovascular deaths, respiratory illnesses, and suicide [3, 4, 9, 22]. The underlying causes of the high mortality from cardiovascular and respiratory disorders are less evident, even if suicide could be seen as a direct result of severe mental illness [1].

2 Material and Method

2.1 *Thirthahalli Is a Taluk of Shimoga District of Karnataka*

2.1.1 Indicators of the Mortality Rate in Karnataka for Schizophrenia Include

The state of Karnataka serves as the administrative hub for the majority of villages and towns [23]. According to the 2011 Census, the town has a population of 14,357, and the Taluk as a whole has 141,453 residents. Patients who live in communities throughout the entire taluk served as the study's subjects. Case identification specifics are covered elsewhere. In a nutshell, the study team used the key informant approach for this goal with assistance from the local health authority. Once a patient has been identified, a skilled psychiatrist will evaluate them and confirm the diagnosis using a mini-international neuropsychiatric interview [24]. The annual rate of

Table 1 Number of incidents between 2005 and 2012

Year	No. of cases
2005	94
2006	225
2007	270
2008	290
2009	310
2010	330
2011	350
2012	370

recruitment grew throughout the first 2 years before beginning to stabilize (Table 1). Each patient is given medication after being diagnosed, coupled with psychoeducation for the patient and their family. There isn't any organized psychological intervention available. Patients and families are encouraged to stay under the study team's care or seek out other mental health specialists of their choosing. With the use of correspondence via letters, telephone calls, and home visits, every effort is being made to maintain the patients under routine follow-up.

Indian Disability Assessment and Evaluation Scale (IDEAS; Rehabilitation Committee of the Indian Psychiatric Society, 2002) [25] and Positive and Negative Syndrome Scale (PANSS) [26] are administered once every 6 months to evaluate the severity of the symptoms and the disability, respectively, during follow-up visits along with the routine assessments. All information is useful in determining how death is related to mental illnesses.

According to Mini-Finland Health Survey, a prior study measured the health status, morbidity, and healthcare needs of Finns aged 30 or older. The conditions that were picked as the primary focus were those that prevented people from working most frequently: mental illnesses, illnesses of the musculoskeletal system and connective tissue, ailments of the cardiovascular and respiratory systems.

The diseases that were selected as the primary targets were those that frequently result in working impairment, including conditions of the cardiovascular and pulmonary systems, mental illnesses, and conditions of the musculoskeletal and connective tissue systems [13].

2.1.2 Participants

Patients with SMD were included in the investigation. Patients with schizophrenia, bipolar disease, or depression with psychotic symptoms are included in this definition of SMD.

As and when deaths occur, the study team continuously updates the data regarding mortality. Accessible medical data and information from family members indicate the cause of death. Only with the family members' permission does this process of investigating the specifics of death take place. For the purposes of this study, we

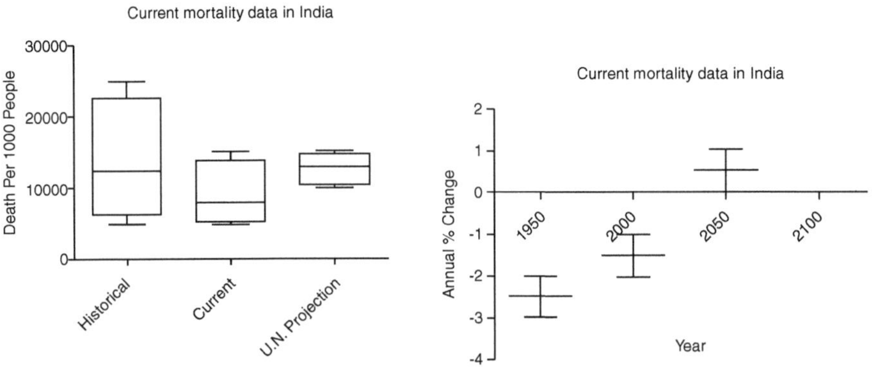

Fig. 1 Current mortality data in IndГia

considered the patient population from 2009 to 2011 when the cohort's patient count stabilized.

2.1.3 Mortality Data

Statistics on mortality were collected from participants and their families for SMD patients, and data was updated as soon as a death was reported. The cause of death was established by the family member interview and further supporting evidence provided by the family members. Hospital records were also used when they were accessible.

Figure 1 displays drop in mortality rates from the previous year in India. The family member interview, additional supporting information offered by the family members and hospital data all helped to establish the below-average death rate [27]. MLA. India Death Rate 1950–2023. www.macrotrends.net. Retrieved 30 Jan 2023.

3 Results

Seventy-four patients died in the patient population between 2011 and 2015. Regarding the SMRs for these years individually, (Table 2) is displayed. SMD's SMR varied from 3.33 in 2011 to 2.76 in 2012 to 2.11 in 2013 to 1.91 in 2014 to 1.89 in 2015. Details about patient mortality are included in (Table 3), which shows that between 2011 and 2015, 83% of deaths were due to natural causes and 18% were not. The majority of deaths from non-natural causes were caused by successful suicide. The average SMR over the course of the 4 years was 2.4, showing a two-fold increased death rate for individuals with SMD. 12.2% of the total patient population die by suicide each year. The correlation between the sociodemographic characteristics and the patients' mortality rates during a 4-year period is shown in

Table 2 South India's mortality ratio for mental illnesses from 2011 to 2015

Year	Total no. of patient with SMR	Crude death rate/1000 population	Expected death	Observed death	SMR
2011	122	8.1	0.9	3	3.33
2012	714	8.2	5.8	16	2.76
2013	1117	8.2	9.4	19	2.11
2014	1168	8.1	9.5	18	1.91
2015	1244	7.6	9.0	18	1.89

SMR Several Mortality Ratio

Table 3 Patients with serious mental illnesses are more likely to die from certain conditions and at what rates

Cause of death	*n* (%)
Natural	62 (83.7)
Unnatural	
Accidental	3 (4.1)
Suicide	9 (12.2)

Table 4 Mortality rates among people with serious mental illnesses and sociodemographic factors

Variables	Alive, *n* (%)	Dead, *n* (%)	*P* (Chi-square test/*t*-test)
Age, Mean (±SD)	42.72 ± 12.36	52.50 ± 16.66	< 0.001
Gender			0.447
Male	643 (51.7)	42 (56.8)	
Female	583 (48.3)	32 (43.2)	

(Table 4). Age, education, and marital status categories, but not gender, statistically distinguish the two groups differently. The mean age of SMD patients who passed away was 52.5, as opposed to 42.72 for those who are still alive. The education span (measured in years) for the former group was 4.82, but it was 6.64 for the patients who are still living. The patients who were still alive had received their education earlier and for a longer period of time than the patients who had passed away.

According to the presence of a severe mental disorder, Fig. 2 displays the percentage of participants who were still alive during follow-up. In comparison to their counterparts, males with serious mental disorders had a shortened life expectancy of 2.8 years (95% confidence interval (CI) = 2.6, 3.0) and an age-adjusted mortality hazard ratio of 2.3 (95% CI = 2.2, 2.4). For men with schizophrenia spectrum, bipolar, depressive, and alcohol-induced disorders, respectively, age-adjusted life expectancy was lowered on average by 2.0 (95% CI = 1.6, 2.3), 1.1 (95% CI = 0.4, 1.9), 2.8 (95% CI = 2.6, 3.1), and 3.1 (2.8, 3.4) years, respectively. The mortality risk linked with any serious mental condition remained virtually unchanged for men who passed away within the first 2 years of follow-up.

For men who had previously been diagnosed with schizophrenia spectrum disorder (Schizophrenia-S), bipolar disorder, depression, or disorders brought on by alcohol, the age-adjusted mortality hazards were 2.0 (95% CI = 1.8, 2.2), 1.5 (95%

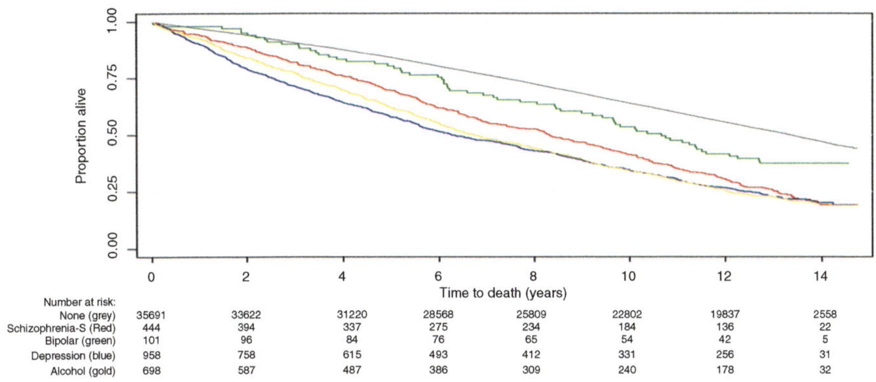

Fig. 2 Sample of older men with or without mental health condition survived up to the period of 14.5 years

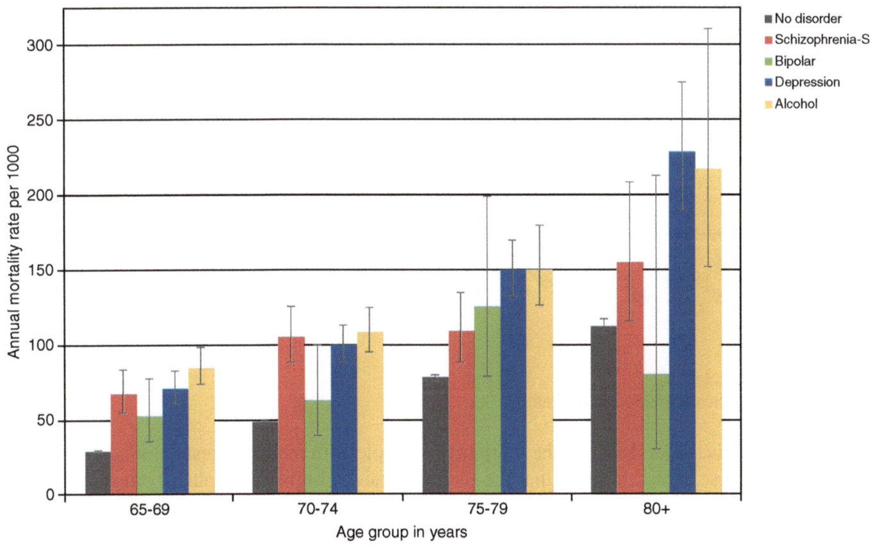

Fig. 3 According to their age category at the time of inclusion, the bars display the mortality rate per 1000 person-years for older men with and without serious mental illnesses

CI = 1.2, 1.9), 2.3 (95% CI = 2.1, 2.5), and 2.6 (95% CI = 2.4, 2.8). https://doi.org/10.1371/journal.pone.0111882.g001.

To determine their death rates for age groups (65–69, 70–74, 75–79, and 80+). The findings of these analyses are presented in Fig. 3 according to the presence of a serious mental condition prior to randomization [28]. A serious mental disorder was consistently associated with a greater annual mortality rate for men than it was for those without it. There were only 6 males with bipolar disorder in this sample, therefore the estimate of the mortality rate for those over 80 was not exact.

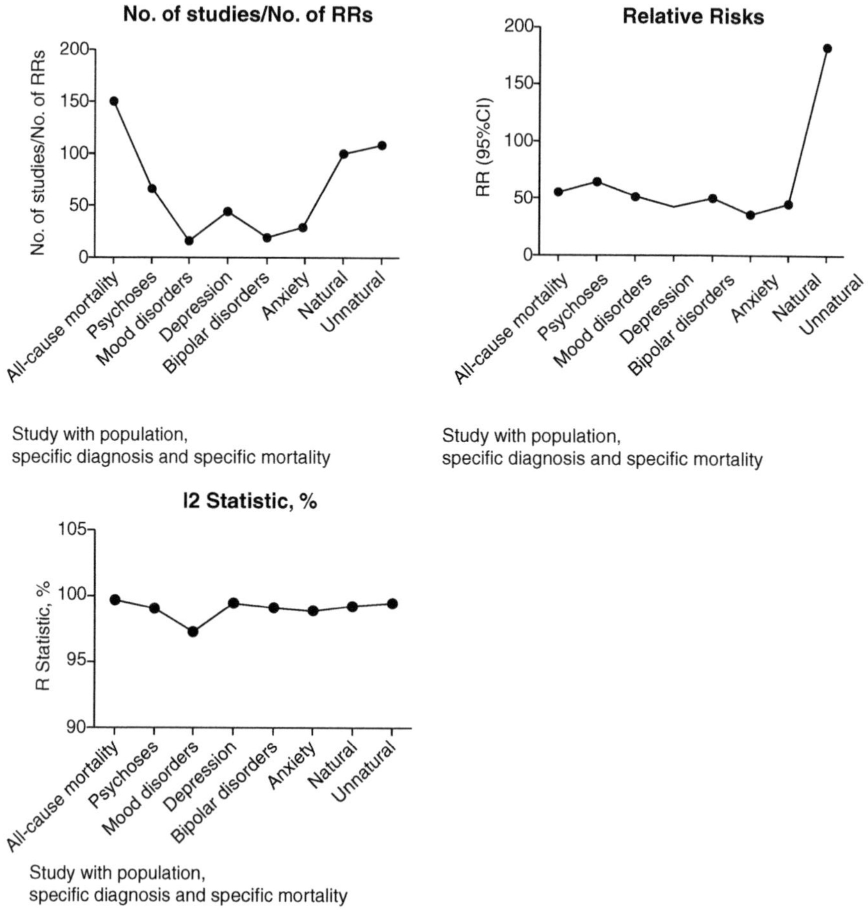

Fig. 4 149 relative risks (RRs) on the mortality of people with mental illnesses for all-cause mortality. 135 of these research found that the mortality rate is higher than other comparator group (Fig. 4) [7].

The 95% confidence intervals for the mean rate are shown by whiskers. Schizophrenia-S: illnesses on the schizophrenia spectrum. The standard deviation was 4.2 and the range from 1 day to 14.7 years, with the mean time to event (death or end of follow-up) being 10.1 years. https://doi.org/10.1371/journal.pone.0111882.g002.

Compares participants' causes of death between those who had and did not have a severe mental condition. Men who had previously been diagnosed with schizophrenia spectrum disorders had higher rates of mortality from diseases such infections, cardiovascular disease, chronic respiratory conditions, mental problems brought on by drugs, diseases of the nervous system, and other conditions. This group did not include any suicides. In comparison to controls, men with a history of bipolar disorder died more often from chronic bronchitis, euthanasia, and psychological disorders (including substance-induced). Men with depression had higher rates of suicide and other fatal causes, as well as cancer, cardiovascular disease, chronic respiratory illnesses, and diseases of the central nervous system. Last but not least, males who had previously been diagnosed with an alcohol-induced problem died more frequently than those without a serious mental illness [28].

Based on competing risks regression models, the risk of particular causes of mortality according to the four severe mental disorder groups (schizophrenia spectrum, bipolar, depression, and alcohol-induced) was examined. These models examine the incident. When competing occurrences are present and prevent the occurrence

Table 5 Death causes for older men with and without significant mental problems over a 14-year period

	No severe mental disorder	Schizophrenia-S	Bipolar	Depression	Alcohol
	N = 35691	*N* = 444	*N* = 101	*N* = 958	*N* = 698
	n (%)	*n* (%)	*n* (%)	*n* (%)	*n* (%)
Cause of death	1 (Reference)	SHR (95% CI)	SHR (95% CI)	SHR (95% CI)	SHR (95% CI)
Alive	17750 (49.7)	101(22.7)	38 (37.6)	211 (22.0)	148 (21.2)
Infection	222 (0.6)	7 (1.6)	0	9 (0.9)	9 (1.3)
		2.4 (1.1, 5.1)	–	1.5 (0.8, 2.9)	2.0 (1.0, 3.9)
Cancer	5976 (16.7)	61 (13.7)	11 (10.9)	185 (19.3)	143 (20.5)
		0.8 (0.6,1.0)	0.6 (0.3, 1.1)	1.2 (1.0, 1.4)	1.2 (1.0,1.5)
Cardiovascular disease	6160 (17.3)	118 (26.6)	23 (22.8)	254 (26.5)	185 (26.5)
		1.6 (1.3, 1.9)	1.4 (0.9, 2.1)	1.6 (1.4, 1.9)	1.6 (1.4, 1.9)
Chronic respiratory disease	1634 (4.6)	44 (9.9)	10 (9.9)	102 (10.6)	86 (12.3)
		2.1 (1.6, 2.9)	2.2 (1.2, 4.1)	2.4 (2.0, 2.9)	2.8 (2.2, 3.4)
Substances induced, mental disorders	432 (1.2)	22 (4.9)	5 (4.9)	14 (1.5)	13 (1.9)
		3.7 (2.4, 5.7)	4.2 (1.7, 10.4)	1.1 (0.7, 1.9)	1.5 (0.9, 2.6)
Nervous system including dementia	702 (2.0)	33 (7.4)	1 (1.0)	44 (4.6)	14 (2.0)
		3.7 (2.6, 5.2)	0.5 (0.1, 3.5)	2.3 (1.7, 3.1)	1.0 (0.6, 1.7)
Suicide	78 (0.2)	0	2 (2.0)	7 (0.7)	1 (0.1)
		–	8.6 (2.1, 35.0)	3.6 (1.7, 7.9)	0.6 (0.1,4.4)
Accidents	249 (0.7)	5 (1.1)	1 (1.0)	7 (0.7)	7 (1.0)
		1.5 (0.6, 3.7)	1.4 (0.2, 10.0)	1.0 (0.5,2.2)	1.4 (0.7, 2.9)
Other	2488 (7.0)	53 (11.9)	10 (9.9)	125 (13.0)	92 (13.2)
		1.7 (1.3, 2.2)	1.4 (0.8, 2.7)	2.0 (1.6, 2.4)	1.6 (1.5, 2.4)

SHR Sub Hazards Ratio from comparing risk regression, *Schizophrenia-S* schizophrenia spectrum disorders, *95%CI* 95% confidence interval of the sub-hazard ratio. https://doi.org/10.1371/journal.pone.0111882.t001 [28]

of the event of interest (for example, death from cardiovascular disease) (e.g., death from cancer, death from a respiratory disease, etc.). In this instance, the risk estimates are expressed as a sub-hazard ratio (SHR) [28] (Table 5).

4 Discussion

According to the study mentioned above, patients with schizophrenia have a significantly higher mortality rate in rural South Indian communities. Patients died 40–116% more frequently overall.

There were 12 total fatalities among the patient population between 2009 and 2011. The information on the SMRs for each of these years is provided in Table 6. Information on the causes of patient mortality is provided in Table 7. These show that for the years 2009, 2010, and 2011, the percentage excess of mortality in patients was 44, 78, and 116, respectively, compared to the mortality experience of the general population. The average SMR over the course of the 3 years was 179.48, which indicates that schizophrenia patients had a roughly two-fold increased death rate.

A noteworthy fact was that 33.3% of patient had died by suicide. Three of them had very little social support; aside from their immediate family members, they had no other source of money or emotional support.

In other words, the patients' mortality rate ranged from 1.42 to 2.16. In wealthy nations with as to be expected top-notch medical and other treatment resources, the SMR for schizophrenia is reported to be 2.8. We had anticipated a significantly

Table 6 Evidence on the 2009–2011 standardized mortality ratios

Year	Total number of cases (patient with schizophrenia)	Crude death rate (CDR) × per 1000 expected death	Expected death	Observed death	Standardized mortality ratio
2009	301	6.9	2.08	3	144.1
2010	317	7.1	2.25	4	177.2
2011	325	7.1	2.31	5	216.4

Table 7 Details regarding cause of death

Causes of death	Frequency
Medical	6 (50)
Suicidal	4 (3.33)
Accidental	1 (8.3)
Unknown	1 (8.3)
Total	12

[a] Medical cause included heart, lung, kidney, and other infections, severe anemia, and other factors (one cause for each patient)

higher SMR for patients, especially for patients living in rural communities, in a nation like India where the treatment gap can reach up to 80%. Although the data show significantly higher patient mortality rates, it should be highlighted that SMR is far lower when compared to wealthy nations. The observation that schizophrenia results are comparatively better in India is further supported by this problem.

In this significant sample of older males from a representative population, the prevalence of severe mental illnesses was 5.8%. 1.2% of people had schizophrenia spectrum disorders, 0.3% had bipolar illness, 2.5% had depression, and 1.8% had disorders brought on by alcohol. Males with serious mental disorders had a mortality risk ratio that was 2.3 times higher than men without significant mental health issues. Age-related increases in mortality rates were accompanied by a roughly consistent difference in rates between males with and without a history of serious mental illness. Our data also revealed that men with severe mental illnesses who volunteered to participate in a clinical examination had various educational, sociodemographic, lifestyle, and clinical backgrounds, even if these factors were insufficient to fully account for the population's increased mortality. Patients' mortality rates for schizophrenia are significantly higher, increasing by 40–116%.

Availability of Data On request, the corresponding author will provide the data that back up the study's conclusions.

Financial Support and Sponsorship Nil.

Conflicts of Interest There are no conflicts of interest.

References

1. Walker ER, McGee RE, Druss BG. Mortality in mental disorders and global disease burden implications. JAMA Psychiatry. 2015;72(4):334–41.
2. Saha S, Chant D, McGrath J. A systematic review of mortality in schizophrenia: is the differential mortality gap worsening over time? Arch Gen Psychiatry. 2007;64:1123–31.
3. Cuijpers P, Smit F. Excess mortality in depression: a meta-analysis of community studies. J Affect Disord. 2002;72(3):227–36.
4. Cuijpers P, Vogelzangs N, Twisk J, Kleiboer A, Li J, Penninx BW. Comprehensive meta-analysis of excess mortality in depression in the general community versus patients with specific illnesses. Am J Psychiatry. 2014;171(4):453–62.
5. Roshanaei-Moghaddam B, Katon W. Premature mortality from general medical illnesses among persons with bipolar disorder: a review. Psychiatr Serv. 2009;60:147–56.
6. Rorsman B, Hagnell O, Lanke J. Mortality in the Lundby study. Natural death in different forms of mental disorder in a total population investigated during a 25-year period. Neuropsychobiology. 1982;8:188–97. https://doi.org/10.1159/000117898.
7. Ojesjo L, Hagnell O, Otterbeck L. Mortality in alcoholism among men in the Lundby community cohort, Sweden: a forty-year follow-up. J Stud Alcohol. 1998;59:140–5. https://doi.org/10.15288/jsa.1998.59.140.
8. Grasbeck A, Rorsman B, Hagnell O, et al. Mortality of anxiety syndromes in a normal population. The Lundby study. Neuropsychobiology. 1996;33:118–26. https://doi.org/10.1159/000119261.

9. Aromaa A, Raitasalo R, Reunanen A, et al. Depression and cardiovascular diseases. Acta Psychiatr Scand Suppl. 1994;377:77–82. https://doi.org/10.1111/j.1600-0447.1994.tb05807.
10. Lawrence D, Almeida OP, Hulse GK, Jablensky AV, Holman CD. Suicide and attempted suicide among older adults in Western Australia. Psychol Med. 2000;30:813–21.
11. Lawrence D, Kisely S, Pais J. The epidemiology of excess mortality in people with mental illness. Can J Psychiatry. 2010;55:752–60.
12. Rehm J, Shield KD. Global burden of disease and the impact of mental and addictive disorders. Curr Psychiatry Rep. 2019;21(2):10.
13. Vigo D, Thornicroft G, Atun R. Estimating the true global burden of mental illness. Lancet Psychiatry. 2016;3(2):171–8. https://doi.org/10.1016/S2215-0366(15)00505-2.
14. Raghavan V, Rao S, Kulandesu A, Karthick S, Gunaselvi S, Senthilkumar S, Rao K, John S, Thara R. Mortality among patients with severe mental disorders from a rural community in South India. Indian Social Psychiatry. 2021;37(4):418–22.
15. Liu NH, Daumit GL, Dua T, Aquila R, Charlson F, Cuijpers P, et al. Excess mortality in persons with severe mental disorders: a multilevel intervention framework and priorities for clinical practice, policy and research agendas. World Psychiatry. 2017;16:30–40.
16. Ringen PA, Engh JA, Birkenaes AB, Dieset I, Andreassen OA. Increased mortality in schizophrenia due to cardiovascular disease—a non-systematic review of epidemiology, possible causes, and interventions. Front Psychiatry. 2014;5:137.
17. Walker ER, McGee RE, Druss BG. Mortality in mental disorders and global disease burden implications: a systematic review and meta-analysis. JAMA Psychiatry. 2015;72:334–41.
18. Joukamaa M, Heliovaara M, Knekt P, Aromaa A, Raitasalo R, et al. Mental disorders and cause-specific mortality. Br J Psychiatry. 2001;179:498–502.
19. Kondo S, Kumakura Y, Kanehara A, Nagato D, Ueda T, Matsuoka T, et al. Premature deaths among individuals with severe mental illness after discharge from long-term hospitalisation in Japan: a naturalistic observation during a 24-year period. BJPsych Open. 2017;3:193–5.
20. Thirthalli J, Venkatesh BK, Kishorekumar KV, Arunachala U, Venkatasubramanian G, Subbakrishna DK, et al. Prospective comparison of course of disability in antipsychotic-treated and untreated schizophrenia patients. Acta Psychiatr Scand. 2009;119:209–17.
21. Almeida OP, Alfonso H, Pirkis J, Kerse N, Sim M, et al. A practical approach to assess depression risk and to guide risk reduction strategies in later life. Int Psychogeriatr. 2011;23:280–91.
22. Stumbrys D, Jasilionis D, Pūras D. The burden of mental health-related mortality in the Baltic States in 2007-2018. BMC Public Health. 2022;22:1776.
23. Government of Tamil Nadu. Birth and death registrars under civil registration system in Tamil Nadu; 2020. https://tn.data.gov.in/catalog/birthanddeathregistrarsundercivilregistration-systemtamilnadu#web_catalog_tabs_block_10. Accessed 18 Aug 2020.
24. Bagewadi VI, Naveen Kumar C, Thirthalli J, Rao GN, Suresha KK, Gangadhar BN. Standardized mortality ratio in patients with schizophrenia—findings from Thirthahalli: a rural south Indian community. Indian J Psychol Med. 2016;38(3):202–6.
25. Indian Disability Assessment and Evaluation Scale. Rehabilitation Committee of Indian Psychiatric Society. 2002.
26. Kay SR, Fiszbein A, Opler LA. The positive and negative syndrome scale (PANSS) for schizophrenia. Schizophr Bull. 1987;13:261–76.
27. Meh C, Sharma A, Ram U, Fadel S, Correa N, Snelgrove JW, Shah P, Begum R, Shah M, Hana T, Fu SH, Raveendran L, Mishra B, Jha P. Trends in maternal mortality in India over two decades in nationally representative surveys. BJOG, 2022;129(4):550–61.
28. Almeida OP, Hankey GJ, Yeap BB, Golledge J, Norman PE, Flicker L. Mortality among people with severe mental disorders who reach old age: a longitudinal study of a community-representative sample of 37,892 men. PLoS One. 2014;9(10):e111882. https://doi.org/10.1371/journal.pone.0111882. PMID: 25360781; PMCID: PMC4216120.

Recent Developments in the Application of Computer-Aided Drug Design in Neurodegenerative Disorders

Kunal Bhattacharya, Biswajit Devanath, Dibyajyoti Das, Nongmaithem Randhoni Chanu, and Atanu Bhattacharjee

Abstract Alzheimer's disease, amyotrophic lateral sclerosis, Parkinson's disease, and Huntington's disease are all examples of neurodegenerative disorders (NDs), which currently do not have a treatment that can reverse their progression. These diseases have an effect on the lives of millions of people all around the world. Researchers from all around the world are facing a tremendous challenge when it comes to the development of medicines that might fulfill this unfulfilled therapeutic requirement. The huge number of possible ligands that need to be examined in biological assays can be reduced by using computer-aided drug design (CADD) methodologies, which in turn reduces the amount of money, time, and effort that is required to generate novel drugs. In this chapter, we provide an introduction to CADD and analyzed the progress that has been achieved in using CADD and other forms of computational studies for NDs. Additionally, we will discuss some of the challenges that have been encountered in this line of research. We offer an up-to-date assessment of prospective therapy targets for a variety of NDs.

Keywords Neurodegeneration · Drug discovery · CADD · Alzheimer's disease · Parkinson's disease · Huntington's disease · Amyotrophic lateral sclerosis

K. Bhattacharya (✉)
Pratiksha Institute of Pharmaceutical Sciences, Guwahati, Assam, India

Royal School of Pharmacy, The Assam Royal Global University, Guwahati, Assam, India
e-mail: kunal@pratiksha-edu.in

B. Devanath · D. Das
Pratiksha Institute of Pharmaceutical Sciences, Guwahati, Assam, India

N. R. Chanu
Pratiksha Institute of Pharmaceutical Sciences, Guwahati, Assam, India

Faculty of Pharmaceutical Science, Assam Downtown University, Guwahati, Assam, India

A. Bhattacharjee
Royal School of Pharmacy, The Assam Royal Global University, Guwahati, Assam, India

G. Battineni et al. (eds.), *Computational Methods in Psychiatry*,
https://doi.org/10.1007/978-981-99-6637-0_12

1 Introduction

Neurodegenerative diseases are becoming more prevalent and more costly for healthcare systems as a result of longer life expectancies. They also pose a steadily rising burden on society as a whole. Targeted, individualized patient care will be required due to genetic and environmental risk factors, which are already foreseeable. To understand the (individual) mechanisms causing neurodegenerative illnesses, it is very important to identify novel pharmacological molecules. The destruction of nerve cells, which results in the loss of cognitive, motor, or sensory functions, is a major characteristic of these diseases. Reactive oxygen species (ROS) and inflammation appear to play a critical role despite the fact that the underlying mechanisms are still unclear [1]. An important strategy for increasing the lifespan and comfort of the life of the patient is the development of novel drugs for the management of neurodegenerative illnesses. The development of therapeutic strategies for NDs represents a significant challenge because current therapies are ineffective and frequently unable to halt or delay the degeneration of the process of a neuron, which is extremely complex and includes a variety of neuropathological conditions and cognitive function losses, such as memory and learning losses. NDs lead to brain aging and loss of neurons, resulting in death. In fact, it has been calculated that brain-related conditions, including Parkinson's disease, amyotrophic lateral sclerosis, Alzheimer's disease, and Huntington's disease, are responsible for more than 25% of global fatalities and impairments [2].

The central nervous system's nerve cells gradually degenerate or die as a result of neurodegenerative disorders (NDs), which are fatal and disabling ailments (CNS). The prevalence of dementia is frighteningly rising worldwide. There were more than 50 million people suffering from dementia in 2020 worldwide, with over 60% of them living in undeveloped and developing nations. By 2050, there will be 152 million people on the planet or roughly twice as many as there are now. In the UK, an estimated 1.14 million people will have dementia by 2025, and that figure is estimated to increase to 2.1 million by 2051, a 40% increase in the next 5 years, and a 157% increase in the following 31 years. The health systems will face enormous financial demands as a result of dealing with a patient population that is still expanding: the WHO estimates that 139 million people worldwide will have dementia by the year 2050, an increase from the current 55 million [3]. Small compounds would at least have cheap production costs, and medication repurposing and preliminary screening using biological sources that have not yet reached their full potential are two possible paths for the discovery of novel therapeutics. Despite the considerable amount of research that has been conducted in the area of drug discovery, only a small portion of the naturally occurring anti-oxidative and anti-inflammatory compounds have been investigated in relation to neurodegenerative diseases [4].

Millions of people throughout the world suffer from neurodegenerative diseases. The two neurodegenerative illnesses with the highest prevalence are Parkinson's and Alzheimer's. According to an estimate from the Alzheimer's Disease Association, 6.2 million people in the US may have Alzheimer's disease by 2022 [5]. According to the Parkinson's Foundation, there are around a million people living with the condition in the United States. When neurons in the brain or peripheral nervous system start losing functionality and finally die, this leads to neurodegenerative illness. Although symptoms of some neurodegenerative disorders may be alleviated by certain treatments, currently, there is no cure and no way to stop the progression of these illnesses. With increasing age, a neurodegenerative disease becomes much more likely to occur. As life expectancy rises, more people may develop neurodegenerative diseases in the ensuing decades. Researchers have discovered that a person's genes and their environment each play a role in determining the likelihood that they will develop a neurodegenerative disease. For example, even if a person has a genome that tends to lead them to Parkinson's disease, their environmental exposures can determine whether, when, and how strongly they are affected. Examining possible exposures that took place prior to a disease diagnosis and comprehending their impact are part of critical research [3].

For many neurodegenerative illnesses, there are few viable therapies currently on the market. It is challenging to find novel, promising treatments for neurodegenerative illnesses using conventional drug discovery methods. Computer-aided drug design (CADD) or computer-assisted molecular design (CAMD) is the name given to the practice of utilizing computers to speed up and facilitate the process of drug discovery in the last one decade. This method is also known as computer-assisted molecular design (CAMD). The use of computer-aided drug design (CADD), which has been shown to be an effective tool for locating prospective lead compounds and aiding in the development of innovative therapies for a variety of ailments, has been widely used in recent years. At this time, the process of locating potentially bioactive chemicals within vast compound libraries makes use of a wide variety of computer methods. The CADD technique for drug discovery is being used more and more frequently. Recent trends in drug development emphasize the rational design of powerful treatments with multiple targets, more efficacies, and fewer side effects, especially in terms of safety [2].

Creating a novel drug is a labor-intensive procedure, but the payoff is worth it. According to the research of Myers and Baker [6], it typically takes over 14 years to bring a new pharmaceutical product to market from the time it is first conceived. A significant amount of money is also invested in this time-consuming process. The developments in genomics, proteomics, and structural genome sequencing may benefit medication development. Technological advancements, like as high-throughput screening and combinatorial chemistry, have been held out as the key to success. A particularly efficient way to accelerate the drug development process is through computer-aided drug design (CADD). Libraries with a large number of chemical compounds for use in lead optimization and discovery can be quickly and easily created using combinatorial chemistry methods. One way to do this is by using computer-aided drug design (CADD), which has been shown to reduce costs and speed up the hunt for new drug leads. There are undeniable advantages to using CADD. Virtual screening (VS) techniques, created to explore large libraries of compounds in silico, often have a much better success rate and yield hits that are more similar to medications than conventional high-throughput screening (HTS). CADD aids in boosting rationality in the drug discovery process. Since CADD relies on mathematical definitions and numerical evaluations, it can be used for virtually all phases of drug development. Using this technique, we can acquire many intricate details about the atomic structure of both small and large molecules, which cannot be done via experimental methods. For the purpose of comprehending the chemistry and biology of the molecules, it makes heavy use of computer programming and utilizes mathematics and physics. The ligand's pharmacological activity at the location of the site is due to the spatial arrangement, electronic make-up, and interactions between the ligand's atoms and their biological counterparts. Understanding the mechanisms behind drug–receptor interactions and assisting medicinal chemists in the discovery of novel therapeutic medicines are both made possible by molecular modeling and computational chemistry. With the development of computer graphics as a cost-effective tool and the availability of sufficient computing power, computational chemistry is no longer constrained by these limitations. The creation of software tools for examining the three-dimensional aspects of specificity has been incited by these developments. Several recent reviews by [7–9] offer more detailed coverage of this area. Each year, a large number of new unexplored compounds are found, necessitating the use of electronic information processing to store this knowledge in databases and improve our understanding of the chemistry that is currently known.

Before beginning a CADD project, it is common to practice to consider the drug target's intricate 3D structure. Novel lead compounds can be developed using either a ligand-based (pharmacophore, QSAR, CoMFA) or a structure-based (de novo ligand design, docking) approach. The most promising strategies will then be put through a cycle of analysis, synthesis, purchasing, activity testing, and CADD feedback. Using crystal structure complexes that depict the ligand features involved in interactions with the target protein and the region around the ligand occupied by the protein, integrated CADD methodologies produce structure-based pharmacophores that reveal the size of the binding cavity and all relevant and significant interactions. One of the biggest issues in structural biology is delving into the energy landscapes to see what it means for things like protein dynamics, aggregation, and folding. A mountain of data on conformational changes on the nanosecond time scale has been generated over the past 30 years via traditional molecular dynamics in Cartesian coordinate space, but this is insufficient to provide a complete answer to the problem. This is because genetic modifications in infectious organisms that alter their interaction with the target protein are the primary mediators of resistance to infectious diseases. Mutation prediction and mechanistic assessments of different sequence- and protein-based computational techniques are also important parts of drug design.

2 Neurodegenerative Diseases

2.1 *Parkinson's Diseases*

Nearly one million Americans are currently affected by Parkinson's disease, a neurological condition. The typical age of onset is around 60 years, and as more Americans are likely to live longer, it is anticipated that illness prevalence will rise. Parkinson's disease advances gradually as small groups of brain cells known as neurons deteriorate. Dopamine, a neurotransmitter that sends signals to the areas of the brain that control muscular movement, is less abundant as a result of the progressive death of those neurons. Symptoms of Parkinson's disease include tremors or shaking in the hands, arms, legs, jaw, and face; rigidity or stiffness in the limbs and trunk; bradykinesia; or slowness of movement; and difficulties with balance, speech, and coordination. In most cases, the symptoms start off mild and gradually get worse [10].

2.2 *Alzheimer's Disease*

Alzheimer's disease is a neurodegenerative disorder that gradually destroys nerve cells in the brain, resulting in a thinning of the brain's tissue. The most common kind of dementia is Alzheimer's disease, which is characterized by a gradual loss of cognitive, behavioral, and social abilities and severely limits a person's capacity for self-sufficiency. 5.8 million Americans aged 65 and more are living with Alzheimer's disease. Around 80% of them are 75 or older. Somewhere between 60 and 70% of the 50 million or so people worldwide with dementia are believed to have Alzheimer's disease. In the early stages of the condition, patients may report a general inability to recall even recent conversations or events. A person with Alzheimer's disease will suffer severe memory loss and an inability to carry out even the most basic of duties as the disease advances. Medications have the potential to alleviate symptoms momentarily or slow their progression. Treatments like this have the potential to improve the quality of life for certain people with Alzheimer's disease and extend the time they can remain independent. Those who suffer from Alzheimer's disease and their carers can find support through a number of organizations and initiatives designed specifically for them. There is currently no approved treatment for Alzheimer's disease that can slow or stop the progression of brain damage. In the later stages, mortality is caused by complications connected to a severe decline in brain function, such as malnutrition, dehydration, or infection [11].

2.3 *Huntington's Disease*

Huntington's disease is a rare genetic illness that leads to the gradual death of brain cells. Huntington's illness, which often causes locomotion, and intellectual and psychological impairments, has a considerable effect on a person's functional capabilities. Although symptoms of Huntington's disease can appear at any age, they are most common in individuals between 30 and 40 years of age. When Huntington's shows well before the age of 20, it is referred to as juvenile Huntington's disease. Juvenile Huntington's has somewhat different symptoms and may progress faster. Medication can assist in alleviating the signs of Huntington's disease. Treatments, however, are not able to reverse the condition's consequences on the mind and behavior [12].

2.4 Amyotrophic Lateral Sclerosis (ALS)

A neurological abnormality that impairs functional capacity and weakens muscles. As a result of condition, the function of the muscles that the nerve cells supply is diminished. There are no recognized common causes. The most noticeable symptom is muscular weakness. Although there is no remedy for ALS, medicines and therapy can help to delay the condition and alleviate symptoms. Some of the typical signs of ALS include muscle weakness, cramps, issues with coordination, tight muscles, loss of muscle, muscle spasms, or hyperactive reflexes. Additionally, there may be issues with lifting the foot, chewing, drooling, restraining, minor cognitive decline, severe constipation, severe accidental weight loss, or breathing difficulties [13].

2.5 Motor Neuron Disease

At ages 60 and 70, motor neuron disease, a rare disorder, damages the brain and neurons. It is brought on by an issue with motor neuron cells and nerves in the brain. With time, these neurons slowly lose their function. Motor neuron disease signs and symptoms develop over time. Early signs can include slurred speech, a shaky grasp, muscle spasms, and loss of weight. Early on in the course of motor neuron disease, a diagnosis might be challenging [14].

3 New Trends in Drug Discovery

The purpose of the time-consuming and expensive drug discovery process is to generate novel treatment alternatives. Computational methods have been used to do this at the preclinical phase of drug discovery. The use of computational tools to create, produce, and assess medications and active substances with identical biological properties is defined as computer-aided drug design (CADD). CADD's main components include homology modeling, virtual screening, molecular docking, quantitative structure-activity relationship (QSAR), and three-dimensional (3D) pharmacophore mapping in general. Virtual screening appears to be the main contributor to CADD among these techniques and has largely replaced experimental high-throughput screening for lead discovery and development as a well-established and popular computational methodology. More than 70 commercially available medications were discovered using some sort of computational technique up to this point. Keep in mind that the initial drug lead was typically found using a CADD approach [15].

It is possible that a rise in research in the field of computational chemistry and the current trend of more multidisciplinary investigation is related to the constant rise in commercial pharmaceuticals obtained through the CADD approach. Virtual screening is a technology used in the development of medications for systematic investigations for new small compounds having pharmacological activity against a protein. It is extremely effective and affordable. Notable advancements support this computational method's foundation in computational algorithms, a sharp rise in the processing power of computers, extensive knowledge of the structural and physicochemical characteristics of molecules in libraries and databases, and a growing understanding of the functional and structural characteristics of protein molecules. Virtual screening uses three-dimensional visuals for easier manipulation and more nuanced information. This technique can be used to screen for synthetic and natural chemical compounds, peptides, or proteins [16]. Virtual screens include two basic types: structure-based and ligand-based. The two paved the way for various supplementary virtual screening methods, such as those based on chemical genomics, accelerated free energy perturbation, fragments, docking, hybrids, homology models, QSAR, pharmacophores, shapes, conformal predictions, retrospectives, and similarities. Virtual screening is crucial for medication repositioning or repurposing as well. This makes it possible to characterize and optimize new therapeutic candidates quickly, which accelerates the design and development of new drugs [5].

In situations when the three-dimensional structure of a protein is available, a technique known as molecular docking has been used extensively in virtual screening in an effort to speed up the research process. In its most basic form, docking can be classified as either ensemble, induced fit, or lock and key docking. There are three types of docking methodologies: flexible ligand and flexible receptor docking, and rigid ligand and rigid receptor docking. To that end, a variety of docking and scoring software applications that use different methods and functions are accessible as internal or open-source apps. Predicting a ligand's bound configuration within a receptor's binding site is the goal of docking. The most effective binding conformations are identified using scoring methods such as descriptor-based, empirical, force-field-based, and knowledge-based [17].

Machine learning and deep learning have also been employed to augment or boost the virtual screening technique. These have been used on their own or in conjunction with various virtual screening processes or as a comparative or benchmark for virtual screening applications. Deep learning and machine learning have been utilized to improve scoring systems for structure-based virtual screening, performance evaluation, and similarity finding in ligand-based virtual screening in a number of virtual screening studies. Improvements in de novo drug design are one area where CADD has benefited from these two approaches. It's an ongoing computational process whereby novel lead compounds are created from scratch while still satisfying fundamental constraints. In order to apply Newtonian mechanics to improve the binding qualities and effectiveness of lead compounds, molecular dynamics simulations are crucial. In addition to using molecular dynamics simulations to supplement virtual screening, some investigations have found that these computations are superior to docking.

Drug discovery efforts should ideally result in commercial or public health successes where measurable outcomes, such as licensed medications, are discernible. Since the invention of computational methodologies, CADD has helped identify several medications that are already available on the market, and many more are still in the process. As a result, virtual screening has become an essential method for finding new drugs [18].

4 Computer-Aided Drug Design Methods

4.1 Drug Targets

Once referred to as drug receptors, they are generally known as drug targets and are divided into different types of receptors, enzymes, ion channels, and other targets. The majority of therapeutic agents used today have an enzyme or a membrane-bound receptor as their site of action. Identifying several unidentified proteins that may serve as new pharmacological targets has been made possible by sequencing the human and animal genomes. However, detailed information about the 3D structure of several membrane proteins is still not known to us. Future collaborative structural genomics programs may seek to determine the three-dimensional (3D) structure of every protein that is currently known using a combination of experimental structural characterization and molecular modeling. A significant number of enzymes and nucleic acids have access to information on the three-dimensional structures of macromolecules in detail (the most recent Brookhaven database has about 290 structures). It is now possible to isolate and clone enough target macromolecules for experimental research as a result of the quick innovation and breakthroughs in the field of genetic engineering. Because of recent developments in nuclear magnetic resonance (NMR) spectroscopy and the high performance and faster reading speed of modern X-ray crystallography detectors, it is now possible to accurately and quickly determine the three-dimensional structure of non-crystalline materials; this gives the discovery of the target's three-dimensional structure a greater emphasis as the starting point for rational drug design. In recent years, it has been seen that support vector machine (SVM) methods have gained significant advancements for predicting druggable proteins. This in silico-based machine learning approach, known as SVM, has been investigated as a novel method for druggable protein prediction using amino acid sequence without any sequence similarity, allowing the identification of druggable proteins with low or no similarity to the targets that are being studied. Identifying a protein's biological function is necessary for determining its potential as a therapeutic target and its use in structure-based drug design. Numerous times, the target protein's amino acid sequence is known, and there are homologous proteins whose three-dimensional structure has been established, where the target structure has been created by combining sidechain substitution and energy minimization with the known structure using computer modeling. When the target's structure is relatively similar to the known structure, one has a higher success rate.

4.2 Statistical Methods

Techniques known as quantitative structure-activity relationships (QSAR) are utilized in an effort to establish a connection between the structural and/or physical properties of the compounds and the biological activities they are involved in. In the past, these descriptors that characterize the topologic, steric, hydrophobic, and electronic properties of a series of molecules were found empirically. However, computational techniques are used these days to make these determinations. Comparative molecular field analysis, also known as CoMFA, is currently one of the most successful and widely used 3D QSAR techniques. Its primary function is to facilitate the production of bioactive molecules. CoMFA relates chemical characteristics to biological activity by computing the lipophilic, steric, and electrostatic properties around the molecules and then using the partial least square approach on the resulting data [19]. Statistical learning methods are being employed more often in order to predict compounds with a specific property and to assess algorithms frequently used to represent the physicochemical and structural features of compounds. Additionally, various statistical learning techniques, such as SVM and neural networks, have been assessed and are frequently used to estimate molecules with greater structural variety than those covered by QSAR and quantitative structure-property relationships (QSPR) [20]. Recent work that examines the techniques, present advancements, and underlying challenges has focused on the use of techniques for predicting compounds using statistical learning with specific pharmacodynamics, pharmacokinetic, and toxicological properties, and it improves the evaluation of drug safety and drug discovery [19].

4.3 Pharmacophore Modeling

A 3D hypothesis on the organization of structural characteristics is called pharmacophore modeling. These models primarily contain aromatic rings, which are hydrophobic groups on compounds that bind to biological targets, and donor and acceptor groups for hydrogen bonds. When one obtains the receptor target's 3D structure, by contrasting them to inactive analogs, one can determine the geometric and steric limitations. Once a pharmacophore model is established, it is possible to do 3D searches in big databases, which significantly increases the number of active analogs. The use of pharmacophore modeling and 3D database searches to enrich screening tests for the discovery of novel bioactive chemicals has proven to be effective. Pharmacophore models that are based on ligands and structures are still essential for the discovery of hits and may help with lead optimization. Structure-based pharmacophores provide for a comprehensive investigation of the binding interactions that take place at a binding site. These pharmacophores also permit the addition of shape and volume data that is immediately derived from the structural data. The search for molecules with chemical functions arranged in a three-dimensional manner (i.e., pharmacophoric features) shared by known active ligands is done using ligand-based pharmacophores, which may prevent the investigation of novel, beneficial interaction patterns that are not satisfied by currently existing ligands. Pharmacophore characteristics contain details on the ionic, hydrophobic, and hydrogen bonding interactions that ligands can have with macromolecules. Pharmacophore searches are commonly employed in the drug development process to identify compounds that may bind to the receptor in a manner that is comparable to that of the known actives but does not have a high degree of sub-structural similarity. Although pharmacophore-based methods can help identify promising hits or leads, further experimental work is required to ascertain their biological activity.

4.4 Virtual Screening

Virtual database screening is a key technique of the computer-aided search for new lead compounds. In the early stages of drug discovery, a great deal of work was put into compressing the early stage of hit-to-lead development in the pharmaceutical business. In particular, in silico-based virtual screening (VS) techniques have developed and largely expanded, whereas high-throughput screening (HTS) and combinatorial chemistry have not had the success that was anticipated. In comparison to the popular HTS technique, VS has emerged as an important method for identifying potential lead structures. In order to distinguish between wanted (supposedly active) and unwanted (presumably inactive) molecules inside compound libraries, VS has now increasingly been recognized as one of the most significant computational techniques. Fundamentally, there are two ways to approach this broad subject: automated docking techniques using virtual screening (VS), which involves understanding the target binding site's 3D structure, and similarity-based virtual screening, which does not require target structure knowledge (instead, compounds that are known to bind the target are used as structural queries) [21]. Open computing grid, a new distributed computing infrastructure that offers secure and robust methods of discovering and accessing remote data resources and software is primarily used in molecular science and engineering. This infrastructure holds great promise for solving significant chemical, pharmaceutical, and material science challenges on a large scale. For instance, an open computing grid-like OpenMolGRID can provide resources for developing QSPR/QSAR models as well as a repository for chemical data. As a result, it is possible to construct molecules with preset chemical properties and biological activity [22]. In the past few years of publications dealing with pharmacophore-based designs [23] published a unique work, the scientists used a ligand-based VS technique that integrated molecular shape descriptors with pharmacophore constraints for database mining to show that some drugs bind to the targets being studied down to the sub-nanomolar concentration level.

4.5 Docking and Molecular Dynamics

The challenges of structural molecular biology and structure-based drug discovery have accelerated the development of the discipline of molecular docking over the past three decades. Molecular docking is one of the most crucial aspects of structural molecular biology and computer-assisted drug development. The goal of ligand-protein docking is to make predictions about the principal binding modes between a ligand and a protein with a known three-dimensional structure. The program is useful for lead optimization since it allows for the virtual screening of vast chemical libraries, rates the results, and suggests structural suggestions for how the ligands block the target. The adaptability of proteins is a significant obstacle for modern drug design because of the difficulty of hitting a complicated flexible protein. In the biotechnology and pharmaceutical sectors, numerous docking programmes are widely employed. Given the enormous demand that flexibility entails, the majority of docking algorithms presumptively assume that the protein is inflexible. The ligands are, however, viewed as flexible molecules by many of the current docking systems. Force field-based techniques like molecular dynamics or Monte Carlo simulations that allow for the movement of ligands and targets are included in the docking algorithms. Programs for docking based on molecular dynamics include QXP38 and ICM39. Programs for docking based on evolutionary approaches include Tabu Search (TB), Evolutionary Programming (EP), and Genetic Algorithms (GA), which have been implemented in PROLEADS40, GOLD43, and AutoDock44. FlexX DOCK 4.0, 42.

5 Stages of Drug Design

Drug design refers to the process of systematically seeking for new compounds with considerable biological activity. Drug research must first begin with the identification and validation of viable targets. New therapeutic molecules that can be used to treat or manage certain diseases are discovered through the process of drug discovery. Starting with a massive chemical compound screening, the best disease targets can be determined. Understanding the structure of the drug receptor is crucial for designing therapeutic compounds that fit snugly into the binding site. In the following parts, we'll go into further depth about the various phases of drug design (Fig. 1):

5.1 Target Identification and Validation

When docking small molecules to a 3D model of a target, the effectiveness of the screening relies on the accuracy of the 3D structure data [24]. The first thing you should do is check the target for places you could attach the binding sites [25]. The initial stage in developing a new drug is generally to identify a druggable target that is associated

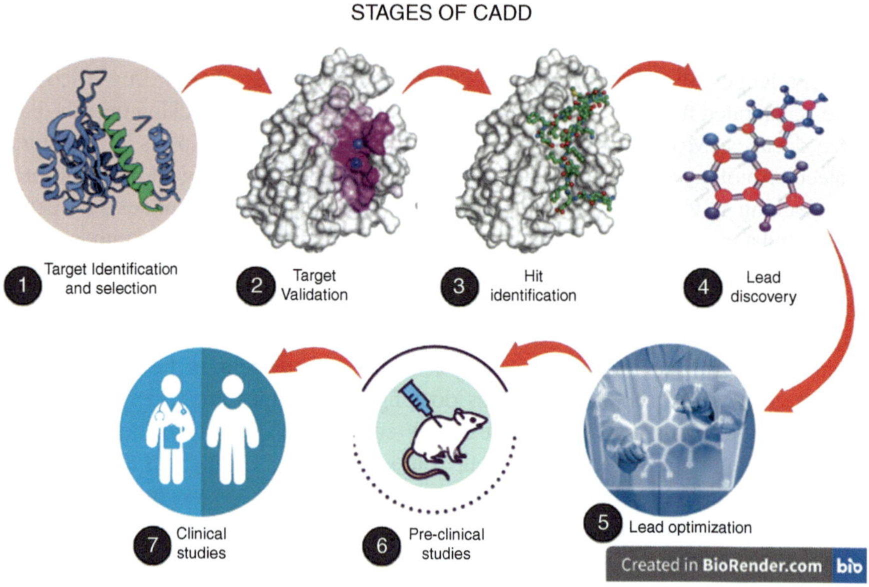

Fig. 1 Stages of computer-aided drug design (Created in Biorender.com)

with the condition of interest. In the face of such targets, researchers search for compounds that can modulate the route in question and cause the desired phenotypic response [26]. In order to do this, researchers often apply in silico methods to analyze known target-ligand co-crystal structures or to discover novel binding sites. The target's topology, structure, ligand-binding sites, key residues, and ligand-binding interactions are all greatly aided by in silico methods. Supporting in vitro investigations for target validation through methods like protein structure elucidation (e.g., X-ray diffraction), alanine scanning, site-directed mutagenesis, and radio ligand binding has become increasingly reliant on in silico methods like homology modeling, molecular docking, and MD simulations. This is supported by the literature ([27–29]. Docking is best initiated once a target structure has been experimentally determined using X-ray crystallography or nuclear magnetic resonance techniques and deposited in the PDB. Integrating the wet lab with computers is greatly aided by chemical and biological databases. Millions of molecules' information, from structural details to chemical formulas to gene and protein sequences, are stored and processed in multiple databases.

5.2 *Hit Identification*

Hit identification is the discovery of compounds having the desired activity against a completely validated target. This is a critical step of the CADD process where the identified small molecules bind to the desired target, usually a protein, and modifies its function. Once the target is identified and validated for a specific disorder, the identification process of hit matter is initiated for compounds that display the desired activity against the target. Robotic technology enabled high-throughput screening (randomly screening hundreds of compounds for biological activity in vitro at once), just as computer technology enabled in silico screening of millions of chemicals. Small chemical sets that were rationally selected from large libraries for biological screening have become more prevalent thanks to the so-called high-throughput virtual screening (or simply virtual screening). A variety of filters are used in virtual screening to gradually narrow down the libraries and eventually offer potential hits for in vitro tests [30]. The computational load and time required to increase significantly as the filters progress from rough to exhaustive, although a smaller library balances this off throughout the steps. Rough filters, which are frequently used at the start of virtual screening campaigns, are an example. They consist of evaluating the presence of drug-like chemicals and PAINS (Pan-assay Interference Compounds) [31, 32]. The entities with non-specific reactive functions and those with potentially poor pharmacokinetics are eliminated because these entities or compounds make up or produce a significant amount of unsuccessful clinical candidates [33]. A ligand- and/or structure-based virtual screening is typically performed after this stage [34].

5.3 *Lead Discovery*

The fundamental steps of the CADD process are lead generation and optimization. Lead compounds can be generated in a variety of ways, and they can be divided into numerous groups based on various techniques and tactics. While there are many different strategies, they may all be roughly divided into two groups: database exploration and de novo design. Comparatively, de novo design creates novel molecules with specific pharmacological activity in the binding region of a target protein, whereas database searching locates pre-existing molecules from libraries of chemical compounds.

5.4 *Structure of Target Protein*

It is crucial to understand the three-dimensional structure of target proteins. De novo design aims to produce innovative pharmaceutically active compounds that are compatible with a specific biological target's binding pattern. Typically, there are two methods to generate the required 3D structures of the particular macromolecules. The most popular method is to access databases. One such database is Protein Data Bank (PDB), which contains a wide range of biological macromolecule crystal structures with high resolution that have been determined experimentally. It is generally acknowledged as the only global database of macromolecular biological structural information and is the main and most trustworthy source for knowledge and information regarding the 3D structures of protein targets [35]. However, the current demand for drug discovery cannot be fully satisfied by the experimentally solved protein structures that already exist. These are the two main causes where there is a large barrier between the number of protein structures, protein sequences and certain proteins, in particular, that have been experimentally determined, cannot be crystallized by X-ray diffraction. On the other hand, several promising new developments have been seen. Experiments known as CASP (critical assessment of protein structure prediction) have been carried out continuously since 1994 and are organized by the Protein Structure Prediction Centre. These experiments have considerably advanced the development of protein modeling. More than 50% sequence similarity is thought to increase the reliability of the projected 3D target sequence model ([6, 36]. On fully automated servers, some of the best CASP-certified performing techniques are put into use (http://predictioncenter.org/). These automated servers, together with the well-known comparative modeling servers Swiss Model and MODELLER, are accessible to the general public.

5.5 *Structure-Based De Novo Design*

De novo ligand design, in general, refers to the development of novel ligands that do not already exist in compound libraries. It is also an effective way to overcome intellectual property constraints. If the target with a high-resolution structure protein is available, it is generally possible to produce a molecule containing the appropriate electrostatic and structural properties compatible with the target protein via molecular fragments connected through computing [37, 38]. A critical initial step in the drug development process is identifying the ligand-binding site of a protein. The location could be quickly located if one or more protein-inhibitor complexes' 3D structures are known. Otherwise, it is necessary to employ computational methods to examine into the target protein's potential binding site [39, 40]. De novo ligand design can commence as soon as the binding site is located. To achieve automated ligand design in binding sites, there are numerous specialized programmes [41, 42]. Combinatorial explosion is an obstacle that is faced by de novo design, and it is essential to significantly reduce the huge search space. Restricting the scope of the structure space to a single class of ligands is an effective strategy for minimizing the search space [37]. Since they can effectively sample the search space and reduce the size of the search space, combinatorial search methods are seen to be the most effective way to solve the combinatorial problem [43]. Simulated annealing ([44, 45]; genetic algorithms [46–48], molecular dynamics [49, 50], evolutionary-based [46, 51] and particle swarm algorithms [52] are well-known combinatorial techniques that are frequently employed in the development of new drugs [42].

5.6 Database Searching

Database searching can be used as a replacement for de novo design. Utilizing the three-dimensional structure of a target protein with a known binding site to screen a database of known compounds, lead compounds could be found. Future efforts to identify new medicines are anticipated to place a greater emphasis on the search of huge commercial and internal libraries, which is currently a major method for generating structure-based lead generation [53]. The DOCK programme is thought to be the earliest virtual screen programme [8, 54] through which the information on receptor binding site for database searching was used for the first time [55]. Surprisingly, compared to HTS, database screening against protein tyrosine phosphatase-1B had a greater hit rate, which has traditionally been the primary method for generating new drug development leads, according to a comparative study by Domain and co-workers [56]. This intriguing result implied that database searching might compete with HTS as a lead-generating strategy [56]. DOCK uses a geometry-based searching algorithm [54]. Spheres produced using SPHGEN [57] are used to represent the binding site's negative image throughout the search process, and ligands are then superimposed on top of the spheres. FRED (Fast Rigid Exhaustive Docking) is another example of a geometry-based algorithm [58]. Gaussian docking functions accurately detect the geometry of the protein binding site [58]. Rejected ligands lack adequate shape complementarity with the binding site. FRED, which is available for free to academic users, is recognized as one of the best database screening methods [59]. Another type of method that is used to identify lead compounds when there is no knowledge of the receptor structure is pharmacophore-based database searching. The 3D configuration of the essential components of a drug is responsible for its biological activity, which is referred to as a pharmacophore [8, 60]. Pharmacophore-based approaches have the clear advantage of being able to offer a variety of lead compounds that may have the appropriate biological activity but have entirely different chemical scaffolds [60]. A few significant computational tools for pharmacophore identification are currently available [60, 61], and numerous effective pharmacophore techniques in the discovery of computational drugs have been described in recent years [8, 21, 53, 62–69].

5.7 Lead Optimization

Just after lead discovery comes the step of lead optimization. Lead compounds that are less potent would then undergo optimization to improve their drug-like characteristics. Increasing a lead compound's drug-like characteristics by making minute changes to the lead structure is the focus at this stage, in accordance with the hypothesis that any incremental (positive or negative) change in the chemical structure generates incremental changes in bioactivity [38]. Bioactivity and ADMET (absorption, distribution, metabolism, excretion, and toxicity) properties are among the characteristics [70].

5.8 Binding Affinity Prediction

It is generally accepted that the biological activity of a given drug has a tight connection to the affinity of that molecule for its respective macromolecular receptor [71]. As a result, from a computational standpoint, it is very necessary to arrive at accurate estimates of the receptor-ligand binding affinities [72]. According to [71]), the primary factors that determine the affinity are the electrostatic interactions that take place between the ligand and the receptor, the role that solvation and desolvation play, the spatial complementarity of both binding partners, the enthalpic and entropic contributions that arise from changes in the number of degrees of freedom, and the conformational alterations that the ligand and the receptor undergo during the formation of the complex.

5.9 Efficient Approaches

An efficient method of estimating binding affinity is to use scoring functions, which are frequently employed in the lead generation phase. By typically summing together the force field scoring functions, which take into account the individual contributions from non-bond interactions like van der Waals and electrostatic interactions, estimate the binding affinity of a protein-ligand complex [73–75]. The test set, which should contain several hundred entries of various types and be appropriately large, significantly impacts how well empirical scoring methods operate. The complexes in the set must also possess binding affinities that span multiple orders of magnitude [76]. Large-scale statistical analyses of protein-ligand complex structures serve as the foundation for knowledge-based scoring functions ([43, 77]. Knowledge-based scoring functions produce better results than force field-based techniques do [71], and these kinds of functions have gained popularity in recent years [43].

Lead optimization, as previously indicated, is conducted to improve the lead compounds' therapeutic potential. If you don't know the structure of the receptor, a quantitative structure-activity relationship (QSAR) model is crucial for lead optimization. The goal of developing a QSAR model is to increase output while simultaneously decreasing turnover. It is important to note that traditional 2D-QSAR approaches can only be used to datasets consisting of structurally related substances [71]. On the other hand, 3D QSAR approaches employ molecular physicochemical and structural traits as descriptors to stand in for biological aspects (e.g., affinity or selectivity). One frequent 3D-QSAR method is the comparative molecular field analysis (CoMFA) strategy. It connects the shapes of ligands to their biological roles through the use of interactive visualizations and statistical analysis [78].

5.10 *Preclinical and Clinical Studies*

In order to acquire vital data about the safety profile and biological effectiveness of a candidate drug before it can be assessed on a target population, namely humans, preclinical studies are carried out using in vitro, in vivo, ex vivo, and in silico models. These models are used during the preclinical phase of drug development. In order to assure the reliability and reproducibility of the outcomes of preclinical research and testing, it is often carried out in line with the GLP and GSP standards (good laboratory practice and good scientific procedures). After the preclinical trial is over, the study is then put through clinical studies, which include research utilizing human participants (sometimes referred to as volunteers) that is meant to further medical knowledge.

Table 1 shows the molecules discovered for neurodegenerative diseases with the help of computational methods.

Table 1 Neurodegenerative diseases with specific molecular targets and selective examples of drugs discovered via computer-aided drug designing methods

Neuro degenerative diseases	Molecules under study	Target	Method	Software	Importance of study	Publication details
Alzheimer's disease	Arecoline, apigenin, chlorogenic acid, curcumin, kaempferol, luteolin, quercetin	MAO-B	Docking	Docking server	According to the study, all selected leads have good target enzyme binding affinity	Sivaraman and Srikanth [79]
Alzheimer's disease	Desoxycordifoline, bahienoside A, bufotenine, (5S)- 5-(1H-indol-3-ylmethyl)imidazolidine-2,4-dione (66), 5-(1H-indol-3-ylmethyl)-2-thioxoimidazolin-4-one (67), 5-(1Hindol-3-ylmethyl)-3-methyl-2-thioxoimidazolidin-4-one (68), and methyl 2-(aminoN-(2-(4-methylcyclohex-3-enyl) propan- 2-yl) methanethioamino)-3-(1H-indol-3-yl)propanoate	AChE, butyrylcholinesterase (BChE), MAO-A&B	Docking	Dock software	New MAO-A inhibitors with neuroprotective effects may be developed using scaffolds containing indolyl-hydantoin and indolylmethyl-thiohydantoin rings	Konrath et al. [80]

Alzheimer's disease	17,194 compounds of the CERMN chemical library	Histamine H3-receptor (H3R) and serotonin 4-receptor (5HT4R)	Pharmacophore modeling and molecular docking	Catalyst software, Schrodinger Glide	The study's findings characterized the benzo[h][1,6] naphthyridine derivatives' strong affinity for the H3R. Previous studies have shown that these ligands acted as antagonists or partial agonists of the 5-HT4R	Lepailleur et al. [81]
Alzheimer's disease	NSC 35839, NSC 80116, NSC 143057, NSC 164472, NSC 281260, NSC 636831, NSC 659829, NSC 702105, NSC 711731 (From NCI database)	AChE	Pharmacophore-based virtual screening and molecular docking	DS V2.5.5 software, LibDock	New inhibitors with the potential to inhibit AChE and protect neurons from Ab toxicity were discovered through research using the NCI database	Lu et al. [82]
Alzheimer's disease	Meridianin analogs 7–56	Dyrk1A	QSAR studies	PHASE module of Schrodinger molecular modeling package	In addition to predicting the Dyrk1A inhibitory activity of natural and synthesized meridianins, the established QSAR model may be useful in synthesizing better compounds with increased Dyrk1A inhibitory activity	Bharate et al. [83]

(continued)

Table 1 (continued)

Neuro degenerative diseases	Molecules under study	Target	Method	Software	Importance of study	Publication details
Alzheimer's disease	1-benzyl-4-[2-(*N*-benzoylamino)ethyl] piperidine derivatives and *N*-benzylpiperidine, benzisoxazoles derivatives	AChE	3D-QSAR (CoMFA)	SYBYL 6.1 molecular modeling software	The steric and electrostatic characteristics of 57 new inhibitors were used in a CoMFA analysis to explain their anti-AChE activity	Tong et al. [84]
Alzheimer's disease	1-Benzyl-1,2,3,4-Tetrahydro-b-Carboline	N-Methyl-D-Aspartate receptors	Molecular modeling	ICM, SWISS-MODEL	The NMDA receptor inhibitor 1-benzyl-1,2,3,4-tetrahydro-b-carboline (1a) was discovered in this research. Based on these findings, it appears that NMDA receptor blockers can be created by making rational modifications to the phenyl group of the scaffold 1-methyl-1,2,3,4-tetrahydro-b-carboline	Espinoza-Moraga et al. [85]

Alzheimer's disease	(*E*)-2-(4-(4-(substitued) piperazin-1-yl)benzylidene)-5,6-dimethoxy-2,3-dihydro-1H-inden-1-one derivatives	AChE, Aβ1–42 peptide	Molecular docking and molecular dynamics simulation	AutoDock 4.2, GROMACS 4.6.5	The IP-9, IP-13, and IP-15 compounds were identified as very effective, multi-purpose agents in the fight against Alzheimer's	Mishra et al. [86]
Alzheimer's disease	Ifenprodil and EVT-101	GluN2B-containing NMDA receptors	Homology modeling, molecular docking, and molecular dynamics simulation	Schrödinger suite	Using chicken embryo forebrain cultures and molecular modeling, the overlapping binding sites of ifenprodil and EVT-101 in GluN2B-containing NMDA receptors were explored	Fjelldal et al. [87]
Parkinson's disease	Kinase inhibitors (9-methyl-N-phenylpurine-2,8-diamine, N-phenylquinazolin-4-amine, and 1,3-dihydroindol-2-one)	Leucine-richrepeatkinase2	Homology modeling, molecular docking	MODELLER, MOE	The acquired docking scores to the LRRK2 ATP binding site correlated with invitro and cellular chemical activity, as shown by receiver operating characteristic plots	Vancraenenbroeck et al. [88]

(continued)

Table 1 (continued)

Neuro degenerative diseases	Molecules under study	Target	Method	Software	Importance of study	Publication details
Parkinson's disease	1-(substituted phenyl)-3-(naphtha [1, 2-d] thiazol-2-yl) urea/thiourea derivatives	Human adenosine A2A receptor	Molecular docking	AutoDock 4.2, MOPAC Ultra 2009	Good binding interactions were observed between AA2AR and 1-(substituted phenyl)-3-(naphtha[1,2-d] thiazol2-yl)urea/ thiourea derivatives in molecular docking studies	Azam et al. [89]
Parkinson's disease	Stimovul, 7,8dihydroxycoumarin, etorphine, propoxyphene, and pentazdine	α-synuclein	Molecular docking	Lead IT suite (flex dock)	Stimovul was determined to be the most promising ligand against the active site of -synuclein, while SER 87 and VAL 95 were identified as the interacting amino acids	Jayaraj et al. [90]
Parkinson's disease	Hesperidin and L-Dopa	A-Synuclein, MAO-B, COMT and UCHL-1	Molecular docking	AutoDock 4.2	Hesperidin was found to have similar binding sites and interactions with synuclein, MAO-B, COMT, and UCHL-1 as L-Dopa	Nagappan and Krishnamurthy [91]

Parkinson's disease	Pyrimidines	Adenosine A2A receptor	Molecular modeling, 3D-QSAR and docking studies	SYBYL X.1.1.1, AutoDock 4.2, LigandScout 3.03	Compound 32, the most effective molecule, served as a model for the structural design of other molecules. Almost all of them significantly boosted A2A receptor activation	Pourbasheer et al. [92]
Amyotrophic lateral sclerosis	A series of 47 N-(benzothiazolyl)-2-phenyl-acetamides	Casein kinase 1 Delta	3D-QSAR using CoMFA, CoMSIA, Auto GPA and molecular docking	Genetic algorithm-based docking program (GOLD), MOE2009.10	The benzothiazole ring's nitrogen atom and the amide group's hydrogen atom interacting with Asp 149, Asn 133, and Lys 38 and 130 were found to be critical for the inhibitory activity of these compounds against the Ck1d enzyme	Makhuri and Ghasemi [93]
Amyotrophic lateral sclerosis	D22G and L35P	Angiogenin	Mutations characterization, molecular dynamics simulation	Amber tools	This study explains the scientific basis for how the loss-of-function of D22G-Angiogenin causes ALS and suggests that people who carry the L35P-Angiogenin mutation are also at increased risk of developing the disease	Padhi et al. [94]

(continued)

Table 1 (continued)

Neuro degenerative diseases	Molecules under study	Target	Method	Software	Importance of study	Publication details
Amyotrophic lateral sclerosis	Riluzole	Nav1.6 sodium channel	Molecular modeling, molecular docking, simulation studies	Esypred3D, PROCHECK, Autodock v4.2, UCSF chimera	Riluzole interacts with the Nav1.6 channel, notably at TYR 1787, LEU 1843, and GLN 1799, suggesting cellular consequences	Sierra Bello et al. [95]
Huntington's disease	N6-(4-hydroxybenzyl) adenine riboside (T1–11)	A2AR and adenosine transporter (ENT1)	Molecular docking	AutoDock tools	T1–11 was found to have dual functions of activating adenosine receptors and blocking adenosine transporter ENT-1	Huang et al. [96]

6 Current Scenario and Future Scope of Computer-Aided Drug Designing in the Management of Neurodegenerative Disorders

The NDs present significant difficulties for medical professionals and researchers since they are incurable. More encouragement is needed to combat NDs because the number of affected people is growing more quickly. In the near future, there will be additional potential to create novel treatments as we gain a deeper knowledge of NDs and the original molecular pathogenesis. By utilizing computational tools, this may be accomplished. By reducing costs and time as well as minimizing the risk of chasing non-viable leads, CADD can significantly influence drug discovery [3].

Predicting the binding of ligands to the target in terms of the binding site and binding energy is one of the primary goals of using in silico drug design. New targets of proteins must be discovered and investigated in order to anticipate possible ligands to treat NDs [97]. The ensuing docking studies must then be verified in vitro and finally in the clinic. Although several medications are available that produce only slight symptom alleviation, there is yet no viable cure for NDs. The BBB, which keeps numerous chemicals out of the parenchyma of the CNS, makes it much more difficult to find treatments that work. As a result, even with encouraging findings from in silico, in vitro, and in vivo studies, a potential drug's clinical success cannot be assured. Future CADD projects may benefit from new experimental techniques such as CRISPR-Cas9 technology, genome-wide association studies (GWAS), organ-on-chip technologies, high-throughput screening (HTS), functional MRI (fMRI), and positron emission tomography (PET), which may expose novel targets of drugs for neurodegenerative disorders [15].

Scientists are creating enormous amounts of data utilizing bioinformatics in this era of Big Data. For target selection, lead identification, optimization, and computational drug design strategies employed bioinformatics techniques and databases. A relatively new and developing interdisciplinary science called bioinformatics seeks to solve biological problems by using computational, mathematical, and statistical methods [98]. Using bioinformatics technologies to design novel drugs has created an entirely new area of study. The requirement for supplementary, low-risk drug design in a very short time is driving up interest in bioinformatics. The use of bioinformatics tools can help create new inhibitors for treating neurological disorders by providing information on potential nucleotide and sequence of a protein, protein expression types, relatives of disease, distinctions, homology, information of map, and structural information [99].

The use of CADD in the current era of drug discovery accounts for the most crucial aspects and offers computational tools and algorithms that lower the danger of identifying non-viable developing leads while saving time, money, and effort. Recent CADD patterns demand a comprehensive study of the molecular and clinical circumstances brought on by diseases in order to find new leads or drugs. For academics and doctors, ND early diagnosis continues to be quite difficult. CADD, however, can help researchers better understand how medications interact with receptors. The pharmacoinformatic technique is used in contemporary drug discovery and supplies a lot of fundamental information on drug–receptor interactions. To advance the CADD approach, new advancements in technology and computer algorithms are necessary since they are expected to produce tools for identifying diseases and screening possible lead compounds. Understanding the neuronal changes related to NDs may be aided by the developing research in the neurological field, which encompasses neurogenomics and neuroproteomics. Additionally, the use of technologies related to neurogenomics, neuroproteomics, next-generation sequencing, and genome-wide association studies may help us find new therapeutic targets and, in turn, enhance our capacity to treat NDs [100].

Despite the numerous successful CADD applications in contemporary drug discovery, it still has several drawbacks. It is not uncommon for compounds generated in silico utilizing computational and theoretical physicochemical to fail to work in real physiological systems. Only 40% of medication candidates successfully complete clinical trials in phase I due to inadequate pharmacokinetics and/or pharmacodynamics. Additionally, every computing method is based on pre-established methods, each of which has drawbacks [101]. Since many compounds that seem to bind in the computational study do not perform as expected in vitro, in silico results must be verified in actual biological systems. Another restriction of CADD is that all strategies for creating and discovering new medications rely on software, which must simplify the underlying chemistry and physics. As a result, these algorithms have a number of drawbacks and must be updated frequently in order to improve accuracy and, ultimately, the production of novel drugs. Additionally, several documented failures have been caused by the lack of investigational data addressing expected ADMET outcomes. Updating and developing new software and associated methodologies, verifying with investigational data, using trustworthy databases, and employing algorithms that offer docking scores that correctly predict in vitro binding are all necessary steps toward overcoming the limitations of CADD and increasing its accuracy. The tools indicated above could therefore be used in the creation of pharmacophores in the future that have the appropriate biological activity [102].

References

1. Singh A, Kukreti R, Saso L, Kukreti S. Oxidative stress: a key modulator in neurodegenerative diseases. Molecules. 2019;24(8):1–20. https://doi.org/10.3390/molecules24081583.
2. Mukherjee S, Madamsetty VS, Bhattacharya D, Roy Chowdhury S, Paul MK, Mukherjee A. Recent advancements of nanomedicine in neurodegenerative disorders theranostics. Adv Funct Mater. 2020;30(35):1–27. https://doi.org/10.1002/adfm.202003054.
3. Wang S, Liu M, Lewin NE, Lorenzo PS, Bhattacharrya D, Qiao L, Kozikowski AP, Blumberg PM. Probing the binding of indolactam-V to protein kinase C through site- directed mutagenesis and computational docking simulations. J Med Chem. 1999;42(18):3436–46. https://doi.org/10.1021/jm990129n.

4. Kins S, Schäfer KH, Endres K. Drug development for neurodegenerative diseases. Biol Chem. 2022;403(1):66482. https://doi.org/10.1515/hsz-2021-0413.
5. Owen MC, Gnutt D, Gao M, Wärmländer SKTS, Jarvet J, Gräslund A, Winter R, Ebbinghaus S, Strodel B. Effects of in vivo conditions on amyloid aggregation. Chem Soc Rev. 2019;48(14):3946–96. https://doi.org/10.1039/c8cs00034d.
6. Myers S, Baker A. Drug discovery—an operating model for a new era. Despite the advent of new science and technologies, drug developers will need to make radical changes in their operations if they are to remain competitive and innovative. Nat Biotechnol. 2001;19(8):727–30. https://doi.org/10.1038/90765.
7. Greer J, Erickson JW, Baldwin JJ, Varney MD. Application of the three-dimensional structures of protein target molecules in structure-based drug design. J Med Chem. 1994;37(8):1035–54. https://doi.org/10.1021/jm00034a001.
8. Guner O, Clement O, Kurogi Y. Pharmacophore modeling and three dimensional database searching for drug design using catalyst: recent advances. Curr Med Chem. 2012;11(22):2991–3005. https://doi.org/10.2174/0929867043364036.
9. Hopfinger AJ. Computer-assisted drug design. J Med Chem. 1985;28(9):1133–9. https://doi.org/10.1021/jm00147a001.
10. Gebreyesus HH, Gebremichael TG. Medical sciences the potential role of astrocytes in Parkinson's disease (PD). 2020.
11. Chakraborty A, Diwan A. Alzheimer and it's possible therapy: a review. 2020;1(4):115–122.
12. Bates GP, Dorsey R, Gusella JF, Hayden MR, Kay C, Leavitt BR, Nance M, Ross CA, Scahill RI. Huntington disease. 2015. pp. 1–21. https://doi.org/10.1038/nrdp.2015.5.
13. Morris J. Amyotrophic lateral sclerosis (ALS) and related motor neuron diseases: an overview. Neurodiagn J. 2015;55(3):180–94. https://doi.org/10.1080/21646821.2015.1075181.
14. Leigh PN, Park C. Motor neuron disease. 1994. pp. 886–896.
15. Alam MZ, Alam Q. Global current trends in drug designing for management of Type-2 diabetes and neurodegenerative disorders. Drug Design Open Access. 2013;2(2):1000e120. https://doi.org/10.4172/2169-0138.1000e120.
16. Islam R, Maji S, Kabiraj S, Habib U, Pal R, Bhattacharya S, Chakraborty S, Bhattacharjee DA. Role of in silico drug design in pharmaceutical sciences. Int J Res Appl Sci Eng Technol. 2022;(5):10, 2358–2367. https://doi.org/10.22214/ijraset.2022.42836.
17. Tripathi A, Misra K. Molecular docking: a structure-based drug designing approach. JSM Chem. 2017;5(2):1042.
18. Kore PP, Mutha MM, Antre RV, Oswal RJ, Kshirsagar SS. Computer-aided drug design: an innovative tool for modeling. Open J Med Chem. 2012;2(4):139–48. https://doi.org/10.4236/ojmc.2012.24017.
19. Andina D, Vega-Corona A, Seijas JI, Alarcòn MJ. Application of neural networks. In: Computational intelligence: for engineering and manufacturing; 2008. pp. 93–108. https://doi.org/10.1007/0-387-37452-3_4.
20. Yap C, Xue Y, Li H, Li Z, Ung C, Han L, Zheng C, Cao Z, Chen Y. Prediction of compounds with specific pharmacodynamic, pharmacokinetic or toxicological property by statistical learning methods. Mini Rev Med Chem. 2006;6(4):449–59. https://doi.org/10.2174/138955706776361501.
21. Lengauer T, Lemmen C, Rarey M, Zimmermann M. Novel technologies for virtual screening. Drug Discov Today. 2004;9(1):27–34. https://doi.org/10.1016/S1359-6446(04)02939-3.
22. Sild S, Maran U, Lomaka A, Karelson M. Open computing grid for molecular science and engineering. J Chem Inf Model. 2006;46(3):953–9. https://doi.org/10.1021/ci050354f.
23. Laggner C, Schieferer C, Fiechtner B, Poles G, Hoffmann RD, Glossmann H, Langer T, Moebius FF. Discovery of high-affinity ligands of σ1 receptor, ERG2, and emopamil binding protein by pharmacophore modeling and virtual screening. J Med Chem. 2005;48(15):4754–64. https://doi.org/10.1021/jm049073+.

24. Fauman EB, Rai BK, Huang ES. Structure-based druggability assessment-identifying suitable targets for small molecule therapeutics. Curr Opin Chem Biol. 2011;15(4):463–8. https://doi.org/10.1016/j.cbpa.2011.05.020.
25. Hajduk PJ, Huth JR, Tse C. Predicting protein druggability. Drug Discov Today. 2005;10(23–24):1675–82. https://doi.org/10.1016/S1359-6446(05)03624-X.
26. Metcalf B, Dillon S. Target validation in drug discovery. 2007;356. pp. 367–377. https://doi.org/10.1016/B978-0-12-369393-8.X5000-7.
27. Agamah FE, Mazandu GK, Hassan R, Bope CD, Thomford NE, Ghansah A, Chimusa ER. Computational/in silico methods in drug target and lead prediction. Brief Bioinform. 2020;21(5):1663–75. https://doi.org/10.1093/bib/bbz103.
28. Anand P, Nagarajan D, Mukherjee S, Chandra N. ABS–scan: in silico alanine scanning mutagenesis for binding site residues in protein–ligand complex. F1000Res. 2014;3:214. https://doi.org/10.12688/f1000research.5165.1.
29. Sahu TK, Pradhan D, Rao AR, Jena L. In silico site-directed mutagenesis of neutralizing mAb 4C4 and analysis of its interaction with G-H loop of VP1 to explore its therapeutic applications against FMD. J Biomol Struct Dyn. 2019;37(10):2641–51. https://doi.org/10.1080/07391102.2018.1494631.
30. Hughes JP, Rees SS, Kalindjian SB, Philpott KL. Principles of early drug discovery. Br J Pharmacol. 2011;162(6):1239–49. https://doi.org/10.1111/j.1476-5381.2010.01127.x.
31. Baell J, Walters MA. 513481a. n.d.. pp. 8–10.
32. Schneider N, Jäckels C, Andres C, Hutter MC. Gradual in silico filtering for druglike substances. J Chem Inf Model. 2008;48(3):613–28. https://doi.org/10.1021/ci700351y.
33. Hazard L. The role of radiation therapy in pancreas cancer. Gastrointest Cancer Res. 2009;3(1):20–8.
34. Katsila T, Spyroulias GA, Patrinos GP, Matsoukas MT. Computational approaches in target identification and drug discovery. Comput Struct Biotechnol J. 2016;14:177–84. https://doi.org/10.1016/j.csbj.2016.04.004.
35. Saur IML, Panstruga R, Schulze-Lefert P. NOD-like receptor-mediated plant immunity: from structure to cell death. Nat Rev Immunol. 2021;21(5):305–18. https://doi.org/10.1038/s41577-020-00473-z.
36. Baker D, Sali A. Protein structure prediction and structural genomics. Science. 2001;294(5540):93–6. https://doi.org/10.1126/science.1065659.
37. Moon JB, Howe WJ. Computer design of bioactive molecules: a method for receptor-based de novo ligand design. Proteins. 1991;11(4):314–28. https://doi.org/10.1002/prot.340110409.
38. Ooms F. Molecular modeling and computer aided drug design. Examples of their applications in medicinal chemistry. Curr Med Chem. 2012;7(2):141–58. https://doi.org/10.2174/0929867003375317.
39. Glick M, Robinson DD, Grant GH, Richards WG. Identification of ligand binding sites on proteins using a multi-scale approach. J Am Chem Soc. 2002;124(10):2337–44. https://doi.org/10.1021/ja016490s.
40. Sung E, Kim S, Shin W. Binary image representation of a ligand binding site: its application to efficient sampling of a conformational ensemble. BMC Bioinformatics. 2010;11:256. https://doi.org/10.1186/1471-2105-11-256.
41. Honma T. Recent advances in de novo design strategy for practical lead identification. Med Res Rev. 2003;23(5):606–32. https://doi.org/10.1002/med.10046.
42. Loving K, Alberts I, Sherman W. Computational approaches for fragment-based and de novo design. Curr Top Med Chem. 2010;10(1):14–32. https://doi.org/10.2174/156802610790232305.
43. Schneider G, Fechner U. Computer-based de novo design of drug-like molecules. Nat Rev Drug Discov. 2005;4(8):649–63. https://doi.org/10.1038/nrd1799.
44. Stahl M, Todorov NP, James T, Mauser H, Boehm HJ, Dean PM. A validation study on the practical use of automated de novo design. J Comput Aided Mol Des. 2002;16(7):459–78. https://doi.org/10.1023/A:1021242018286.

45. Todorov NP, Dean PM. Evaluation of a method for controlling molecular scaffold diversity in de novo ligand design. J Comput Aided Mol Des. 1997;11(2):175–92. https://doi.org/10.1023/A:1008042711516.
46. Dey F, Caflisch A. Fragment-based de novo ligand design by multi-objective evolutionary optimization. Supporting information. J Chem Inf Model. 2008;48(3):679–90.
47. Douguet D, Munier-Lehmann H, Labesse G, Pochet S. LEA3D: A computer-aided ligand design for structure-based drug design. J Med Chem. 2005;48(7):2457–68. https://doi.org/10.1021/jm0492296.
48. Pegg SCH, Haresco JJ, Kuntz ID. A genetic algorithm for structure-based de novo design. J Comput Aided Mol Des. 2001;15(10):911–33. https://doi.org/10.1023/A:1014389729000.
49. Amaro R, Li W. Emerging methods for ensemble-based virtual screening. Curr Top Med Chem. 2010;10(1):3–13. https://doi.org/10.2174/156802610790232279.
50. Jorgensen WL, Ruiz-Caro J, Tirado-Rives J, Basavapathruni A, Anderson KS, Hamilton AD. Computer-aided design of non-nucleoside inhibitors of HIV-1 reverse transcriptase. Bioorg Med Chem Lett. 2006;16(3):663–7. https://doi.org/10.1016/j.bmcl.2005.10.038.
51. Liu Q, Masek B, Smith K, Smith J. Tagged fragment method for evolutionary structure-based de novo lead generation and optimization. J Med Chem. 2007;50(22):5392–402. https://doi.org/10.1021/jm070750k.
52. Hartenfeller M, Proschak E, Schüller A, Schneider G. Concept of combinatorial de novo design of drug-like molecules by particle swarm optimization. Chem Biol Drug Des. 2008;72(1):16–26. https://doi.org/10.1111/j.1747-0285.2008.00672.x.
53. Horvath D. Pharmacophore-based virtual screening. Methods Mol Biol. 2011;672(973):261–98. https://doi.org/10.2174/092986708784049630.
54. Schneidman-Duhovny D, Nussinov R, Wolfson HJ. Predicting molecular interactions in silico: II. Protein-protein and protein-drug docking. Front Med Chem. 2010;3:585–613. https://doi.org/10.2174/978160805206610603010585.
55. Kindt T, Morse S, Gotschlich E, Schluederberg A, Kuntz ID. Human retroviruses and AIDS 1989, A compilation and analysis of nucleic and amino acid sequence. Rev Infect Dis. 1989;345(August):270.
56. Doman TN, McGovern SL, Witherbee BJ, Kasten TP, Kurumbail R, Stallings WC, Connolly DT, Shoichet BK. Molecular docking and high-throughput screening for novel inhibitors of protein tyrosine phosphatase-1B. J Med Chem. 2002;45(11):2213–21. https://doi.org/10.1021/jm010548w.
57. Kuntz ID, Blaney JM, Oatley SJ, Langridge R, Ferrin TE. A geometric approach to macromolecule-ligand interactions. J Mol Biol. 1982;161:269.
58. McGann MR, Almond HR, Nicholls A, Grant JA, Brown FK. Gaussian docking functions. Biopolymers. 2003;68(1):76–90. https://doi.org/10.1002/bip.10207.
59. Mcgaughey GB, Sheridan RP, Bayly CI, Culberson JC, Kreatsoulas C, Lindsley S, Maiorov V, Truchon J, Cornell WD. Comparison of topological, shape, and docking methods in virtual screening. J Chem Inf Model. 2007;47:1504–19.
60. Dror O, Shulman-Peleg A, Nussinov R, Wolfson HJ. Predicting molecular interactions. 2004. pp. 71–90.
61. Wolber G, Seidel T, Bendix F, Langer T. Molecule-pharmacophore superpositioning and pattern matching in computational drug design. Drug Discov Today. 2008;13(1–2):23–9. https://doi.org/10.1016/j.drudis.2007.09.007.
62. Chiang YK, Kuo CC, Wu YS, Chen CT, Coumar MS, Wu JS, Hsieh HP, Chang CY, Jseng HY, Wu MH, Leou JS, Song JS, Chang JY, Lyu PC, Chao YS, Wu SY. Generation of ligand-based pharmacophore model and virtual screening for identification of novel tubulin inhibitors with potent anticancer activity. J Med Chem. 2009;52(14):4221–33. https://doi.org/10.1021/jm801649y.
63. Chou K-C, Wei D-Q, Du Q-S, Sirois S, Zhong W-Z. Progress in computational approach to drug development against SARS. Curr Med Chem. 2006;13(27):3263–70. https://doi.org/10.2174/092986706778773077.

64. Kan WM, Chang C, Wang KC. Phytochemistry. 2001;44(23).
65. Michaux C, de Leval X, Julémont F, Dogné JM, Pirotte B, Durant F. Structure-based pharmacophore of COX-2 selective inhibitors and identification of original lead compounds from 3D database searching method. Eur J Med Chem. 2006;41(12):1446–55. https://doi.org/10.1016/j.ejmech.2006.07.017.
66. Murumkar PR, Zambre VP, Yadav MR. Development of predictive pharmacophore model for in silico screening, and 3D QSAR CoMFA and CoMSIA studies for lead optimization, for designing of potent tumor necrosis factor alpha converting enzyme inhibitors. J Comput Aided Mol Des. 2010;24(2):143–56. https://doi.org/10.1007/s10822-010-9322-z.
67. Oprea TI, Matter H. Integrating virtual screening in lead discovery. Curr Opin Chem Biol. 2004;8(4):349–58. https://doi.org/10.1016/j.cbpa.2004.06.008.
68. Schuster D, Nashev LG, Kirchmair J, Laggner C, Wolber G, Langer T, Odermatt A. Discovery of nonsteroidal 17β-hydroxysteroid dehydrogenase 1 inhibitors by pharmacophore-based screening of virtual compound libraries. J Med Chem. 2008;51(14):4188–99. https://doi.org/10.1021/jm800054h.
69. Seifert MHJ, Wolf K, Vitt D. Virtual high-throughput in silico screening. Drug Discov Today Biosilico. 2003;1(4):143–9. https://doi.org/10.1016/s1478-5382(03)02359-x.
70. Patel H, Bodkin MJ, Chen B, Gillet VJ. Knowledge-based approach to de novo design using reaction vectors. J Chem Inf Model. 2009;49(5):1163–84. https://doi.org/10.1021/ci800413m.
71. Gohlke H, Klebe G. Approaches to the description and prediction of the binding affinity of small-molecule ligands to macromolecular receptors. Angew Chem Int Ed Engl. 2002;41(15):2644–76. https://doi.org/10.1002/1521-3773(20020802)41:15<2644::AID-ANIE2644>3.0.CO;2-O.
72. Jorgensen WL. Efficient drug lead discovery and optimization. Acc Chem Res. 2009;42(6):724–33.
73. Ewing TJA, Makino S, Skillman AG, Kuntz ID. DOCK 4.0: search strategies for automated molecular docking of flexible molecule databases. J Comput Aided Mol Des. 2001;15(5):411–28. https://doi.org/10.1023/A:1011115820450.
74. Pang YP, Perola E, Xu R, Prendergast FG. EUDOC: A computer program for identification of drug interaction sites in macromolecules and drug leads from chemical databases. J Comput Chem. 2001;22(15):1750–71. https://doi.org/10.1002/jcc.1129.
75. Sanchez G. Las instituciones de ciencia y tecnología en los procesos de aprendizaje de la producción agroalimentaria en Argentina. In: El Sistema Argentino de Innovación: Instituciones, Empresas y Redes. El Desafío de La Creación y Apropiación de Conocimiento. 2013;14(2006):659–664. https://doi.org/10.1002/prot.
76. McConkey BJ, Sobolev V, Edelman M. The performance of current methods in ligand-protein docking. Curr Sci. 2002;83(7):845–56.
77. Stouten PFW, Kroemer RT. Docking and scoring. In: Comprehensive medicinal chemistry II. 2006;4(20), 255–279. https://doi.org/10.1016/b0-08-045044-x/00253-4.
78. Xiang M, Cao Y, Fan W, Chen L, Mo Y. Computer-aided drug design: lead discovery and optimization. Comb Chem High Throughput Screen. 2012;15(4):328–37. https://doi.org/10.2174/138620712799361825.
79. Sivaraman D, Srikanth J. Discovery of novel monoamine oxidase-b inhibitors by molecular docking approach for Alzheimer's and Parkinson's disease treatment. Int J Pharm Sci Rev Res. 2016;40(1):245–50.
80. Konrath EL, Nurisso A, Carrupt PA, Oliveira CMA, Kato L, Henriques AT. Indole alkaloids and semisynthetic indole derivatives as multifunctional scaffolds aiming the inhibition of enzymes related to neurodegenerative diseases—a focus on Psychotria L. genus. Curr Top Med Chem. 2014;14:1056–75. https://doi.org/10.2174/1568026614666140324142409.
81. Lepailleur A, Freret T, Lemaître S, Boulouard M, Dauphin F, Hinschberger A, Dulin F, Lesnard A, Bureau R, Rault S. Dual histamine H3R/serotonin 5-HT4R ligands with antiam-

nesic properties: pharmacophore-based virtual screening and polypharmacology. J Chem Inf Model. 2014;54(6):1773–84. https://doi.org/10.1021/ci500157n.
82. Lu SH, Wu JW, Liu HL, Zhao JH, Liu KT, Chuang CK, Lin HY, Tsai WB, Ho Y. The discovery of potential acetylcholinesterase inhibitors: a combination of pharmacophore modeling, virtual screening, and molecular docking studies. J Biomed Sci. 2011;18(1):8. https://doi.org/10.1186/1423-0127-18-8.
83. Bharate SB, Yadav RR, Vishwakarma RA. QSAR and pharmacophore study of Dyrk1A inhibitory meridianin analogs as potential agents for treatment of neurodegenerative diseases. Med Chem. 2013;9(1):152–61. https://doi.org/10.2174/1573406411309010152.
84. Tong W, Collantes ER, Chen Y, Welsh WJ. A comparative molecular field analysis study of N-benzylpiperidines as acetylcholinesterase inhibitors. J Med Chem. 1996;39(2):380–7. https://doi.org/10.1021/jm950704x.
85. Espinoza-Moraga M, Caballero J, Gaube F, Winckler T, Santos LS. 1-Benzyl-1,2,3,4-Tetrahydro-β-Carboline as channel blocker of N-methyl-d-aspartate receptors. Chem Biol Drug Des. 2012;79(4):594–9. https://doi.org/10.1111/j.1747-0285.2012.01317.x.
86. Mishra CB, Kumari S, Manral A, Prakash A, Saini V, Lynn AM, Tiwari M. Design, synthesis, in-silico and biological evaluation of novel donepezil derivatives as multi-target-directed ligands for the treatment of Alzheimer's disease. Eur J Med Chem. 2017;125:736–50. https://doi.org/10.1016/j.ejmech.2016.09.057.
87. Fjelldal MF, Freyd T, Evenseth LM, Sylte I, Ring A, Paulsen RE. Exploring the overlapping binding sites of ifenprodil and EVT-101 in GluN2B-containing NMDA receptors using novel chicken embryo forebrain cultures and molecular modeling. Pharmacol Res Perspect. 2019;7(3):1–15. https://doi.org/10.1002/prp2.480.
88. Vancraenenbroeck R, De Raeymaecker J, Lobbestael E, Gao F, De Maeyer M, Voet A, Baekelandt V, Taymans JM. In silico, in vitro and cellular analysis with a kinome-wide inhibitor panel correlates cellular LRRK2 dephosphorylation to inhibitor activity on LRRK2. Front Mol Neurosci. 2014;7:51. https://doi.org/10.3389/fnmol.2014.00051.
89. Azam F, Prasad MVV, Thangavel N, Ali HI. Molecular docking studies of 1-(substituted phenyl)-3-(naphtha [1, 2-d] thiazol-2-yl) urea/thiourea derivatives with human adenosine A2A receptor. Bioinformation. 2011;6(9):330–4. https://doi.org/10.6026/97320630006330.
90. Jayaraj RL, Ranjani V, Manigandan K, Elangovan N. Insilico docking studies to identify potent inhibitors of alpha-synuclein aggregation in Parkinson disease. Asian J Pharm Clin Res. 2013;6(Suppl. 4):127–31.
91. Nagappan P, Krishnamurthy V. Structural prediction and comparative molecular docking studies of hesperidin and L-Dopa on A-Synuclein, MAO-B, COMT and UCHL-1 inhibitors. Int J Pharm Clin Res. 2015;7(3):221–5.
92. Pourbasheer E, Shokouhi Tabar S, Masand VH, Aalizadeh R, Ganjali MR. 3D-QSAR and docking studies on adenosine A2A receptor antagonists by the CoMFA method. SAR QSAR Environ Res. 2015;26(6):461–77. https://doi.org/10.1080/1062936X.2015.1049666.
93. Makhuri FR, Ghasemi JB. Computer-aided scaffold hopping to identify a novel series of casein kinase 1 delta (CK1d) inhibitors for amyotrophic lateral sclerosis. Eur J Pharm Sci. 2015;78:151–62. https://doi.org/10.1016/j.ejps.2015.07.011.
94. Padhi AK, Banerjee K, Gomes J, Banerjee M. Computational and functional characterization of angiogenin mutations, and correlation with amyotrophic lateral sclerosis. PLoS One. 2014;9(11):e111963. https://doi.org/10.1371/journal.pone.0111963.
95. Sierra Bello O, Gonzalez J, Capani F, Barreto GE. In silico docking reveals possible Riluzole binding sites on Nav1.6 sodium channel: implications for amyotrophic lateral sclerosis therapy. J Theor Biol. 2012;315:53–63. https://doi.org/10.1016/j.jtbi.2012.09.004.
96. Huang NK, Lin JH, Lin JT, Lin CI, Liu EM, Lin CJ, Chen WP, Shen YC, Chen HM, Chen JB, Lai HL, Yang CW, Chiang MC, Wu YS, Chang C, Chen JF, Fang JM, Lin YL, Chern Y. A new drug design targeting the adenosinergic system for Huntington's disease. PLoS One. 2011;6(6):e20934. https://doi.org/10.1371/journal.pone.0020934.

97. Sliwoski GR, Meiler J, Lowe EW. Computational methods in drug discovery prediction of protein structure and ensembles from limited experimental data view project antibody modeling, antibody design and antigen-antibody interactions view project. Comput Methods Drug Discov. 2014;66(1):334–95.
98. Gill S, Christopher A, Gupta V, Bansal P. Emerging role of bioinformatics tools and software in evolution of clinical research. Perspect Clin Res. 2016;7(3):115. https://doi.org/10.4103/2229-3485.184782.
99. Somberg JC. Drug discovery and development. In: Cardiovascular drug development: protocol design and methodology. 2016. https://doi.org/10.3109/9780203909522-4.
100. Ikezu T, Gendelman HE. Neuroimmune pharmacology. In: Neuroimmune pharmacology; 2016. pp. 1–1035. https://doi.org/10.1007/978-3-319-44022-4.
101. Lin JH, Lu AYH. Role of pharmacokinetics and metabolism in drug discovery and development. Pharmacol Rev. 1997;49(4):403–49.
102. Muratov EN, Amaro R, Andrade CH, Brown N, Ekins S, Fourches D, Isayev O, Kozakov D, Medina-Franco JL, Merz KM, Oprea TI, Poroikov V, Schneider G, Todd MH, Varnek A, Winkler DA, Zakharov AV, Cherkasov A, Tropsha A. A critical overview of computational approaches employed for COVID-19 drug discovery. Chem Soc Rev. 2021;50(16):9121–51. https://doi.org/10.1039/d0cs01065k.

Student Stress Detection in Online Learning During Outbreak

Asmita Ray, Vishal Goyal, and Samir Kumar Bandyopadhyay

Abstract Stress is a state of mental strain for a specific person experiencing issues with their social and environmental well-being, which can result in a variety of illnesses. Young age is a crucial stage since it is a time when youth experience many changes in their lives. They are anticipated to be the social elite. Thus, in order to have a healthy life once they are integrated into society, individuals should improve their stress management skills. The newly infectious disease COVID-19 became the pandemic and due to this government around the world has closed all the educational institutions to stop the spread of COVID-19. The sudden shift from physical class room to virtual space has created the direct impact on students, educators, and institutions. This study explored and analysed the academic stress level experienced by students during online education which arose due to COVID-19 pandemic with regard to mental health of students during social isolation. Our study intends to define and characterise how the COVID-19 pandemic and the development of new technology affect an individual's stress levels. This research employed deep learning algorithms such as Convolutional Neural Networks (CNN) and Multilayer Perceptron (MLP) and machine learning algorithms support vector machine (SVM), K-Nearest Neighbour (K-NN), Decision Tree (DT) to quickly and accurately identify stress in a large population. To achieve the best accuracy rate, a comparative study between the machine and deep learning algorithms has been performed. The results exhibited that CNN the deep learning algorithm outperformed than non-deep learning methods and MLP. As a result, CNN, a deep learning technique, might serve as a more accurate predictor for the identification of stress level. In order to prevent stress from endangering those millions of people's lives, this paper aims to raise their awareness of early stress diagnosis and treatment. Finally, the report clarifies how policies on stress and preventative measures for stress will be rebuilt by policymakers in the school sector and general industry sector.

Keywords COVID-19 · Online education · Academic stress · Pandemic · Supervised and unsupervised machine learning

A. Ray (✉) · V. Goyal · S. K. Bandyopadhyay
GLA University, Mathura, Uttar Pradesh, India

G. Battineni et al. (eds.), *Computational Methods in Psychiatry*,
https://doi.org/10.1007/978-981-99-6637-0_13

1 Introduction

Stress is a state of physical or mental tension or worry that a person may experience as a result of inescapable events or any thinking that causes them to feel restless, irate, or frustrated. A person's physical, mental, or emotional responses are the result of the body's response to whatever change it encounters. Simply said, when expectations predicted and actuality experienced are not in sync, a person feels stressed. This causes them to become restless and tight [1]. Stress can be good if it keeps a person alert, energised, and prepared for any danger. On the other hand, if the stressors (i.e. stress-related elements) persist for prolonged periods of time without relief or waiting until a breakdown occurs, stress may have a general detrimental effect on an individual. We are well aware that stress cannot be completely eradicated, but we can at least recognise and deal with the numerous elements of stress in people from diverse vocational fields. We are fully aware that stress cannot be completely eliminated, but we can at least recognise and deal with the numerous elements of stress in people from diverse vocational fields. Consequently, overcoming the stresses is crucial to creating a stress management strategy that works [2]. In recent years, there have been many developments in the field of stress. Stress level increased during the COVID-19 pandemic for different factors like online classes and assignments and covid infection [3].

Novel Corona Virus (COVID-19) is the deadliest virus that claim the lives of million people around the globe. Corona virus belongs to family of coronavirus. It is zoonotic virus. The main reason of zoonotic virus is transmission of pathogen from animal to human. Virus outer covering is crown-like spikes so it is called coronavirus. Coronavirus rapidly spread by droplets at the time of talking, coughing, and sneezing as droplets can only propagate via direct contact [4]. It is known from the recent research that COVID-19 virus can exist in air up to 3 h, 4 h on copper, 72 h on plastic and stainless steel. In March 2020, COVID-19 spread across several countries, and World Health Organization (WHO) declared COVID-19 as pandemic [5, 6]. Online learning is the only way at social distancing period for all levels of education and teaching. In distance learning, learning and teaching took place through electronic medium. This virtual environment was the main medium of interaction between learners and educators [7].

Online education is not the new concept but COVID-19 pandemic make this online education as global need. Adapting the new teaching methodology due to the transition to online learning was a challenging task. So, all the countries were not able to handle this challenge. Research showed that 85% of institutions transfer the learning procedure from in person online learning and 29% of African institution can cope with online education [8]. Stress is defined as body's response which changes the mental state that is the cause of physical, emotional, or psychological strain. Stress requires attention or action. Stress is very crucial mediator which relates the stressful events to health. Perceived a very important tool is used to assess the student's stress level [9]. Different learning method has introduced in China. In early Feb 2020, this online-based learning platform accomplishes the objective of suspending classes without suspending learning [10]. To alleviate the education issues, in Jordan, online teaching was started [11].

Online learning though introduces students to various resources across the world yet it also comes with a lot of challenges as enormous time is consumed for strategizing goals plans required for proper utilisation of available resources. Apart from its problems in students' engagement, coupled with lack of motivation to maintain proper online routine cannot be ruled out. One of the main issues of online learning is mission out the traditional and time-tested classroom experiences. It is also pertinent to mention that a lack of adequate internet access for the downtrodden is also a hindrance for scale implementation of online learning [12]. This pandemic affects globally in social, emotional, and psychological way. Due to this pandemic outbreak, lot of students faced psychological problems that affected not only academics but also all over personality.

Psychological problems such as depression, stress, and anxiety students during their school and college year COVID-19 pandemic have aggravated the problems to a larger scale. COVID-19 pandemic has introduced online classes for students which have also had a devastating effect on the mental health of students as they were detached from the interaction of fellow students causing enormous mental health issues and it had a direct impact on the social life. Limitations on online learning due to lack infrastructure also played a huge role in it [13]. Lockdown life had great impact on the mental health of everyone as it effects on three parameters: autonomy, competency, and connectedness. During lockdown, people could not meet their near and dear ones and perform their day-to-day activities.

A recent study on "The psychological impact of quarantine and how to reduce it" by Samantha K Brooks presents as to how COVID-19 was having a huge impact on people during lockdown. Symptoms like sadness, insomnia, anger, confusion, post-traumatic stress, emotional disturbance, and exhaustion were very common. Stress can be defined as a non-specific response of the body to any demand [14]. Every single person at some point of time experienced stress which makes them shaky or frightened. Stress if continued for a longer period of time damages people's health and it affects their quality of their daily life. These days stress becomes very common for everyone irrespective of age and genders while it cannot be denied that stress if is given on a right scale can sharpen the mind, reflexes and encourage for change and growth. The major shift in communication due to COVID-19 pandemic not only affects our physical health, but it also creates a great impact on mental health [15–18]. Students bear more pressure due to this recent change in education domain resulting the government around the world close all the educational institutions to stop the spread of deadly disease among the students, educators, and all associated people [19, 20].

The major movement in teaching from physical to virtual classroom creates a severe disruption on students, and it suddenly entirely changed the lives and perspectives of all people. The current online education has brought a lot of shocks for students as well as parents [21–24]. Parents have to spend more time to monitor their children and motivate them to continue their study as home confinement and distance learning may have adverse effect on students' physical and mental health.

Different types of issues like fear of contagion, frustration, boredom, inadequate information increase due to this disease outbreak, and that impacted individual mental health and well-being. The communication shifted from face to face to virtual due to this outbreak [25]. Academic stress, separate the students from their class mates' that effect on students' behaviour. COVID-19 outbreak has emerged the problems like change of eating and sleeping habits, conflicting family schedules, loneliness may have adverse impact on the mental health of students [26–28].

The aim of the study is to identify the three main stressors which are directly influence impact on the mental health of students such as academic workload, separation from school, and fear of contagion [29]. This study also focuses to analyse the perception of academic stress experienced by students due to online education. Analysing the coping strategy of students using emotional intelligence is the objective of this study. Our study provides a list of many stress-related variables, causes of stress, and the effects of technological apprehension on stress. The paper will present a perspective for educators and students to develop appropriate solutions and maintain best practises of stress management in schools, colleges, and universities.

2 Degree of Stress

Acute stress: It is a very common form of stress which has a positive as new as a negative effect. It arises in answer to unexpected energies. However it does not lead to serious health issue. If it is does not liger on for a considerable period of time, there is nothing to worry about. Some common sign of acute stress includes stomach pain, chest pain, headache, and increasing blood pressure.

Episodic stress: It is a continuous stress. It is accompanied by a constant worry. The symptoms of episodic stress are almost similar to that of acute stress but it extends for a longer period of time. Episodic stress is most seen in people who display so-called Type A personality. This people are often ambitious, organised, proactive, and carrier oriented in nature. People affected by episodic stress remain unaware of how bad effect of episodic stress can be.

Chronic acute active stress: This stress has a feeling of never-ending stress. It often arises in response to situation that a person finds himself in an utterly hopeless position like a trouble marriage or poverty.

2.1 Stress Classification

Stress can be experienced, in four main varieties: time, anticipatory, situational, and encounter. This type of stress can be experienced in different situation from home to work place. Students are facing this type of stress.

Time stress: When someone feels constantly shortage of time to do any unnecessary task, the stress cause is known as time stress.

Anticipatory stress: Anxiousness of finishing a task in hand is crux of this type of stress. This kind of stress is more predominant among students.

Situational stress: When someone cannot control an alarming situation, then situational stress occurs. The two essential characteristics of this kind of stress are as follows: (a) it happens suddenly, (b) it happens without any anticipation and warning.

Situational stress: When the situation is not under control like present situation and that the cause of stress and upset is called situational stress. This type of stress occurs suddenly.

Encounter stress: Encounter stress occurs when a person is not comfortable to stay alone or in a group or feel anxious to see certain people. Students experience this situation when they meet unfamiliar classmates or intimidating professors.

2.2 *The Impact of Stress on Human Body*

Stress is a typical physical and psychological response to experience throughout life. Everybody occasionally displays signs of stress. Stress can be brought on by anything, from regular obligations like job and family to significant life events like a new illness, war, or the loss of a loved one. Stress can be good for your health in conditions that are urgent and short term. It can assist you in handling potentially dangerous circumstances. Stress causes your body to release hormones that quicken your heartbeat and breathing as well as prepare your muscles for action.

However, if your stress response doesn't slow down and your stress levels remain high for a lot longer than is necessary for survival, it could negatively impact your health. Numerous symptoms and your general well-being might be brought on by chronic stress. Chronic stress has the following symptoms:

- Irritability
- Anxiety
- Depression
- Headaches
- Insomnia

Stress can affect the function of different body parts. Some of them are listed below.

2.2.1 Respiratory Systems

The respiratory system eliminates carbon dioxide waste from the body and delivers oxygen to cells. Air enters the body through the nose, travels down the trachea through the larynx in the throat, and then enters the lungs through the bronchi. Red blood cells are subsequently given oxygen by the bronchioles so they can circulate. As the airway between the nose and the lungs narrows under stress and under the influence of intense emotions, respiratory symptoms including shortness of breath and fast breathing might manifest. Psychological stressors can exacerbate breathing issues for people with pre-existing respiratory diseases like asthma and chronic obstructive pulmonary disease, but this is typically not a problem for people without respiratory disease because the body can manage the additional work to breathe comfortably (COPD; includes emphysema and chronic bronchitis). According to studies, a sudden stressor, like losing a loved one, might actually cause asthma attacks. In addition, someone who is prone to panic attacks may experience a panic attack due to the rapid breathing—or hyperventilation—caused by stress. It can be beneficial to acquire relaxation, breathing, and other cognitive behavioural techniques with the assistance of a psychologist.

2.2.2 Cardiovascular System

The cardiovascular system is made up of the heart and blood arteries, which together transport nutrients and oxygen to the body's organs. The body's reaction to stress is likewise coordinated by the functioning of these two components. The stress chemicals adrenaline, noradrenaline, and cortisol serve as messengers for these effects in acute stress, which is instantaneous or short-term stress such as meeting deadlines, getting stopped in traffic, or abruptly slamming on the brakes to escape an accident. Additionally, the blood arteries that carry blood to the heart, large muscles, and other major organs of the body expand, boosting blood flow to these areas of the body and raising blood pressure. The fight-or-flight reaction is another name for this. The body returns to normal after the acute stress episode has ended.

Chronic stress, or persistent stress that lasts for a long time, can cause heart and blood vessel issues in the long run. The body can suffer from the constant and continuous increase in heart rate, as well as the high levels of stress hormones and blood pressure. The risk of hypertension, heart attacks, and stroke may rise as a result of this long-term, continuing stress. This is one mechanism that is believed to link stress to heart attack. Repeated acute stress and persistent chronic stress may both lead to inflammation in the circulatory system, especially in the coronary arteries. Additionally, it seems that a person's reaction to stress can influence cholesterol levels.

Depending on whether a woman is premenopausal or postmenopausal, her risk of heart disease from stress seems to vary. Premenopausal women with higher oestrogen levels tend to have better blood vessel response to stress, which helps their body cope with stress better and guards against heart disease. Due to the decrease of oestrogen after menopause, postmenopausal women are less protected from the effects of stress on heart disease. Cardiovascular is impacted by stress hormones. You breathe more quickly when under stress in an effort to immediately deliver oxygen-rich blood to your body. Stress can exacerbate respiratory issues, such as asthma or emphysema, if you already have them. Your heart also beats more quickly when under stress. Your blood vessels narrow as a result of stress hormones, which increases the amount of oxygen delivered to your muscles and gives you more power. But doing this also makes you more hypertensive. Therefore, sustained or ongoing stress will cause your heart to beat too quickly and forcefully, the likelihood of experiencing a heart.

2.2.3 Endocrine System

The hypothalamic-pituitary-adrenal (HPA) axis, which is the main regulator of the endocrine stress response, starts a cascade of events when someone views a situation as difficult, dangerous, or unpredictable. As a result, the synthesis of steroid hormones known as glucocorticoids—among which is cortisol, also known as the "stress hormone"—increases.

The HPA Axis

The pituitary gland, which is placed above the kidneys, receives signals from the hypothalamus, a group of nuclei that connects the brain and endocrine system, telling it to make a hormone, which then tells the adrenal glands to produce more cortisol. By releasing glucose and fatty acids from the liver, cortisol raises the amount of energy fuel that is readily available. Over the day, cortisol is frequently created in variable amounts; it typically rises in concentration before awakening and gradually falls throughout the day, creating a regular cycle of energy. During a stressful situation, a rise in cortisol can give you the energy you need to handle a protracted or difficult challenge.

The immune system and inflammation are controlled by glucocorticoids, which include cortisol. The communication between the immune system and the HPA axis can become hindered under chronic stress, despite the fact that this is helpful under stressful or hazardous circumstances where harm may result in enhanced immune system activation. Chronic fatigue, metabolic diseases (such as diabetes and obesity), depression, and immunological disorders have all been related to the future emergence of a wide range of physical and mental health conditions.

2.2.4 Gastrointestinal System

The fact that one can feel "butterflies" in the stomach is due to the hundreds of millions of neurons that make up the gut. These neurons can operate somewhat autonomously and are in constant communication with the brain. This brain-gut connection can be hampered by stress, which makes it easier to experience pain, bloating, and other stomach discomfort. Millions of bacteria reside in the gut, and their health, as well as the health of the brain, which affects thinking and emotion, can have an impact on both. Gut bacterial alterations brought on by stress have been linked to changes in mood. Thus, the neurons and bacteria in the stomach have a significant impact on the brain and vice versa. Early life stress can alter how the nervous system develops and how the body responds to stress. The likelihood of developing subsequent gastrointestinal illnesses or dysfunction can rise as a result of these alterations.

Exophages

People may eat significantly more or significantly less than usual when under stress. Heartburn or acid reflux can be brought on by eating more or different types of meals, increasing your alcohol or smoke intake, or both. The intensity of chronic heartburn pain can also be exacerbated by stress or weariness. Infrequently, severe stress can cause oesophageal spasms, which are frequently mistaken for heart attacks. Stress can also make it more difficult to swallow food or cause you to swallow more air, which causes more burping, gassiness, and bloating.

Stomach

Stress may make it easier to feel pain, bloating, nausea, and other stomach discomfort. Vomiting could happen if the stress is too great. Stress might also result in an unneeded increase or decrease in appetite. Unhealthy diets may worsen a person's mood in turn. Contrary to popular perception, stress does not make the stomach produce more acid or lead to ulcers. The latter are actually brought on by an infection with bacteria. Ulcers may be more unpleasant when under stress.

Bowel

Additionally, stress can make it easier to detect pain, bloating, or discomfort in the intestines. It may slow down or speed up digestion, which may result in diarrhoea or constipation. Additionally, stress may cause uncomfortable gut muscular spasms. Digestion and the nutrients the intestines receive might be impacted by stress. It's possible that gas generation from nutrient absorption will rise. The body is shielded from (most) food-related bacteria by the tight barrier that exists in the intestines. Stress can weaken the intestinal barrier, allowing the body to absorb bacteria from the gut. Although the majority of these germs are quickly eliminated by the immune system and do not harm humans, the ongoing, minimal demand for inflammatory response can result in long-lasting moderate symptoms. Chronic bowel illnesses like inflammatory bowel disease and irritable bowel syndrome are particularly affected by stress. This might be caused by more sensitive gut nerves, altered gut bacteria, altered rates of food transit through the gut, or altered gut immunological responses.

2.2.5 Nervous System

The nervous system is divided into two main groups: the central group, which includes the brain and spinal cord, and the peripheral group, which includes the somatic and autonomic nervous systems. The sympathetic nervous system (SNS) and the parasympathetic nervous system are two components of the autonomic nervous system that directly affect how the body reacts to stress (PNS). The SNS plays a role in the "fight or flight" response that occurs when the body is under stress. The body redirects its energy resources in order to defend itself or run away from an aggressor. Adrenalin (epinephrine) and cortisol are released by the adrenal glands in response to signals from the SNS. These hormones drive the heart to beat more quickly, the breathing rate to rise, the blood vessels in the arms and legs to widen, the digestive process to alter, and the blood glucose levels (sugar energy) to rise in response to the emergency.

To get the body ready to react to an emergency scenario or acute stress—short-term stressors—the SNS response is rather quick. The body often returns to its pre-emergency, unstressed state after a crisis has passed. The PNS, which often has opposite effects to the SNS, aids in this recuperation. However, excessive PNS activity can potentially exacerbate stress responses by, for instance, encouraging bronchoconstriction (as in asthma) or increased vasodilation and weakened blood circulation. The immune system, which can also control stress reactions, is strongly influenced by both the SNS and the PNS. Since the central nervous system controls the autonomic nervous system and is crucial in evaluating environments as potentially dangerous, it plays a significant role in inducing stress reactions.

Chronic stress, or being exposed to stressors for an extended length of time, can have a lasting negative impact on the body. The body experiences wear and tear as the autonomic nervous system continues to create bodily reactions. Chronic stress affects the neurological system, but what the nervous system does to other bodily systems when it is constantly activated is what causes problems.

2.2.6 Male Reproductive System

The neurological system has an impact on the male reproductive system. While the sympathetic portion of the nervous system generates arousal, the parasympathetic portion causes rest. The fight-or-flight reaction, commonly known as the autonomic nervous system, is what causes arousal and produces testosterone in the male anatomy. It also stimulates the sympathetic nervous system. The hormone cortisol, which is made by the adrenal glands, is released by the body in response to stress. Blood pressure management and the healthy operation of various bodily systems, such as the cardiovascular, circulatory, and male reproductive systems, depend on cortisol. The male reproductive system's typical biochemical operation can be hampered by high cortisol levels.

Sexual Desire

The production of testosterone can be affected by chronic stress, which is persistent stress for an extended length of time. This can lead to a loss in libido and sex drive, and it may even result in erectile dysfunction or impotence.

Reproduction

Chronic stress can hinder sperm maturation and production, making it difficult for couples who are trying to get pregnant. In comparison to males who had no stressful life events, researchers discovered that men who had two or more stressful life events in the previous year had lower percentages of sperm that were motile (able to swim) and had normal morphology (size and shape).

Diseases of the Reproductive System

Stress can weaken the immune system, making the body more susceptible to illness. Infections of the testicles, prostate, and urethra in the male anatomy can interfere with normal male reproductive function.

2.2.7 Female Reproductive System

Menstruation

Teenage girls' and women's menstruation may be impacted by stress in a variety of ways. For instance, excessive levels of stress may be linked to menstrual cycle absence or irregularity, painful periods, and variations in cycle duration.

Sexual Desire

Over the course of their lives, women balance a variety of pressures including financial, professional, family, and personal obligations. Particularly when women are also caring for small children or other sick family members, managing chronic medical issues, feeling depressed, experiencing marital troubles or abuse, managing challenges at work, etc., stress, distraction, weariness, etc., may impair sexual desire.

Pregnancy

The plans a woman has for getting pregnant might be significantly impacted by stress. A woman's ability to conceive, the health of her pregnancy, and her postpartum adjustment may all be severely impacted by stress. The most common problem with pregnancy and postpartum adjustment is depression. The probability of experiencing depression and anxiety during this period is increased by excessive stress. Maternal stress can interfere with bonding with the infant in the days and weeks after birth as well as significantly affect foetal and ongoing childhood development.

Premenstrual Syndrome

Premenstrual symptoms can be distressing for many women, and stress can make premenstrual symptoms worse or harder to manage. These signs and symptoms include mood changes, irritability, bloating, and cramping as well as fluid retention and cramps.

Menopause

Hormone levels dramatically change as menopause approaches. These alterations are linked to stress, mood fluctuations, and unpleasant feelings. Therefore, menopause itself may be a source of stress. It can be challenging to deal with some of the physical changes brought on by menopause, especially hot flashes. In addition, mental distress may exacerbate the physical symptoms. For instance, women who are more worried may have more hot flashes overall, as well as more frequent hot flashes that are more strong or severe.

Diseases of the Reproductive System

When stress is high, there is increased chance of exacerbation of symptoms of reproductive disease states, such as herpes simplex virus or polycystic ovarian syndrome. The diagnosis and treatment of reproductive cancers can cause significant stress, which warrants additional attention and support.

3 Stress Characteristics and Impact of Technology Rise

Stress affects everyone but it effects on a different scale for each. The symptoms and signs of stress vary from one person to another person which is very important to understand. Be that as it may there are some common signs and symptoms which can be classified into four different heads like physical, emotional, cognitive, and behavioural symptoms. A physical symptom of stress includes but not limited to irregular bowl movement, missed periods and reduces libido. Emotional symptoms may include impatience, depression, and restlessness and reduce desire for activities. Cognitive symptoms incorporate impaired concentration, amnesia, chronic distress reduce judgemental capacity. Behavioural symptoms encompass change in appetite and sleeping habits.

Human lives have been made easier by modern communication technologies. Exchanges that used to take weeks to complete may now be completed in a matter of minutes or seconds on the other side of the globe. They have, nevertheless, accelerated their pace of movement. Modern technology has become so ingrained in our lives that it is simple to develop a dependence on it to the point that it begins to negatively affect us on a variety of levels. This study would examine how technology has changed our lives and contributed to an increase in people's general levels of stress. First of all, it has been shown that people who use information and communication technology, or ICT, experience stress, concern, and tension as a result of using the technology. This condition is known as techno anxiety. In addition, users may encounter psychological affects that can undermine their confidence. Such situations can produce powerless and uncomfortable feelings, as well as aversion or dread of using computers, a syndrome called as technophobia. Third, over use of ICTs might result in a disorder called techno-addiction [30].

Last but not least, technological stress is a condition of the modern day brought on by the incapacity to adapt to new computing technology in a healthy and productive way [31]. According to research [32], using social media sites excessively—defined as more than 2 h per day—is associated with poor mental health, increased psychological distress, and suicidal thoughts in addition to being potentially dangerous and addictive for a very small percentage of people. The COVID-19 pandemic has been a problem since early 2020. The state implemented a number of emergency measures. These included the methods used by both public and private companies to access home-based remote work. Without sacrificing the services, they provided, the government sought to reduce crowding and restrict movement around the national territory [33, 34].

Despite this, workers were able to adjust to the quick, drastic change due to the rapid growth of ICTs. There was a fear of technology despite expectations that employees would react to it favourably and quickly. Lack of readiness and technical readiness were concerns in the educational sector. Patients were continually concerned about any data that revealed significant diseases or inaccurate diagnosis in the medical and healthcare fields. However, in the banking industry, there is apprehension because of how clients view technology. Customers are concerned about making mobile payments and sharing their info. The fear of technology and the growing amount of family duties have led to reduced focus on technology use in families [35, 36].

Teachers are increasingly expected to integrate the usage of technology into their teaching approaches in the classrooms due to the rising workload [31]. For teachers, this results in an excessive workload, a challenge, and stress. The lack of time and the rising expectations of the schools and colleges cause teacher's constant struggle.

It has been extremely demanding and difficult for the teachers to keep up with the emerging technologies and the advances related to them. Even though teachers may view technology as a tool for lesson planning, information delivery, or student acquisition, many lack the necessary skills and competences to put this positive use of technology into practise [31]. The pandemic is making it difficult for students to concentrate due to their emotional state, which can also affect their ability to learn independently and their health [37].

Perceived fear and expectation confirmation were found to be important predictors of willingness to use mobile learning. Additionally, prior research demonstrated how employing mobile learning (ML) in the educational setting during the pandemic presented a potential benefit for both teaching and learning. The dread of losing friends, a stressful home environment, and the worry about future academic performance may lessen this effect [38]. As previously mentioned, the development of technology has facilitated the simplification of daily living. Despite the fact that using technology made it easier to work, coordinate, and teach, it did contribute to raising stress levels for both in the classroom and at employment. Speaking of social media, the younger age was already absorbed in it, but now everyone staying at home during the pandemic had joined them. Additionally, it was noted that the general mood on social media was indifferent [39, 40].

3.1 Distinct Challenging Stressor Among Students During COVID-19

People around the world experienced stress during COVID-19. In the current study, prevalent stress factors are discussed.

Academics: This kind of stress is very common prime type of stress for all type of students. This is very long-term stress during the students' life as this stress is inevitable. Students who are already in depression this stress imposes more anxiety. During the pandemic, the stress level increases undoubtedly. This type of stress is becoming an escalating nerve-racking problem and both teachers and student face the consequence. It seems that this type of stress will be controlled easily, but if it IS not managed it will create an adverse effect on student's performance. The reason of this stress among students is completely imperative to realise, and it plays a major role to create a great impact of their effective learning.

Classes time table and credit load: If class schedule is not prepared based on desire after a couple of weak, teacher get frustrated not only that one, if the scheduling of classes of different subjects may also the cause of stress. The solution to handle this type of stress is to prepare the schedule based on the requirement and that flexibility reduce mental stress. Academic performance is another factor that create pressure on students as good result helps to fulfil the desired career. In respect of teachers balancing the workload with the personal life and social life is very hard die to the increase of workload and difficulty of courses. Completely discard the school related stress is very difficult as students surrounded by the stressors and stressed classmates. Few points are addressed in this study to overcome the stress level of students.

(a) Seriousness in learning is the cause of good performance so study properly and take the preparation for examination seriously.
(b) Focus an exam at a time that helps to get a good result.
(c) Do not visualise the exam during studies.
(d) To clear the concept, take help of tutor.
(e) Avoid thinking of examination.

Future: For many students, schools are very comfortable zone. So, after entering into to college due to the unfamiliar and unknown environment, life gets stressed. The stress level will increase if that student experienced that his/her friends and peers are more confident in study and for their future plan. That situation makes that student feel anxious if he does not have any plan for future. Unemployment and poor opportunity for employment after finishing the course also the cause of stress and anxiety of their carrier choice and future prospects.

3.2 Strategy for Future Planning to Avoid Stress

Future uncertainty is very hard to manage. So, taking advice for career and proper guidance for future from councillors, family, friends, professors helps to show the path of success. Aptitude test also plays a crucial role to take the right decision for choosing career.

Necessary steps to maintain the student's health:

(a) To avoid the particular illness around the campus and community, the best way is to avoid contact with anyone and take the precautionary instruction.
(b) Another reason of stress is not achieving the social intimacy. Interpersonal relationship could not be developed due to lack of time.
(c) Make lifelong friends where student/s can invest their time and that friendship really matter to them.
(d) It is seen that education cost has risen now in days and that is the cause of stress for students over their finance when they are in school.

So overcome this situation, positive thinking is the best way to improve the physical well-being and that positive thinking produces lower feelings of depression and distress. Education is the worth investment that believe can lead to better job opportunity after the completion of study.

3.2.1 Recommended Approach for Managing Stress

Stress is inevitable. So realising the cause and kind of stress helps to respond productively. There are many ways to handle the stress, and different people have different ways of coping with it. How to overcome the stress is very important to learn and cope with it productively. It is not possible to control the stressors but it is very crucial to grasp hoe to respond to them.

There are several reasons of academic stress such as new responsibilities, challenging classes, low grade, increase in workload over insufficient time, etc.

3.2.2 Social Stress

Creating a new social network, separation from home, living with roommate are the major cause of this type of stress.

3.2.3 Others Stress

Financial crisis, long study, hard hours, waking up early for attending classes are the major causes of stress.

There are two ways to handle the stress:

(a) Healthy
(b) Unhealthy

Smoking, drinking and the use of drugs, over and under eat, spend compulsively are the unhealthy way to manage the stress.

Confront the stressor, time management, being organised, exercise, proper nutrition, and sleep, spend time with loved one are the healthy ways to handle the stress.

4 Research Methodology

The block diagram of proposed method is shown in Fig. 1.

The proposed module consists of three steps (a) data collection, (b) preprocessing, (c) feature extraction, (d) classification, (e) performance evaluation

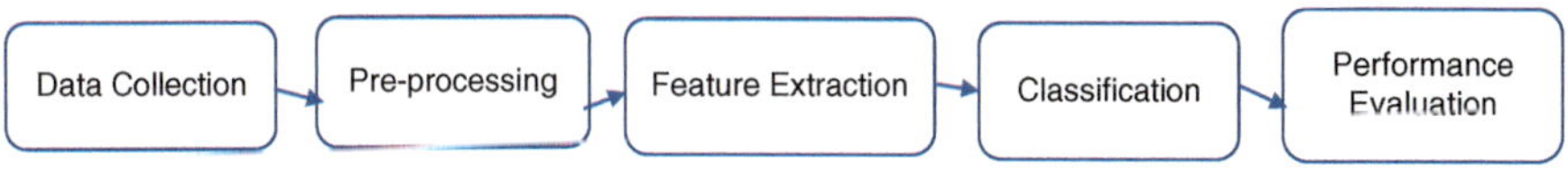

Fig. 1 Block diagram of proposed method for stress detection

4.1 Data Collection

Data have been collected from a large number heterogeneous group of students. Google form has been used for this purpose. Three elements were found to be the most crucial in this online study.

1. Socio-demographic characteristics that include age, gender, educational qualification, and location of residence.
2. Perceived Stress Scale (PSS) of Sheldon Cohen, this scale consists of ten questions to measure the stress level experienced by the students over the past months.
3. A question has included regarding the emotions and concern during the outbreak.

Three hundred sixty-seven participants, including both male and female students, had their data collected using the Galvanic Skin Response (GSR) and Electrocardiogram (ECG) sensors.

The mean, median, standard deviation, minimum reading, maximum reading, max ratio, and min ratio are extracted to acquire the best features after pre-processing the raw data. Processed data was analysed and classified using machine and deep learning algorithm, to predict the stress.

4.2 Machine Learning Algorithms

(a) **Support Vector Machine (SVM):** One of the most widely utilised supervised learning algorithms, Support Vector Machine, or SVM, is used to solve classification and regression problems. However, it is largely employed in machine learning classification issues. The SVM algorithm's objective is to establish the best line or decision boundary that can divide n-dimensional space into classes, allowing us to quickly classify fresh data points in the future. A hyperplane is the name given to this optimal decision boundary. SVM selects the extreme vectors and points that aid in the creation of the hyperplane. Support vectors, which are used to represent these extreme instances, form the basis for the SVM method. Take a look at the diagram below, where a decision boundary or hyperplane is used to categorize two distinct categories.

Hyperplane: In n-dimensional space, there may be several lines or decision boundaries used to divide classes; however, the optimal decision boundary for classifying the data points must be identified. The hyperplane of SVM is a name for this optimal boundary. The dataset's features determine the hyperplane's dimensions, therefore if there are just two features (as in the example image), the hyperplane will be a straight line. Additionally, if there are three features, the hyperplane will only have two dimensions. We always build a hyperplane with a maximum margin, or the greatest possible separation between the data points.

Support Vectors: Support vectors are the data points or vectors that are closest to the hyperplane and have the greatest influence on where the hyperplane is located. These vectors are called support vectors because they support the hyperplane.

(b) **K-Nearest Neighbour (K-NN)**: One of the simplest machine learning algorithms, based on the supervised learning method, is K-Nearest Neighbour. The K-NN algorithm makes the assumption that the new case and the existing cases are comparable, and it places the new instance in the category that is most like the existing categories. A new data point is classified using the K-NN algorithm based on similarity after all the existing data has been stored. This means that utilising the K-NN method, fresh data can be quickly and accurately sorted into a suitable category. Although the K-NN approach is most frequently employed for classification problems, it can also be utilised for regression. Since K-NN is a non-parametric technique, it makes no assumptions about the underlying data. It is also known as a lazy learner algorithm since it saves the training dataset rather than learning from it immediately. Instead, it uses the dataset to perform an action when classifying data. The K-NN method simply saves the information during the training phase, and when it receives new data, it categorises it into a category that is quite similar to the new data.

(c) **Decision Tree:** A supervised learning method called a decision tree can be used to solve classification and regression problems, but it is typically favoured for doing so. It is a tree-structured classifier, where internal nodes stand in for dataset's features, branches for the decision-making process, and each leaf node for the classification result.

The decision node and leaf node are the two nodes of a decision tree. While leaf nodes are the results of decisions and do not have any more branches, decision nodes are used to create decisions and have numerous branches. Classification and regression issues can be resolved using the supervised learning technique known as a decision tree, however this approach is frequently preferred. It is a tree-structured classifier, where each leaf node represents the classification outcome and inside nodes represent the features of a dataset.

The two nodes in a decision tree are the decision node and leaf node. Decision nodes are used to make decisions and have many branches, whereas leaf nodes are the outcomes of decisions and do not have any more branches.

4.3 Deep Learning Algorithm

(a) **Convolutional Neural Networks (CNN):** A neural network type called a convolutional neural network, or CNN or ConvNet, is particularly adept at processing input with a grid-like architecture, like an image. A binary representation of visual data is a digital image. It is made up of a grid-like arrangement of pixels, each of which has a pixel value to indicate how bright and what colour it should be. Deep learning techniques are based on neural networks, a branch of machine learning. They are made up of node levels, each of which includes an input layer, one or more hidden layers, and an output layer. Each node has a threshold and weight that are connected to one another. Any node whose output exceeds the defined threshold value is activated and begins providing data to the network's uppermost layer. Otherwise, no data is transmitted to the network's next tier. There are three basic categories of CNN: (a) convolutional layer, (b) pooling layer, (c) fully connected (FC).

- Convolutional layer: The central component of a CNN is the convolutional layer, which is also where the majority of computation takes place. It needs input data, a filter, and a feature map, among other things.
- Pooling layer: Dimensionality reduction, sometimes referred to as downsampling or pooling layers, lowers the amount of factors in the input. The pooling process sweeps a filter across the entire input, much like the convolutional layer does, however this filter doesn't contain any weights.
- Fully connected (FC) layer: The full-connected layer is exactly what its name implies. In partially connected layers, there is no direct connection between the input image's pixel values and the output layer. In contrast, every node in the output layer of the fully connected layer is directly connected to a node in the layer above it. Based on the features that were retrieved from the preceding layers and their various filters, this layer conducts the classification operation.

(b) **Multilayer Perceptron (MLP):** The feed forward neural network is supplemented by the multilayer perceptron (MLP). The input layer, output layer, and hidden layer are the three different types of layers that constitute it. The input layer is where the input signal for processing is received. The output layer completes the necessary task, such as classification and prediction. The real computational engine of the MLP consists of an arbitrary number of hidden layers that are sandwiched between the input and output layers. Data flows from the input to the output layer of an MLP in the forward direction, much like a feed forward network.

4.4 Performance Evaluation

The performance of the stress detection model will be assessed using a number of performance evaluation measures. The metrics accuracy, precision, recall, and F1 score are displayed below:

Accuracy: The percentage of correctly classified data instances over all data instances is known as accuracy.

$$Accuracy = \frac{TP + TN}{TP + FP + FN + TN}$$

Precision: A classification model's capacity to isolate only the necessary data points. Precision is calculated by dividing the total number of true positives by the total number of true positives + false positives.

$$Precision = \frac{TP}{TP + FN}$$

Recall: The capacity of a model to locate all pertinent instances in a data source. Recall is calculated mathematically as the product of the number of true positives divided by the sum of the true positives and false negatives.

$$Recall = \frac{TP}{TP + FN}$$

F1-score: The definition of the F1 score, a metric that considers both recall and precision, is as follows.

$$F1 = 2 * \frac{Precession * Recall}{Precession + Recall}$$

5 Result and Discussion

The main objective of this paper is to detect the stress level of students for online learning during outbreak. We have done a socio-demographic analysis, that represents the stress level of different age group, gender, and educational level like intermediate school, secondary school, and university. We have classified the stress level into three categories: low, moderate, and high.

5.1 Statistical Analysis

Statistical Package for the Social science (SPSS) version 23.0 software has been used to perform for statistical analysis. Chi-square test was used for comparison of perceived stress level. Three hundred sixty-seven students have participated in this survey. The students have average age 17.39 ± 2.33 years. Numbers of female responders from secondary schools are more than male. The value of p will be considered when it will be less than 0.05.

In Table 1, the demographic details of the sampled population are shown. The survey received 367 responses in total from students. The majority of respondents (74.7%) were female and enrolled in high school (79.8%). Stress level has been estimated based on age, gender, and educational levels stress levels. There are three categories for stress levels: low, moderate, and high. To compare the perceived

Table 1 Socio-demographic analysis

	Low stress (%)	Moderate stress (%)	High stress (%)	Total ($n = 367$) (%)	P-value
Age group					
13–15 years	11.7	47.4	43.9	16.3	0.007
16–18 years	18.6	57.4	26.2	72.4	
>18 years	4.2	53.2	43.9	14.3	
Gender					
Female	14.1	52.6	34.9	75.7	0.022
Male	18.4	62.4	18.4	26.3	
Educational levels					
Intermediate school	14.7	41.2	46.1	13.5	0.024
Secondary school	17	56	26	78.8	
University	0	59.6	39	6.4	

Table 2 Comparison result of machine learning and deep learning algorithms

Classifier	Accuracy (%)	Precision (%)	Recall (%)	F1 score
SVM	80	82	76	77
K-NN	83	79	78	79
Decision tree	87	85	88	86
MLP	92	93	92	91
CNN	96	97	97	97

stress scale, the Chi-square test was utilised. The differences were deemed statistically significant when the p-values were less than 0.05.

In our study, we have used both machine learning and deep learning algorithms. The dataset is divided into a training dataset which contains 70% of data and testing dataset contains 30% of data. In our experiment, we have used SVM, K-NN, DT, the machine learning algorithms, and MLP and CNN as deep learning algorithms. Deep learning algorithms achieve satisfactory performance in comparison to machine learning algorithms.

The result shown in Table 2 demonstrates that CNN, the deep learning algorithm has the highest performance in terms of accuracy, precision, recall, and F1 score. This paper presented an approach of comparison study between machine learning and deep learning algorithms to identify the stress level. CNN, the deep learning algorithm achieves the best performance among all deep learning and non-deep learning algorithms in terms of accuracy, precession recall, and F1 score.

6 Conclusion

COVID-19 affected everyone worldwide. Lockdown imposed during pandemic caused immense disturbance in the mental state of the students. As a result of which there is a substantial increase of stress level on them cause due to various factors like academics, environment, and family. Academic problems are the biggest contributors of stress-related issues of students which needs to be addressed urgently. Specific and targeted measures like students' welfare programs, student's friendly atmosphere coupled with regular extra-curricular activities should be introduced within a short period of time. Feedback from the students with regard to the aforesaid steps should be taken, reviewed periodically. Regular study habits, peaceful sleep, stress free environment, adequate extra-curricular activities should help students to avoid stress and lead a normal healthy and enjoyable life.

Students all over the globe face a serious level of stress arising out of many academic as well as non-academic aspects. Environmental, socio-cultural, and psychological factors are considered as non-academic aspects. Stress actually put heavy pressure on students. This study showed high to moderate level of stress among students. To manage the stress and coping, the strategy online stress management program is recommended. Different types of psychiatric disorders such as depression and anxiety play a crucial role in this purpose.

References

1. Parslow RA, Jorm AF, Christensen H, Broom DH, Strazdins L, D'Souza RM. The impact of employee level and work stress on mental health and GP service use: an analysis of a sample of Australian government employees. BMC Public Health. 2004;4:41.
2. Amanvermez Y, Zhao R, Cuijpers P, de Wit LM, Ebert DD, Kessler RC, et al. Effects of self-guided stress management interventions in college students: a systematic review and meta-analysis. Internet Interv. 2022;28:100503.
3. Vogel EA, Zhang JS, Peng K, Heaney CA, Lu Y, Lounsbury D, et al. Physical activity and stress management during COVID-19: a longitudinal survey study. Psychol Health. 2022;37(1):51–61.
4. Banerjee A, Kulcsar K, Misra V, Frieman M, Mossman K. Bats and Coronaviruses. Viruses. 2019;11(1):41.
5. World Health Organization. Coronavirus disease (Covid-19) outbreak: rights, roles and responsibilities of health workers, including key considerations for occupational safety. World Health Organization [Internet]. 2019:1–3. https://www.who.int/docs/default-source/coronaviruse/who-rights-roles-respon-hw-covid-19.pdf?sfvrsn=bcabd401_0.
6. Coronavirus disease (COVID-19) advice for the public. Geneva: World Health Organization. 2020.
7. Martinez PJ, Aguilar FJ, Ortiz M. Transitioning from face-to-face to blended and full online learning engineering master's program. IEEE Trans Educ. 2020;63(1):2–9.
8. Wang C, Pan R, Wan X, Tan Y, Xu L, Ho CS, et al. Immediate psychological responses and associated factors during the initial stage of the 2019 coronavirus disease (COVID-19) epidemic among the general population in China. Int J Environ Res Public Health. 2020;17:1729.

9. Mirna F, Ali S. E-learning: depression, anxiety, and stress symptomatology among Lebanese university students during COVID-19 quarantine. Nurs Forum. 2021;56(1):52–7.
10. Le HT, Lai AJX, Sun J, Hoang MT, Vu LG, Pham HQ, et al. Anxiety and depression among people under the nationwide partial lockdown in Vietnam. Front Public Health. 2020;8:589359.
11. Cedeño TDD, Rocha ICN, Ramos KG, Uy NMC. Learning strategies and innovations among medical students in the Philippines during the COVID-19 pandemic. Int J Med Stud. 2021;9(1):77–9.
12. Chang J, Yuan Y, Wang D. Mental health status and its influencing factors among college students during the epidemic of COVID-19. Nan Fang Yi Ke Da Xue Xue Bao. 2020;40(2):171–6.
13. Saddik B, Hussein A, Sharif-Askari FS, Kheder W, Temsah MH, Koutaich RA, et al. Increased levels of anxiety among medical and non-medical university students during the COVID-19 pandemic in the United Arab Emirates. Risk Manag Healthc Policy. 2020;13:2395–406.
14. Kelly H. The classical definition of a pandemic is not elusive. Bull World Health Organ. 2011;89:469–544.
15. Gao W, Ping S, Liu X. Gender differences in depression, anxiety, and stress among college students: a longitudinal study from China. J Affect Disord. 2020;263:292–300. PMID: 31818792.
16. Hurst CS, Baranik LE, Daniel F. College student stressors: a review of the qualitative research. Work Stress. 2013;29:275–85. PMID: 23023893.
17. Taylor MR, Agho KE, Stevens GJ, Raphael B. Factors influencing psychological distress during a disease epidemic: data from Australia' s first outbreak of equine influenza. BMC Public Health. 2008;8:347.
18. Centers for Disease Control and Prevention. Information for healthcare professionals about coronavirus (COVID 19) [Internet]. 2020 [cited 2020 June 23].
19. Kingdom's Government Sets Preventive. Precautionary measures to prevent COVID 19 infection transmission, interior ministry says. Riyadh: Saudi Press Agency; 2020.
20. Jing G, Zhong Y, Hao Y, Zhou D, Tsui H, Hao C, et al. Preventive behaviors and mental distress in response to H1N1 among university students in Guangzhou, China. Asia Pac J Public Health. 2015;27(2):NP1867–79.
21. Chen Q, Liang M, Li Y, Guo J, Fei D, Wang L, et al. Mental health care for medical staff in China during the COVID-19 outbreak. Lancet Psychiatry. 2020;7:e15–6.
22. Seligman LD, Wuyek LA. Correlates of separation anxiety symptoms among first-semester college students: an exploratory study. J Psychol. 2007;141:135–45.
23. Hsiang S, Allen D, Annan-Phan S, Bell K, Bolliger I, Chong T, et al. The effect of large-scale anti-contagion policies on the COVID-19 pandemic. Nature. 2020;584:262–7.
24. Corsano P, Majorano M, Champretavy L. Psychological well-being in adolescence: the contribution of interpersonal relations and experience of being alone. Adolescence. 2006;41:341–54.
25. Brewster ME, Moradi B, DeBlaere C, Velez BL. Navigating the borderlands: the roles of minority stressors, bicultural self-efficacy, and cognitive flexibility in the mental health of bisexual individuals. J Couns Psychol. 2013;60:543–56.
26. Akgun S, Ciarrochi J. Learned resourcefulness moderates the relationship between academic stress and academic performance. Educ Psychol. 2003;23:287–94.
27. Subramani C, Kadhiravan S. Academic stress and mental health among high school students. Indian J Anim Res. 2017;7:404–6.
28. Wang Y, Wang Y, Chen Y, Qin Q. Unique epidemiological and clinical features of the emerging 2019 novel coronavirus pneumonia (COVID-19) implicate special control measures. J Med Virol. 2020;92:568–76.
29. Dwivedi YK, Hughes DL, Coombs C, Constantiou I, Duan Y, Edwards JS, et al. Impact of COVID-19 pandemic on information management research and practice: transforming education, work and life. Int J Inf Manag. 2020;55:102211.
30. la Torre G, Esposito A, Sciarra I, Chiappetta M. Definition, symptoms and risk of technostress: a systematic review. Int Arch Occup Environ Health. 92:13–35. Springer.

31. Dong Y, Xu C, Chai CS, Zhai X. Exploring the structural relationship among teachers' technostress, technological pedagogical content knowledge (TPACK), computer self-efficacy and school support. Asia Pacific Educ Res. 2020;29(2):147–57.
32. Chauhan T, Palivela H. Optimization and improvement of fake news detection using deep learning approaches for societal benefit. Int J Inform Manag Data Insights. 2021;1(2):100051.
33. Király O, Potenza MN, Stein DJ, King DL, Hodgins DC, Saunders JB, et al. Preventing problematic internet use during the COVID-19 pandemic: consensus guidance. Compr Psychiatry. 2020;100:152180.
34. Molino M, Ingusci E, Signore F, Manuti A, Giancaspro ML, Russo V, et al. Wellbeing costs of technology use during Covid-19 remote working: an investigation using the Italian translation of the technostress creators scale. Sustainability. 2020;12(15):5911.
35. Alhumaid K, Habes M, Salloum SA. Examining the factors influencing the mobile learning usage during COVID-19 pandemic: an integrated SEM-ANN method. IEEE Access Pract Innov Open Solutions. 2021;9:102567–78.
36. Chakraborty A, Kar AK. How did COVID-19 impact working professionals—a typology of impacts focused on education sector. Int J Inform Learn Technol. 2021;38(3):273–82.
37. Shirish A, Chandra S, Srivastava SC. Switching to online learning during COVID-19: theorizing the role of IT mindfulness and techno eustress for facilitating productivity and creativity in student learning. Int J Inf Manag. 2021;61:102394.
38. Sciagrà R, Martini AL, Allocca M. The brain connection between stress and heart: a convincing research opportunity to reduce risk and gender disparity in cardiovascular disease. J Nucl Cardiol. 2021;28(2):433–5.
39. Sharma A, Sanghvi K, Churi P. The impact of instagram on young adult's social comparison, colourism and mental health: Indian perspective. Int J Inform Manag Data Insights. 2022;2(1):100057.
40. Stone JA, Can SH. Gendered language differences in public communication? The case of municipal tweets. Int J Inform Manag Data Insights. 2021;1(2):100034.

Emotional Recognition and Expression Based on People to Improve Well-Being

E. J. G. S. Appuhamy, B. G. D. A. Madhusanka, and H. M. K. K. M. B. Herath

Abstract The elderly and disabled population in Sri Lanka has been growing for a while. Some people include the country's protracted conflict, traffic accidents, a low labor force, and tiny family structures. As a result, caregivers must provide physical and mental aid to the elderly and people with disabilities. The demand for caregivers will worsen as a result of these hectic lives. In the future, this service robot may be utilized to address this issue. Most of the researchers work to create various types of service robots, particularly with voice recognition, facial recognition, etc., to replace caregivers. However, they could be more effective for those who are disabled. In order to care for people based on their gait, a new way is needed to recognize emotional experiences. As a result, research efforts are concentrated on creating an interactive service robot eye that can recognize and display emotions based on human movements. Acknowledging and understanding people's emotions and assisting them in adequately expressing and managing them, identifying emotional recognition and expression seek to comprehend and enhance people's emotional well-being. These people enable the development of systems and apps that support emotional understanding and improve mental health and well-being. This chapter explains how people's well-being influences emotional recognition. It investigates if a single physiological signal may improve the current approach to emotional recognition. There is still a great deal of emotional strain present, far more than Sri Lankans deem healthy. According to studies, time management may seriously

E. J. G. S. Appuhamy
Faculty of Engineering Technology, Department of Mechanical Engineering, Open University of Sri Lanka, Nugegoda, Sri Lanka

B. G. D. A. Madhusanka (✉) · H. M. K. K. M. B. Herath
Faculty of Engineering, Department of Mechanical and Mechatronics Engineering, Sri Lanka Technological Campus, Padukka, Sri Lanka
e-mail: achintham@sltc.ac.lk; kasunkh@sltc.ac.lk

G. Battineni et al. (eds.), *Computational Methods in Psychiatry*,
https://doi.org/10.1007/978-981-99-6637-0_14

impair people's ability to improve their health. Increased health awareness is correlated with better emotional and physical health and emotional recognition. An experiment was carried out in the selected residential setting with several users to test the effectiveness of the created intelligent system. During set up, several items are put in the nearby area. By removing several unnecessary factors, the robot eye could correctly discern human emotions during robot eye implementation, according to the experiment's results. By using additional datasets, it is possible to establish the fundamental behavior of the robot eye with high precision and under various lighting situations.

Keywords Emotional recognition · Convolutional neural network · Human activity recognition · Activities of daily living

1 Introduction

Emotional recognition and expression are essential for improving well-being because they allow individuals to understand better and manage their emotions, communicate effectively with others, and build stronger relationships. Emotional recognition involves being able to identify and understand one's own emotions, as well as the emotions of others [1]. This skill is essential for developing self-awareness and empathy, which can lead to better communication and social interactions. Emotional expression involves being able to communicate one's emotions effectively to others. This can help individuals build stronger relationships and foster greater understanding and empathy. Several techniques and tools can improve emotional recognition and expression [2]. These include mindfulness practices, meditation, journaling, therapy, and social skills training. Emotion recognition software and wearable devices can also monitor and track emotional states [3]. Improving emotional recognition and expression can significantly benefit individuals and society, including better mental health, stronger relationships, and improved communication and understanding.

Robotic eyes are being developed to recognize and express emotions to improve human–robot interaction and facilitate more effective communication between humans and machines [4]. These robotic eyes use computer vision technology and machine learning algorithms to analyze facial expressions and body language [5, 6]. They can recognize and interpret various emotions, including happiness, sadness, anger, fear, and surprise [7]. The development of robotic eyes for emotional recognition and expression has many potential applications. For example, they could be used as robotic assistants or caregivers for the elderly or individuals with disabilities, where recognizing and responding to emotions can improve the quality of care [8, 9]. They could also be used in education or therapy settings to help assess and improve emotional regulation and communication skills. Additionally, robotic eyes could facilitate more natural and intuitive communication between humans and robots. By allowing robots to express and respond appropriately to human emotions, people may be more likely to accept and trust them as partners in various tasks and activities. However, there are concerns about using robotic eyes for emotional recognition and expression. Some worry that such technology could further break down human–human communication and emotional connection. There are also concerns about privacy and the potential for the misuse of emotional data collected by these devices. While the development of robotic eyes for emotional recognition and expression has potential benefits, it is essential to consider the ethical implications and ensure they are used to promote human well-being and social connection.

Activities of Daily Living (ADLs) can be applied to emotional recognition and expression to help individuals better understand and manage their emotions [10–13]. ADLs refer to daily activities, such as bathing, dressing, and eating. The ADLs concept can also be extended to emotional activities, such as recognizing and expressing emotions. Individuals can better understand and regulate their emotions by breaking emotional recognition and expression down into smaller, more manageable tasks. For example, recognizing and naming emotions is an important ADL for emotional recognition and can be practiced by identifying and labeling emotions in oneself and others. Expressing emotions appropriately is another ADL that can be practiced through activities such as journaling or role-playing. The concept of ADLs for emotional recognition and expression can also be used in therapy or counseling to help individuals develop these skills [14]. Individuals can build emotional intelligence and improve well-being by identifying and practicing specific emotional ADLs. In addition, technology such as wearable devices or mobile applications can be used to support ADLs for emotional recognition and expression. For example, apps that help users identify and label emotions or wearable devices that monitor physiological indicators of emotion can help individuals better understand and manage their emotions. Overall, the ADLs concept can be a helpful framework for improving emotional recognition and expression. It can help individuals develop the skills to regulate emotions and communicate more effectively with others.

Interactive features of emotion recognition and expression based on human motion refer to the ability of technology to detect and respond to human movements and expressions in real time [15–17]. This can be accomplished through various methods, including computer vision, motion tracking, and machine learning algorithms. One example of interactive emotion recognition and expression is gesture-based interfaces in virtual or augmented reality environments. Users can interact with virtual objects and environments in these settings using natural gestures and movements. The system can detect and respond to users' emotional states based on their movements and expressions. Another example is motion sensors in wearable devices to track physiological indicators of emotion, such as heart rate or skin conductance. This information can then provide feedback or prompts to the wearer, such as suggesting a relaxation exercise or notifying them when they are stressed. Interactive emotion recognition and expression can also be used in robotics, where robots can detect and respond to human emotions based on their movements and expressions. This can help improve human–robot interaction quality and facilitate more natural and intuitive communication.

Overall, the interactive features of emotion recognition and expression based on human motion have many potential applications, including healthcare, education, and entertainment [18]. By detecting and responding to human emotions in real time, these systems can improve emotional regulation and communication and help individuals better understand and manage their emotions.

The rest of this chapter is organized as follows. Section 2 presents an approach to emotional expression based on implicit intention understanding. Section 3 describes recognizing activities of daily living to understand emotion recognition and expression to improve well-being. Section 4 describes the emotion recognition robot eye based on human motion. Section 5 describes the experimental results of emotion recognition. Finally, Sect. 6 presents the most relevant conclusions of the chapter.

2 Approach to Emotional and Expression Based on Implicit Intention Understanding

The aging and disabled population in Sri Lanka has indeed increased in recent decades [19]. This is due to several factors, including improvements in healthcare that have increased life expectancy and better access to education and awareness about disability issues. According to the World Bank, the proportion of the population aged 60 years and over in Sri Lanka increased from 9.7% in 2000 to 14.5% in 2020. This trend is expected to continue, with projections indicating that the proportion of the population aged 60 years and over could reach 22% by 2050. In addition to the aging population, there are significant numbers of people with disabilities in Sri Lanka. According to the World Health Organization, an estimated 8.2% of Sri Lanka's population has a disability. This includes physical, sensory, intellectual, and mental disabilities. The increasing number of disabled people in Sri Lanka presents various challenges, including providing adequate healthcare and social services, ensuring accessibility and inclusivity in public spaces, and addressing poverty and social isolation issues. However, there are also opportunities to promote greater understanding and support for these populations and to leverage their skills and experiences to contribute meaningfully to society.

Caring for elderly family members is an essential aspect of Sri Lankan culture. Family members, especially children, and grandchildren are expected to provide care and support to their elderly relatives. This includes providing for their physical needs and ensuring they are emotionally and socially connected. Traditionally, Sri Lankan families have been significant and multi-generational, with grandparents playing an essential role in grandchildren's upbringing. Even today, many Sri Lankan families continue to live together in multi-generational households, which makes it easier for elderly family members to receive care and support from their loved ones. In addition to family care, Sri Lanka has a network of government-funded elderly care homes and day-care centers that provide services for elderly citizens who may not have family support or require specialized care [20]. However, the preference for family care is still strong in Sri Lankan society, and many older adults may resist living in a care home. Overall, the culture of caring for elderly family members is an important part of Sri Lankan society. It reflects the values of respect for elders and the importance of intergenerational connections. However, as the population of older adults in Sri Lanka continues to grow, there may be a need to explore additional options for providing care and support to this vulnerable population.

A caregiver is a person who helps other individuals with impairment with their activities of day-to-day activities. Caregivers can be unpaid or paid persons. Receiving care from professional caregivers are paid persons [21]. Unpaid persons can be mostly family members, friends, and neighbors. Caregivers devote much time, energy, focus, and financial resources to care for elders and people with disabilities. But if the caregiving responsibilities become too demanding, they become exhausted and stressed over time. As a result, they try to increase their pay rate or leave the caregiving jobs. As a result, they find that well-trained caregivers also have challenging tasks. So, the shortage of caregivers will become a severe problem shortly. It is time to pay concerted attention to this question. Because most of the elder and disabled need physical and cognitive assistance from caregivers. Service robots are developed to solve the crisis of caregivers with the rapid rise of the disabled and elderly population in busy lifestyles. Anyone can get care from service robots without any expert knowledge about them. These robots can also be used in domestic environments. They are expected to support daily tasks such as cooking, cleaning, and taking care of health care.

Many researchers try to invent different kinds of service robots to replace caregivers, especially with voice recognition. But it couldn't use for deaf people. Deaf and dump persons can't give a voice response to the service robots. In this case, when they try to communicate with others, they are unable. Because they have no speaking and listening power, they can communicate easily with others from different body postures, facial expressions, etc. Facial expression is also an excellent method to recognize a person's emotional state. Still, it is not helpful to care for elders and people with disabilities because the least amount of information can gain from facial expressions. The service robot of emotion recognition must interact with a person except for recognition of the emotional state. Emotional expression from human motion with a whole body is the best method because deaf people can use their legs, arms, faces, etc., to express their emotions.

Therefore, the robot eye is essential for the service robot to interact with people at the most suitable times. The robot's accuracy also depends on the robot's vision [22, 23]. The technology of the robot eye is still developing. Many researchers are ongoing about robot eyes. Most of them are developed to detect the skeleton angles of humans by using kinetic sensors. This is not a more human-like manner. They only check the skeleton of humans without background colors. But in the future, they might develop technologies which the same as human eyes to make more human-like service robots. Therefore, we need to find a new method to identify the emotional experiences that focus on the deaf and dump person's emotional states as more human-like robot eyes.

Several emotion recognition and expression approaches are based on the human motion [15]. One common practice is to use computer vision and machine learning algorithms to analyze the movements and expressions of individuals in real time. This involves using cameras or other sensors to capture video or motion data and then processing this data to identify patterns or features corresponding to specific emotional states. Another approach is to use physiological sensors to detect changes in heart rate, skin conductance, or other indicators of emotional arousal [24–26]. These sensors can be integrated into wearable devices or other systems that can provide feedback or prompts to the user based on their emotional state. In addition, some approaches to emotion recognition and expression based on human motion rely on specific postures or gestures associated with particular emotions [23]. For example, the "power pose" has been associated with increased confidence and empowerment, while the "defeated pose" has been associated with ness and sadness. Overall, the approach to emotion recognition and expression based on human motion will depend on the specific context and application. In some cases, it may be more effective to use physiological sensors, while in other cases, computer vision and machine learning may be more appropriate. Regardless of the approach, it is essential to consider the ethical implications and ensure that the technology promotes human well-being and social connection.

The research project aims to develop interactive service robot eyes capable of emotional recognition and expression based on human motion in a more human-like manner. Mainly there are three objectives for the research project—first, the design and development of a robot eye with pan-tilt movement in a domestic environment. Second, develop intelligent systems to understand the emotional state. Finally, develop the human–robot interaction and test for selecting emotional states in a domestic environment.

Also, this research is focused on detecting only three emotion types. They are happiness, sadness, and relaxation. Because they are widely accepted and recognized by elders and people with disabilities. Typically, service robots detect only one person's emotional stage at a time. Therefore, this research focuses on detecting only one person's emotional stages in the domestic environment. This robot's eyes can get maximum accuracy from the chosen domestic environment. All the emotion classifiers are trained in that environment. Therefore, this experiment was conducted in a domestic environment with constant illumination.

Emotions are limited in the trained, intelligent system. Mainly there are two types of trained emotions. Namely, they are a person who sits on a chair and stands in the environment. The intelligent robot system recognizes different emotions with the position of hands, legs, faces, etc. [27]. All the emotions are detected according to them. The emotions are classified according to those body postures. Figures 1, 2, and 3 show all body postures related to emotions detected by the intelligent system under relaxed, sad, and happy moods, respectively.

To get the maximum result from the robot eye, the person must wear a short-arm t-shirt. Using many negative and positive images of different person's body postures may help get a more accurate result from the intelligent system. Due to lack of time, this intelligent system was trained only for two person's body postures and only a few types of body postures for each emotional state which was about 1500 positive and 5000 negative images.

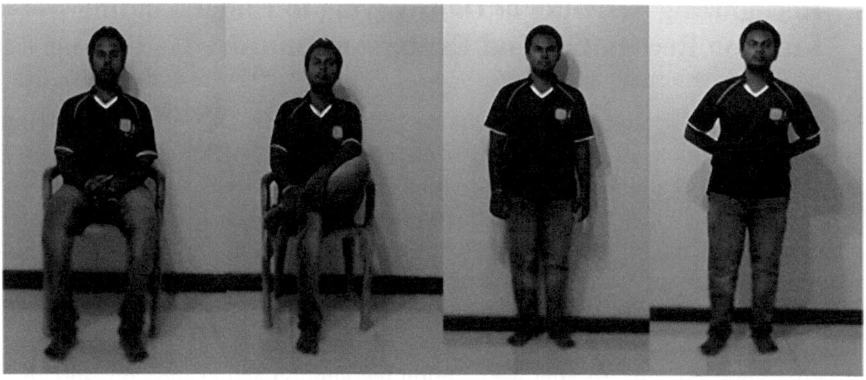

Fig. 1 All the types of body postures that are trained for a relaxed mood

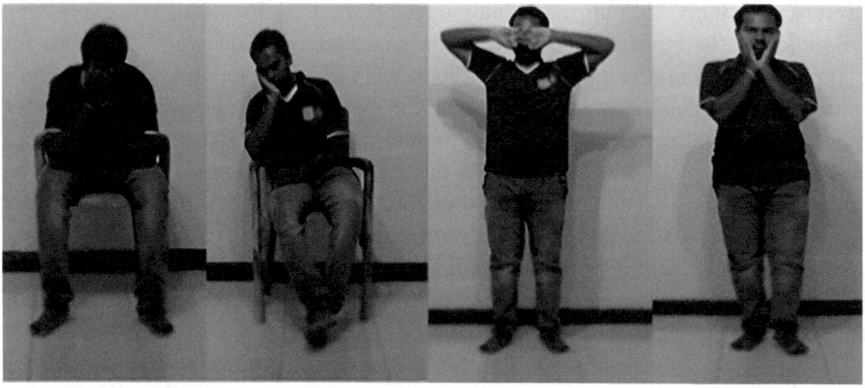

Fig. 2 All the types of body postures that trained for sad mood

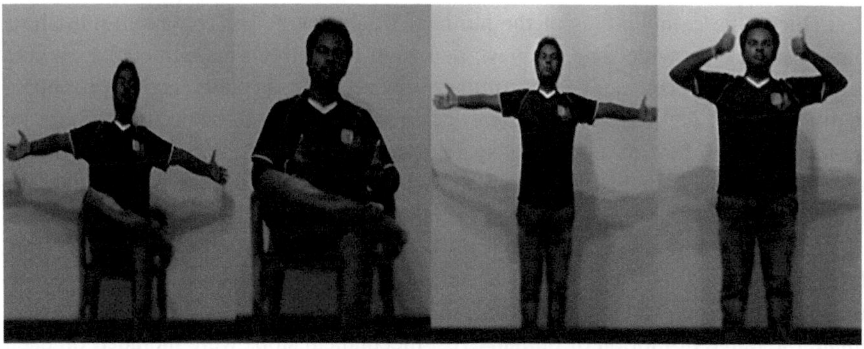

Fig. 3 All the types of body postures that trained for a happy mood

3 Recognizing Activities of Daily Living to Understanding Emotion Recognition and Expression Improve Well-Being

Recognizing ADLs can be a helpful framework for understanding and improving emotion recognition, expression, and overall well-being. ADLs are essential for daily life, such as bathing, dressing, grooming, and eating. By recognizing and performing these activities, individuals can better maintain their physical health and independence. Similarly, identifying and expressing emotions are essential to emotional health and well-being. Individuals can better understand and regulate emotional responses by recognizing and labeling them. Individuals can improve communication with others and build stronger relationships by expressing their emotions appropriately. To improve emotion recognition and expression, applying the concept of ADLs to emotional activities can be helpful. For example, recognizing and labeling emotions can be treated as an ADL, with specific practices and exercises designed to help individuals develop these skills. Similarly, expressing emotions can be treated as an ADL, with particular techniques and strategies for communicating emotions effectively. Technology can also support ADLs for emotion recognition and expression, such as through wearable devices that monitor physiological indicators of emotion or mobile applications that provide exercises and activities to help individuals develop emotional regulation skills. Recognizing daily living activities can provide a useful framework for improving emotional recognition and expression and, ultimately, promoting overall well-being. By breaking down expressive activities into manageable tasks and practicing them regularly, individuals can develop more robust emotional intelligence and improve their ability to navigate complex emotional situations.

3.1 Robot Eye Mechanism

To achieve the complexities of the human visual system, the robot eye must be a binocular, active, wide field of view, and high-resolution area. Binocular camera arrangement is necessary to discriminate objects with disparity and approximate depth [28, 29]. A vibrant eye helps to get a more human-like speed and range of motion. As with human vision, the system should also have field of view to depict motion and objects in the far fields with high-resolution capability. A good pan and tilt movement of a robot eye gives an excellent opportunity to achieve these factors.

To mimic human eye movements, each eye can rotate about a vertical axis (pan DOF) and a horizontal axis (tilt DOF). Human eyes have more than two degrees of freedom, but the pan and tilt DOFs are sufficient to scan the visual space. To approximate the range of motion of human eyes, mechanical stops were included on each eye to permit a 120-degree pan rotation and a 60-degree tilt rotation. This information has been used to design the research robot eye model.

Fig. 4 Robot eye model

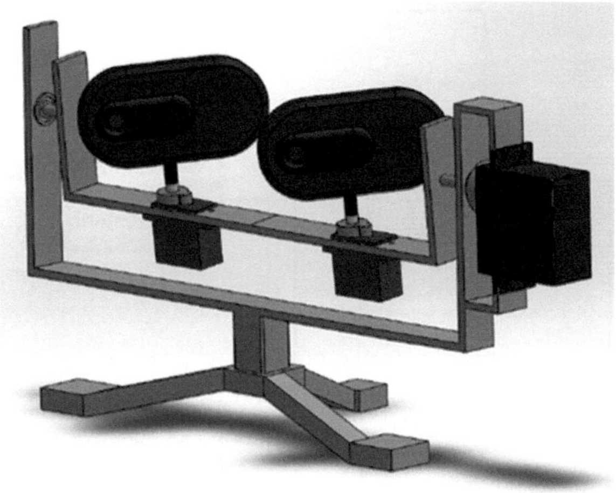

The eye model was constructed with three degrees of freedom in a more human-like manner. Two web cameras were used as the eyes of the robot to give input signals to the PC. Movements of eyes are achieved by using three servo drivers. Both eyes have individual pan movements and a common tilting movement as human eyes. The eye model was designed to place directly into a service robot. Figure 4 shows the mechanical drawing of the robot eye model.

As shown in Fig. 4, the cameras have been mounted on top of the two servo motors, and their common tilting axis goes through the center of each camera lens. The panning axis coincided with the rotational axis of the respective servo drives. The common tilting movement has been achieved using another servo motor.

The research is done to apply a robot eye to the service robot area. So, the eye must be applied to the robot directly. Therefore, the research design is done for the average human range of motion for each degree of freedom to be more human-like. The range of speeds achieved in each degree of freedom was used according to the specifications of the servo motors. Additionally, the design was fine-tuned to fit the pan-tilt engines purchased and eliminate collisions and vibration of components while in motion. Most researchers try to apply stereo vision by using two web cameras to capture useful data in three-dimensional space. Using two web cameras, objects' depth can also be analyzed.

3.2 Design of Electrical and Control Systems

This research project focuses on recognizing the emotions from using live video streaming. Because the model is made directly set for a service robot, therefore, using live video streaming, the service robot can get an idea about the live emotional state and react according to it. So, using video streaming, the web cameras can give

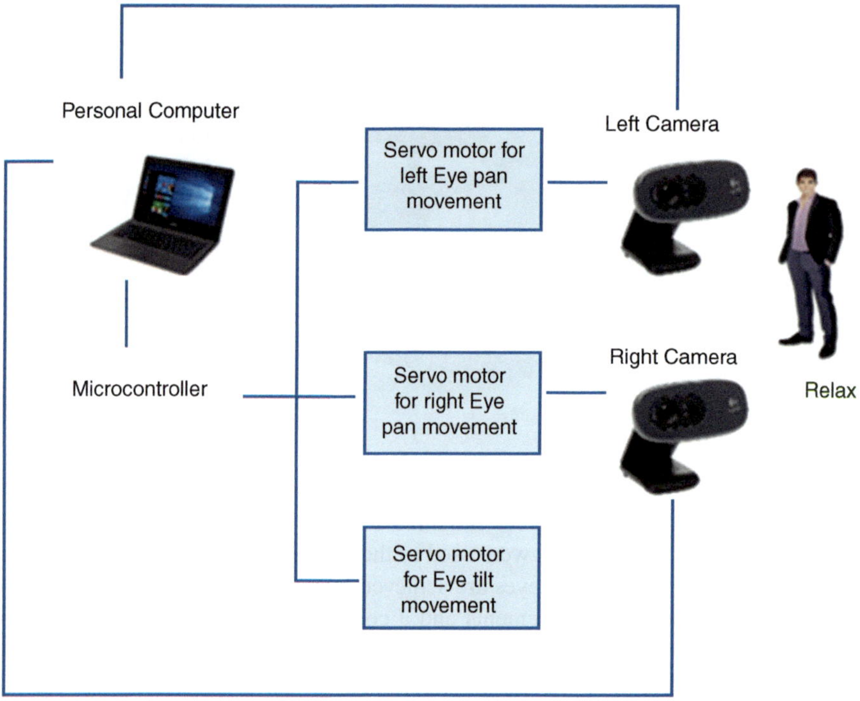

Fig. 5 A controlling mechanism for the robot eye

highly accurate inputs to the PC for the intelligent part of the robot eye. Typically, the human eye is not a fixed one. It has several complex movements, including pan and tilt movements. To reach the activities, we have to use suitable actuators for the eye model. The electrical system should be capable of supplying sufficient power to all the actuators of the robotic eyes while facilitating flexible control of those actuators. The controlling mechanism for the robot eye can be seen in Fig. 5.

Figure 5 shows three DC servo motors that implement three degrees of freedom to control the robot eye's pan and tilt movements. Personal computer with high performance used to implement the research project. It is essential that regular processors like Raspberry Pi cannot give the required high-performance speed to project implementation. Because the image processing techniques used with artificial intelligence must have high-performance processing speed. PC communicates with the microcontroller and the web cameras through the software part to control the eye mechanism to recognize emotion. The communication between the PC and the microcontroller allows passing data from the PC to the microcontroller to provide commands and position information calculated by image processing functions in some operational modes and for monitoring different variables controlled via the microcontroller using the PC interface.

4 Emotion Recognition Robot Eye Based on Human Motion

An emotion recognition robot eye based on human motion is an artificial intelligence system that uses computer vision and machine learning algorithms to analyze the human face's and body's movements to recognize emotional expressions. The system is typically designed to interpret human emotions based on the direction of facial muscles and body language, such as changes in posture, gestures, and other physical cues. The system typically involves data collection, labeling, feature extraction, training, and testing and validation to build an emotion recognition robot eye based on human motion. Once fully developed and validated, the system can be integrated into a robot's eye to recognize human emotions based on facial and body movements. This can have various applications, such as improving human–robot interactions by allowing the robot to respond appropriately to the user's emotional state.

4.1 System Overview

An emotion recognition system is an artificial intelligence system designed to recognize and classify human emotions based on various modalities, such as facial expressions, speech, physiological signals, and body language [30]. Overall, an emotion recognition system integrates multiple components to collect and process data from various modalities and uses machine learning algorithms to classify the user's emotional state. The system can have numerous applications, such as improving human–robot interactions, enhancing user experience in virtual environments, and aiding in medical diagnosis and treatment.

Figure 6 shows the system overview for the research project implementation. Robot's emotional state control module is excellent for successfully recognizing emotions. The robot's emotional state control module is the intelligent system of the robot's eye [31]. All admitted emotional states are classified as sad, relaxed, and happy in this context. Intelligent systems recognize emotional states according to the classification in context memory and communicate with robot eyes to detect persons. Vision output from the robot eye is controlled using pan and tilt movement of the servo motors in the robot eye through the Arduino microcontroller. Therefore, the serial communication between the PC and the Arduino microcontroller helps communicate the robot's eye with the emotional state control module. A person's body posture is the vision output from the robot eye after the data classifying in the intelligent system; the output signal can be given from the PC screen through a GUI after completing several machine vision applications.

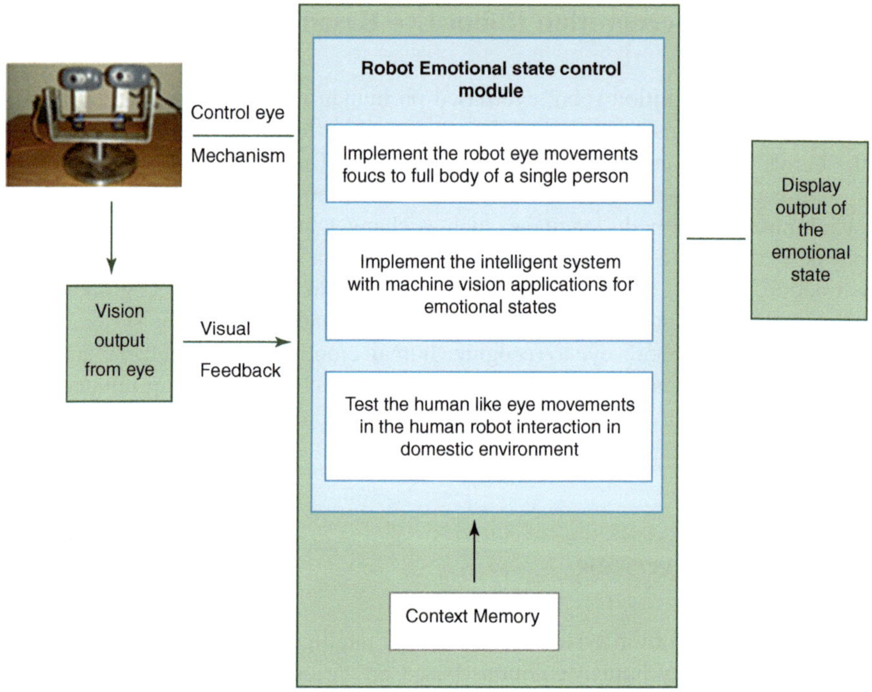

Fig. 6 System overview during implementation

4.2 An Emotion of a Person Searching and Detecting

It's difficult to determine a person's emotional state based solely on searching and detecting. However, here are some emotions that a person might experience in searching and detecting, such as curiosity, frustration, determination, anxiety, and satisfaction. Overall, a person's emotional state of searching and detecting can vary widely depending on the context and the individual's personal experiences and mindset.

The robot eye is designed for a service robot that helps care for deaf or dumb persons. Usually, people are unique. People change their emotions, positions, and body language occasionally. The time can be from milliseconds to hours. Therefore, the developed robot eye should be able to detect the person using pan-tilt movements like human behavior. Developed robot eye model continuously searching for a person's emotion to detect his emotional state. Always the robot eye tries to find an emotional state according to train Haar classifiers. The program of intelligent system always communicates with the microcontroller for the task. Therefore, the robot eye only rotates with the pan axis till the detection of emotion with ROI.

Various types of intelligent systems are used to classify human emotional states globally. Haar classifier training, artificial neural networks, and fuzzy logic are the most common methods. According to the research project requirement, a suitable intelligent system can be swung. Stergiou and Signals state that an Artificial Neural Network (ANN) is an information-processing method inspired by how biological nervous systems, such as the brain, process information [32]. The critical element of this method is the novel structure of the information-processing system. It is composed with the help of many highly interconnected processing elements working in unison to solve specific problems. An ANN is most suitable for particular applications, such as pattern recognition or data classification, through the learning process. Rouse, in 2016 states that Fuzzy logic is a method of computing based on "degrees of truth" rather than the usual "true or false" (1 or 0) on which the modern computer is based. It is closer to the way our brains work. Fuzzy logic is essential for developing human-like capabilities such as AI, sometimes called artificial general intelligence. Haar Cascade classifier training is also a suitable method for beginners. It is an easy and popular method among the research community. This classifier is helpful for normal object detection purposes. The most practical applications, like fuzzy logic or ANN, must be used if the application is complex.

The developed research is focused on detecting human emotion and displaying the emotional state using body posture. But it does not calculate emotional state in percentage. Therefore, Haar cascade classifiers can be easily used to perform the task. It is also a machine learning-based approach where a cascade function is trained from many positive and negative images. Then it can be used to detect objects in other images. Therefore, this research can implement the help of negative and positive photos of a particular emotion type and can use it to detect similar positive emotion types from a live video stream.

4.3 Haar Classifier Algorithm for Training Emotional States

Haar classifier algorithm is a machine learning-based approach for object detection, including facial feature detection [33]. While it is not specifically designed for training emotional states, it can be used for emotion recognition by detecting facial features associated with specific emotions.

Overall, the Haar classifier algorithm can be used as a part of the emotion recognition system to detect specific facial features associated with different emotions. This can be a useful approach to training emotion recognition systems in a more automated way. Still, it requires a large and diverse dataset of facial images to recognize different emotional states accurately. Positive and negative data sets are used for the data preparation process. Creating a cascade is important through data set training method for emotion recognition in developing algorithms. These cascades are train-boosted cascades of weak classifiers based on the positive and negative datasets.

These 1400 positive picture samples of emotions must be stored in a specific PC folder. Figure 7 shows some positive pictures used during classifier training for relaxing feelings. The size of the image can vary. It is important that if a classifier has more than one emotion type, like sitting and standing, then the classifier training

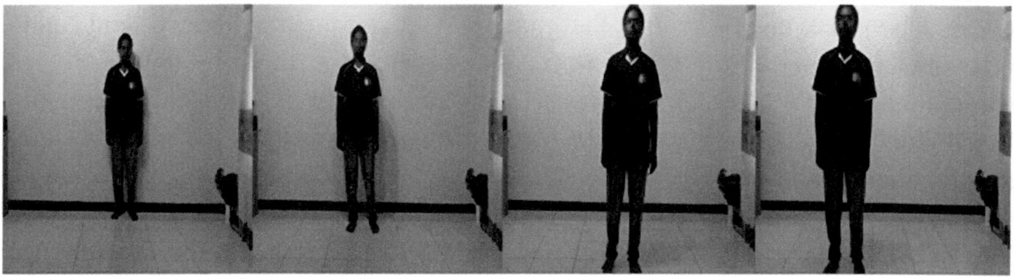

Fig. 7 Collection of positive images

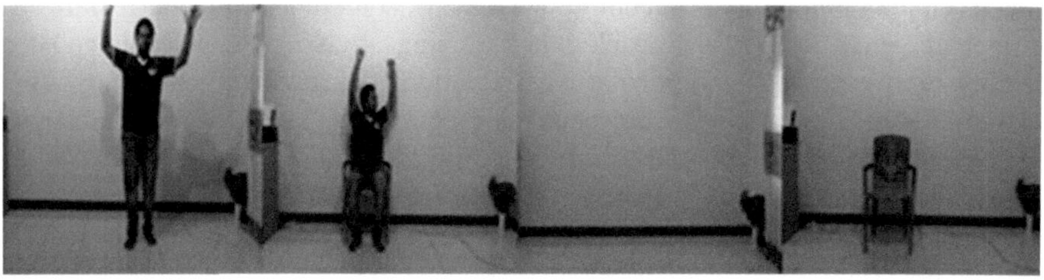

Fig. 8 Collection of negative images

time will increase. Also, many positive picture samples must make a robust classifier XML file.

Negative images could be anything that does not contain positive samples. It can be anything like a chair or table. This at helpful in differentiating and detecting the object from the real world. During the research purpose, the background photos of the environment without the person and pictures of a person with emotions, except the classifying emotion, are added to the 5000 negative photo set. Figure 8 shows some picture collections of negative photos.

4.4 Intelligent System to Recognize the Emotions

An intelligent system that recognizes emotions is an artificial intelligence system designed to identify and classify human emotions based on various modalities, such as facial expressions, speech, physiological signals, and body language. Several approaches to building such systems include rule-based, feature-based, and machine-learning-based approaches. An intelligent system recognizing emotions involves integrating various components to collect and process data from various modalities and using machine learning algorithms to classify the user's emotional state. The system can have various applications, such as improving human–robot interactions, enhancing user experience in virtual environments, and aiding in medical diagnosis and treatment.

From identifying persons' emotions domestically, an idea can be gotten for body postures in person according to different emotions. To recognize this, legs, hands,

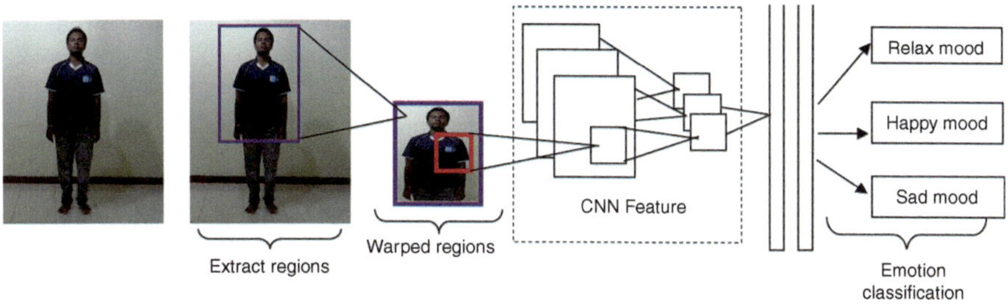

Fig. 9 Regions with CNN features

and faces can be selected. First, emotions are classified according to body postures. These classifiers have about 1400 images with the same pattern to classify that pattern type. After that, the intelligent system continuously checks the image pattern of the live video stream. If a trained image pattern in the classifier detects, then the ROI is shown with the image pattern as detecting emotions. The image pattern is getting according to emotions. Therefore, the emotion type can be seen in the output if there is any image pattern.

It is possible to use a Convolutional Neural Network (CNN) to identify emotional states from various input modalities such as images, videos, and audio recordings [34]. However, the accuracy of such models depends on several factors, including the quality and quantity of the training data, the design of the model architecture, and the selection of appropriate features for the input modality.

A deep artificial neural network is CNN, for example. It functions using the principles of the nervous system of humans. It is well suited for object recognition in photos using information from multiple arrays of different modalities. Numerous applications of this strategy have been executed successfully. Software with the appropriate versions must be chosen for CNN training. To surround the areas that CNN features would process during the emotion identification process, the robot eye extracts continuous input pictures during the installation of the intelligent system. Based on the presented ROI and emotional likelihood percentage, CNN classifies the image as happy, calm, or sad, as shown in Fig. 9.

The intelligent system can detect only the happy, sad, relaxation body postures related to each emotion. Table 1 summarizes the classifier training process for each emotion type mentioned above.

According to Table 1, the Haar classifier training was done for emotions which include 12 types of body postures. Images of two persons were used to construct every classifier. The above table shows the number of positive and negative images in each known person in an intelligent system to construct classifiers. Background images without persons are also included in negative images. It also consists of the periods which make positive ROI ranges in each classifier in positive images and the period it takes to train that classifier.

The intelligent system needs a large number of positive and negative images. Therefore, taking photos one by one is impossible. So, an OpenCV algorithm takes

Table 1 Summary of the classifier training process for each emotion type

Classifier	No. of positive images		Total no. of positive images	No. of negative photos			Total no. of negative images	Required time to crop the positive images (h)	Required time for training classifier (h)
	Known person 1	Known person 2		Known person 1	Known person 2	Only background			
Relax type 1	750	750	1500	1800	1800	1000	4600	3	5
Relax type 2	750	750	1500	1800	1800	1000	4600	3	5
Relax type 3	750	750	1500	1800	1800	1000	4600	3	5
Relax type 4	750	750	1500	1800	1800	1000	4600	3	5
Sad type 1	750	750	1500	1800	1800	1000	4600	3	5
Sad type 2	750	750	1500	1800	1800	1000	4600	3	5
Sad type 3	750	750	1500	1800	1800	1000	4600	3	5
Sad type 4	750	750	1500	1800	1800	1000	4600	3	5
Happy type 1	750	750	1500	1800	1800	1000	4600	3	5
Happy type 2	750	750	1500	1800	1800	1000	4600	3	5
Happy type 3	750	750	1500	1800	1800	1000	4600	3	5
Happy type 4	750	750	1500	1800	1800	1000	4600	3	5

pictures with 30 fps from the web camera to store images in a hard drive. Each trained classifier has a particular process to train—the cropping part of Haar training helps to set positive ROI for the classifiers. During the classifier training process, the ROI size is unimportant. But the shape of it is an essential thing for detecting emotions. To make a successful, intelligent system, a good collection of cropped images is important with the correct ROI range and helps make an accurate emotion classifier.

5 Experiment Results of the Emotion Recognition

The experiment conducted environment is shown in Fig. 10. There are some unnecessary things in the environment, like chairs, a table, a curtain, and a flower vase. But during the implementation, the intelligent system detects and focuses only on person's emotional state according to the body posture while rejecting the other things in the environment.

5.1 Speed of Robot Eye Rotation

Servo motor rotation speed is an important factor affecting the robot eye's behavior. During the high-speed eye rotation using servo motors, there can be some vibrations of the robot eye and missing ROI ranges during implementation due to not focusing ROI range according to body postures. It will harm the robot eye's visual feedback to the intelligent system. Table 2 shows the angles per step and the rotation speed of the servo motors for those steps. As a result, the robot eye is developed using the slowest speed of servo motors. It also helps to detect emotional states accurately by correctly focusing on the person's emotional state.

Fig. 10 Experiment setup in the domestic environment

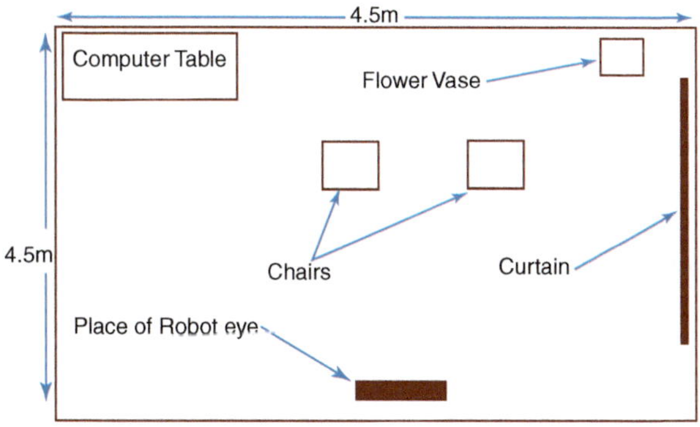

Table 2 Servo motor rotation speeds during implementation

Angles per each step (degree)	Time for cycle (s)		Speed of rotation (degree/s) (Pan axis)	Speed of rotation (degree/s) (Tilt axis)
	Pan axis	Tilt axis		
1	8.0	6.9	8.75	8.6
2	4.0	3.5	17.5	17
3	2.6	2.3	26.9	25.4
4	2.0	1.8	35	33.2

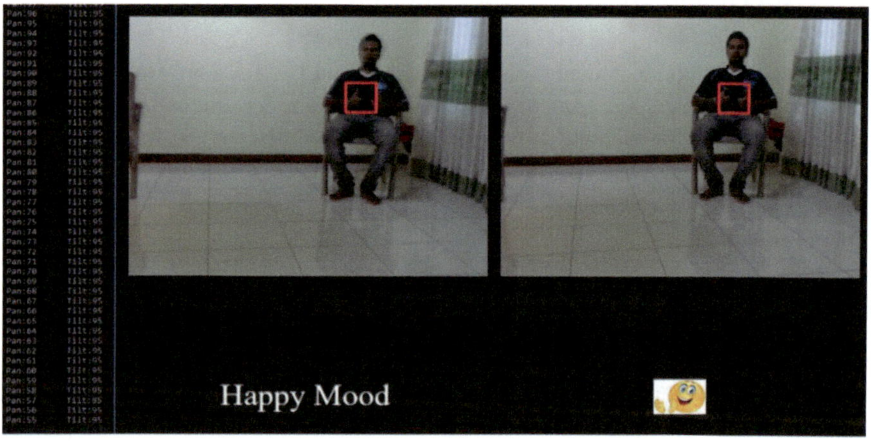

Fig. 11 Emotion classification: Happy mood of known person 1 *(T = 4 s)*

5.2 *Results of the Emotion Recognition*

A simple experiment was conducted to ensure the success of the robot eye in emotion recognition. The sample experiment includes two happy emotion body postures, two sad emotion body postures, and two relaxing emotion body postures. Three persons are selected for the experiment, including two known persons in the intelligent system and one unknown person in the intelligent system. Detection of emotions in GUI and the rotation angles during implementation is shown in Figs. 11, 12, 13, 14, 15, and 16.

Figure 17 shows the servo angle rotation of the robot eye during implementation. This experiment was conducted in a 50s period. Classifiers detected emotions only for the trained body postures. If not detecting a trained classifier, the robot eye always tries to find an emotional state. Six places have constant rotation angles in the pan motor rotation. The robot eye detects the person's emotions

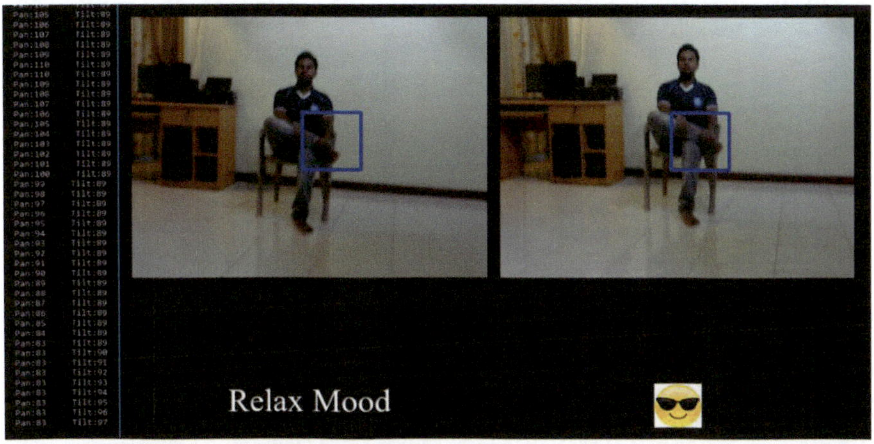

Fig. 12 Emotion classification: Relax mood of known person 1 *(T = 13 s)*

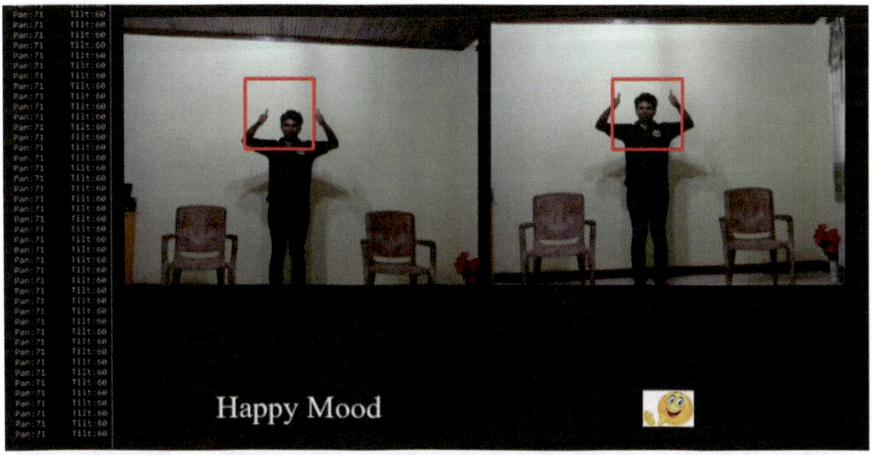

Fig. 13 Emotion classification: Happy mood of known person 2 *(T = 21 s)*

during that period, which is the period when body postures are similar to trained emotion classifiers. After detecting the emotion type, pan and tilt motors try to focus it on the middle of the window. Therefore, the tilt motor rotation angle is also stable in each case. There is also some period in high gradients. It means that during that period, the robot eye tried to find an emotional state using the pan and tilt movement.

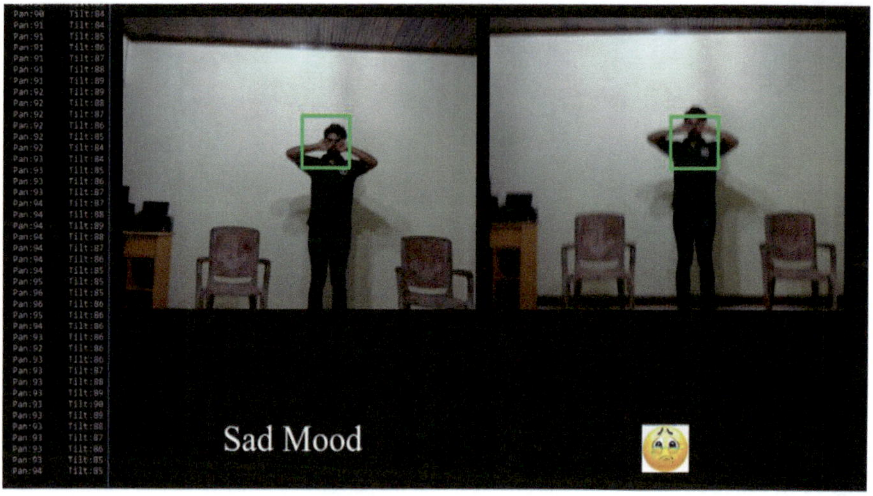

Fig. 14 Emotion classification: Sad mood of known person 2 *(T = 31 s)*

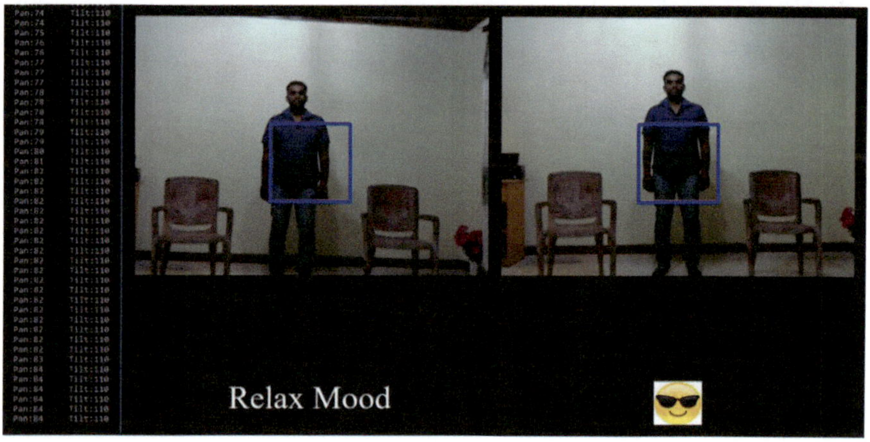

Fig. 15 Emotion classification: Relax mood of unknown person *(T = 37 s)*

5.3 Accuracy of the Intelligent System for Detecting Human Emotion

As a result of this experiment, the emotions are detected successfully. Table 3 shows the summary of experimental results with the accuracy of each classifier.

This experiment was done in a particular domestic environment. Therefore, the room size is limited to $20.25\ m^2$. The table includes the average distances between the robot eye and the person to detect emotions in each classifier. During the

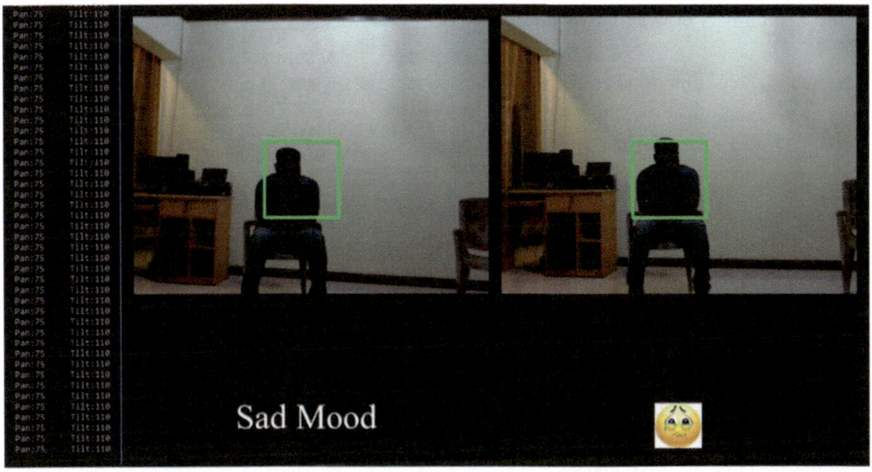

Fig. 16 Emotion classification: Sad mood of unknown person *(T = 46 s)*

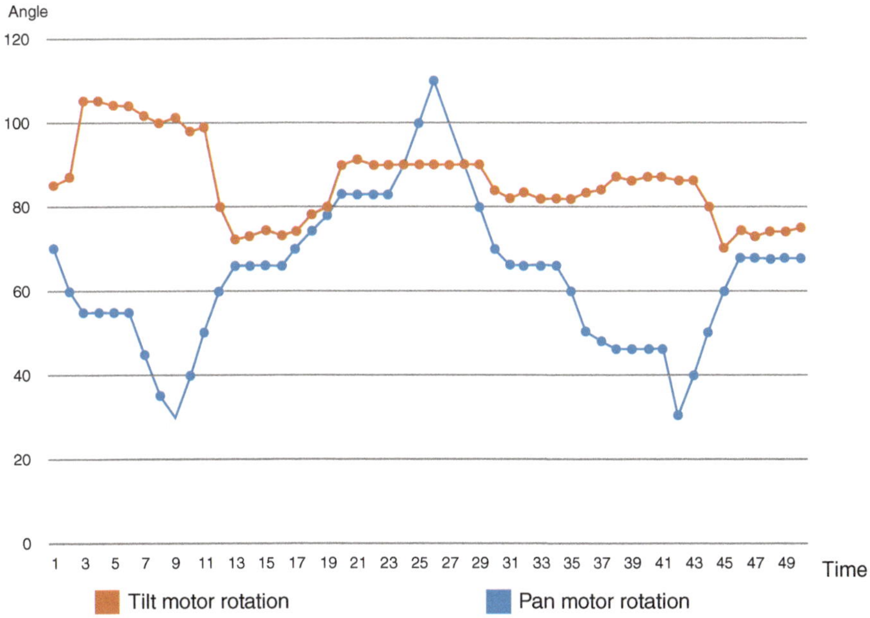

Fig. 17 Servo angle rotation of the robot eye during the experiment

experiment, the person is changed to 40 positions in the environment. Therefore, the accuracy of each classifier states separately. Finally, the overall accuracy of the intelligent system was calculated for each person. According to Table 3, the trained classifier detects emotions accurately for known persons in the intelligent system.

Table 3 Summary of experimental results with accuracy of each classifier

Emotion type	Emotion detecting the distance from the robot eye (m)	Accuracy of system with known person 1 (%)	Accuracy of system with known person 2 (%)	Accuracy of system with unknown person 1 (%)
Relax in a chair	3.0	82.5	85.0	69.0
Relax in standing	3.6	80.0	77.5	82.5
Happy in a chair	3.0	78.0	80.0	81.5
Happy in standing	3.6	82.5	79.5	79.5
Sad in a chair	3.0	79.0	81.5	78.0
Sad in standing	3.6	87.5	82.5	80.0
The overall accuracy of the intelligent system for each person		**81.58**	**81.00**	**80.08**

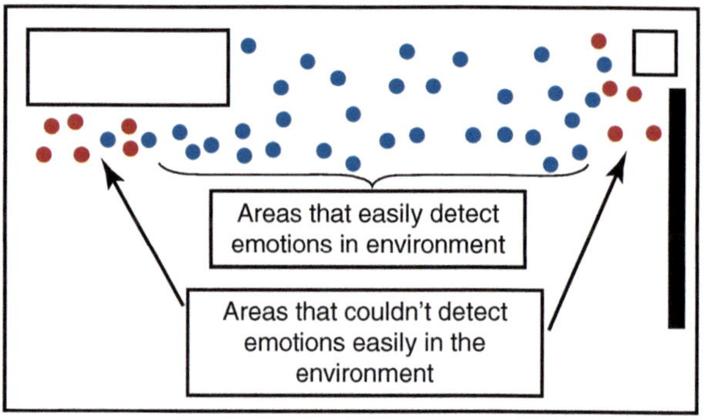

Fig. 18 Limitation of the service area

The result of an unknown person is lower than known persons in an intelligent system. By analyzing the results during implementation, some places couldn't identify emotions accurately due to some disturbance in the domestic environment. Changing light illumination of corners of the experiment conducted room and limited field of view of the robot eye are the disturbances for the intelligent system. Figure 18 shows the result of the experiment by using the detected and undetected areas during implementation.

In the middle of the room has a wall with white background. Therefore, a weak classifier also can detect emotions easily by using those areas in the intelligent system. But corners of the room resist recognizing emotions from the weak classifier due to the abovementioned disturbances, but the emotions are detected with low accuracy in those areas. Each classifier in the intelligent system is trained using about 2000 positive and 4500 negative images. This experiment was done by using three persons. Two are known persons in the intelligence system, and one is unknown in an intelligence system. A robust classifier can be made by using more images using different light illuminations and images of other persons to get a maximum result from the intelligent system.

6 Conclusion

The robot eye is designed for service robots to replace caregivers. As the first step of human–robot interaction, it must identify the emotional states of the human. After recognizing emotion, algorithms can develop the interaction part of the service robot. Therefore, robot eye development is an essential factor in service robot design. Some factors should be considered to increase the accuracy of the developed system during designing, tracking, and focusing the robot eye. They are camera selection, actuators selection, material selection for the robot eye design, and software selection to develop the intelligent system. Each Haar classifier training takes about 4 h to train each experimental classifier. It depends on the data set provided to the classifiers. Light illumination is a factor in classifier training. Suppose the lighting condition changes during the capture images to the Haar training process. In that case, the data set should have more images to train a successful emotion classifier and spend more than 4 h. Therefore, the maximum accuracy of the robot eye can be obtained only in a particular domestic environment where the intelligent system was trained. Emotion types are trained using two people's images in the intelligent system. A robust classifier can make by using different person images with different color illumination backgrounds. It also increases the classifier accuracy. The robot eye would thus be capable of accurately identifying human emotions wherever people live. The developed robot eye has been tested in various situations by changing a person's emotional state. According to the results of this experiment, the Haar classifier training approach is better than other algorithms for locating and monitoring significant emotions based on the body positions of old and disabled people. More images might be added to the Haar classifier training process to produce more reliable classifiers, enhancing the system. The proposed robotic eye is a foundation for adding more interactive features. The robot sight might need some substantial enhancements. Testing should be done to see whether the robot eye for service robot can be utilized for its intended purpose before looking at the entire design, materials, and manufacturing processes and optimizing them for the expected number of robots. The generated robot eye model's size does not correspond to that of the human eye. The outside of the robot eye might be designed to resemble human eyes with the right design. The robot eye looks better with an excellent exterior cover. Designing an outside cover using molding techniques and lightweight materials is preferred. The robot eye's architecture will interact effectively if more sensors are included. As a result, the research study has been improved. The robotic eye may be used as a study platform to implement various control techniques, such as artificial intelligence systems and machine learning strategies, to make the emotion recognition process more human like.

References

1. Brackett MA, Rivers SE, Salovey P. Emotional intelligence: implications for personal, social, academic, and workplace success. Soc Personal Psychol Compass. 2011;5(1):88–103.
2. Sebe N, Cohen I, Huang TS. Multimodal emotion recognition. In: Handbook of pattern recognition and computer vision, 2005. pp. 387–409.

3. Kutt K, Nalepa GJ, Giżycka B, Jemiolo P, Adamczyk M. Bandreader—A mobile application for data acquisition from wearable devices in effective computing experiments. In: 2018 11th international conference on human system interaction (HSI). IEEE. 2018. pp. 42–48.
4. Saunderson S, Nejat G. How robots influence humans: a survey of nonverbal communication in social human–robot interaction. Int J Soc Robot. 2019;11:575–608.
5. Dautenhahn K. Socially intelligent robots: dimensions of human–robot interaction. Philos Trans R Soc B Biol Sci. 2007;362(1480):679–704.
6. Sciutti A, Mara M, Tagliasco V, Sandini G. Humanizing human-robot interaction: on the importance of mutual understanding. IEEE Technol Soc Mag. 2018;37(1):22–9.
7. Herath HMKKMB, Karunasena GMKB, Mittal M. Monitoring the impact of stress on facial skin using affective computing. In: Predictive analytics of psychological disorders in healthcare: data analytics on psychological disorders. Singapore: Springer Nature; 2022. p. 55–85.
8. Martinez-Martin E, del Pobil AP. Personal robot assistants for elderly care: an overview. In: Personal assistants: emerging computational technologies; 2018. pp. 77–91.
9. Decker M. Caregiving robots and ethical reflection: the perspective of interdisciplinary technology assessment. AI Soc. 2008;22:315–30.
10. Madhusanka BGDA, Ramadass S. Implicit intention communication for activities of daily living of elder/disabled people to improve well-being. In: IoT in healthcare and ambient assisted living; 2021. pp. 325–342.
11. Edemekong PF, Bomgaars DL, Sukumaran S, Levy SB. Activities of daily living. In: StatPearls [internet]. StatPearls Publishing; 2021.
12. Barber SJ, Lee H, Becerra J, Tate CC. Emotional expressions affect perceptions of younger and older adults' everyday competence. Psychol Aging. 2019;34(7):991.
13. Madhusanka BGDA, Ramadass S, Rajagopal P, Herath HMKKMB. Attention-aware recognition of activities of daily living based on eye gaze tracking. In: Internet of things for human-centered design: application to elderly healthcare. Singapore: Springer Nature; 2022. p. 155–79.
14. McKenna J. Emotional intelligence training in adjustment to physical disability and illness. Int J Ther Rehabil. 2007;14(12):551–6.
15. Zacharatos H, Gatzoulis C, Chrysanthou YL. Automatic emotion recognition based on body movement analysis: a survey. IEEE Comput Graph Appl. 2014;34(6):35–45.
16. Castellano G, Villalba SD, Camurri A. Recognising human emotions from body movement and gesture dynamics. In: Affective computing and intelligent interaction: second international conference, ACII 2007 Lisbon, Portugal, September 12–14, 2007 Proceedings 2. Berlin: Springer; 2007. pp. 71–82.
17. Mittal M, Sharma RK, Singh VP. Modified single pass clustering with variable threshold approach. Int J Innov Comput Inform Control. 2015;11(1):375–86.
18. Mohammed SN, Hassan AKA. A survey on emotion recognition for human robot interaction. J Comput Inf Technol. 2020;28(2):125–46.
19. Vodopivec M, Arunatilake N. Population aging and labour market participation of old workers in Sri Lanka. J Popul Ageing. 2011;4:141–63.
20. Mittal M, Kaur I, Pandey SC, Verma A, Goyal LM. Opinion mining for the tweets in healthcare sector using fuzzy association rule. EAI Endorsed Trans Pervasive Health Technol. 2018;4(16):e2.
21. Boaz RF, Muller CF. Paid work and unpaid help by caregivers of the disabled and frail elders. Med Care. 1992;30(2):149–58.
22. Moladande MWCN, Madhusanka BGDA. Implicit intention and activity recognition of a human using neural networks for a service robot eye. In: 2019 international research conference on smart computing and systems engineering (SCSE). IEEE; 2019. pp. 38–43.
23. Sanjeewa EDG, Herath KKL, Madhusanka BGDA, Priyankara HDNS, Herath HMKKMB. Understanding the hand gesture command to visual attention model for mobile robot navigation: service robots in domestic environment. In: Cognitive computing for human-robot interaction. Academic; 2021. pp. 287–310.

24. Healey JA, Picard RW. Detecting stress during real-world driving tasks using physiological sensors. IEEE Trans Intell Transp Syst. 2005;6(2):156–66.
25. Kyriakou K, Resch B, Sagl G, Petutschnig A, Werner C, Niederseer D, et al. Detecting moments of stress from measurements of wearable physiological sensors. Sensors. 2019;19(17):3805.
26. Seshadri DR, Li RT, Voos JE, Rowbottom JR, Alfes CM, Zorman CA, Drummond CK. Wearable sensors for monitoring the physiological and biochemical profile of the athlete. NPJ Digit Med. 2019;2(1):72.
27. Noroozi F, Corneanu CA, Kamińska D, Sapiński T, Escalera S, Anbarjafari G. Survey on emotional body gesture recognition. IEEE Trans Affect Comput. 2018;12(2):505–23.
28. Lebreton P, Raake A, Barkowsky M, Le Callet P. Evaluating depth perception of 3D stereoscopic videos. IEEE J Select Topics Signal Process. 2012;6(6):710–20.
29. Tian X, Liu R, Wang Z, Ma J. High quality 3D reconstruction based on fusion of polarization imaging and binocular stereo vision. Inform Fusion. 2022;77:19–28.
30. Marechal C, Mikolajewski D, Tyburek K, Prokopowicz P, Bougueroua L, Ancourt C, Wegrzyn-Wolska K. Survey on AI-based multimodal methods for emotion detection. In: High-performance modelling and simulation for big data applications, 2019;11400:307–324.
31. Adams B, Breazeal C, Brooks RA, Scassellati B. Humanoid robots: a new kind of tool. In: IEEE intelligent systems and their applications. 2000;15(4):25–31.
32. Grosan C, Abraham A, Grosan C, Abraham A. Artificial neural networks. In: Intelligent systems: a modern approach. 2011. pp. 281–323.
33. Sharma V, Mir RN. A comprehensive and systematic look up into deep learning based object detection techniques: a review. Comp Sci Rev. 2020;38:100301.
34. Nguyen TL, Kavuri S, Lee M. A multimodal convolutional neuro-fuzzy network for emotion understanding of movie clips. Neural Netw. 2019;118:208–19.

Applications of 4.0 Technologies in Healthcare

Anwar Ahmed Khan, Shama Siddiqui, and Indrakshi Dey

Abstract The 4.0 industrial revolution, also known as Industry 4.0, is characterized by the integration of advanced technologies such as artificial intelligence, Internet of Things, cloud computing, augmented/virtual reality, and big data into various industries, including healthcare. The application of Industry 4.0 technologies in healthcare domain is referred as healthcare 4.0; adoption of these technologies can lead to improved patient outcomes, enhanced operational efficiency, while reducing costs. When it comes to mental healthcare delivery, the 4.0 technologies are expected to bring a revolution due to facilitating diagnoses as well as therapies. Some of the most prominent aspects that are expected to be affected by 4.0 technologies include predictive analytics, telemedicine, personalized medicine, and improved clinical decision-making by using decision support systems. In most of the healthcare scenarios, advanced sensing and analytics solutions can be used for providing early diagnosis and developing efficient care plans. This chapter presents a detailed analysis of applications of emerging 4.0 technologies in the healthcare domain.

Keywords Mental health · 4.0 technologies · Patient experience

A. A. Khan
Department of Computer Science, Millennium Institute of Technology and Entrepreneurship, Karachi, Pakistan

S. Siddiqui
Department of Computer Science, DHA Suffa University, Karachi, Pakistan

I. Dey (✉)
Walton Institute for Information and Communications System Science, Waterford, Ireland
e-mail: indrakshi.dey@mu.ic

G. Battineni et al. (eds.), *Computational Methods in Psychiatry*,
https://doi.org/10.1007/978-981-99-6637-0_15

1 Introduction

The scope of connected devices and systems has extended far beyond automated manufacturing. Today, healthcare 4.0 technologies have been realized to ensure safe and reliable healthcare service delivery for the patients, regardless of their physical location or lack of resource [1]. Conventionally, healthcare has been delivered via simple interaction between the patient and a single clinician, where the diagnosis and treatment plan were solely dependent on the discretion of clinician. In major healthcare facilities, instead of relying on a single healthcare provider, multiple teams, clinicians, and healthcare facilities participate to provide the healthcare service. However, in such settings, the diagnosis is mostly based on the history provided by the patients, which may be inaccurate, biased, and misinterpreted [2]. In comparison to the physical health, the patients are more likely to provide falsified information about their mental health due to social taboos, emotional distress, and lack of medical knowledge [3]. Therefore, the use of computational technologies has been highly recommended for mental healthcare domain.

Wearables and cyber-physical systems are the basic elements of healthcare 4.0, including wearables, the Internet of Things (IoT), RFID, intelligent sensors, and medical robots [4]. These solutions are integrated with 4.0 technologies of IoT, big data analytics, machine learning, cloud computing, and decision support systems. Healthcare 4.0 connects the healthcare facilities, equipment/devices, and patient's homes and communities. To maintain the confidentiality, specific protocols have been developed to share patient-related information such as diagnosis, medication history, treatment plans, lab results, insurance, billing claims, etc. [5].

This chapter first presents a brief review of the 4.0 technologies that have been heavily adopted in the healthcare domain. Second, the applications of these technologies for specific domains of healthcare have been discussed. Finally, the emerging trends of using novel 4.0 technologies for healthcare applications are reviewed.

2 Healthcare 4.0 Technologies

2.1 Artificial Intelligence

Artificial Intelligence (AI) is the simulation of human intelligence in machines that are designed to think and act like humans. It deals with the development of algorithms and statistical models that enable computers to perform tasks that typically require human intelligence, such as visual perception, speech recognition, decision-making, and language translation. AI systems use advanced techniques such as machine learning, deep learning, and natural language processing to process large amounts of data, learn from it, and make predictions or decisions based on that information. The goal of AI is to create systems that can perform tasks that would normally require human intelligence, making them faster, more accurate, and more scalable.

Artificial Intelligence (AI) has the potential to revolutionize the healthcare industry by improving the accuracy and efficiency of medical diagnosis, treatment, and overall patient care. Firstly, AI algorithms can assist medical professionals in analysing medical images, such as X-rays, CT scans, and MRI images, to identify and diagnose conditions. Secondly, AI can be trained to assist in medical diagnosis by analysing large amounts of patient data to identify patterns and predict potential diseases. This can help medical professionals in developing more effective treatment plans both for physical and mental health.

In addition to providing decisions based on the patient's physiological parameters taken from sensors and other connected equipment, AI can integrate well with other clinical information systems. For example, AI algorithms can be integrated into electronic health records (EHRs) to provide real-time recommendations for patient care based on the latest medical research and best practices. Similarly, AI can help healthcare organizations to predict patient outcomes and develop personalized treatment plans based on individual patient characteristics, such as age, gender, and medical history. In the era of predictive and precision medicine, AI helps to customize the drugs for patients based on their individual mental health state. AI can be used to analyse vast amounts of biological data to identify new targets for drug development and to optimize existing drugs for improved efficacy and safety.

The major applications of AI for mental health have been illustrated in Fig. 1 and described below:

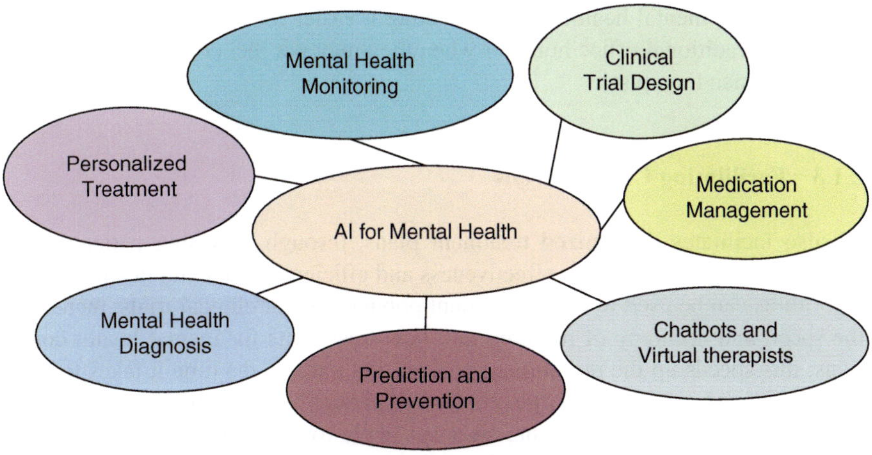

Fig. 1 Applications of AI for mental healthcare management

2.1.1 Mental Health Diagnosis

First and foremost, AI algorithms can monitor patients for symptoms and signs of mental health conditions, providing real-time data to mental health providers for informed decision-making. AI can be used to track symptoms and monitor changes over time, providing healthcare providers with valuable insights into a patient's mental health status. AI can assist with the analysis of medical images, such as MRI scans, to identify structural changes in the brain that may be associated with mental health conditions. Secondly, these algorithms can help diagnose mental health conditions based on medical history and demographic information. These algorithms may analyse patterns in data and predict future health outcomes, enabling mental health providers to intervene before a problem becomes more serious.

2.1.2 Chatbots and Virtual Therapists

AI-powered chatbots and virtual therapists can provide a convenient, accessible, and low-stakes way for people to get support and resources for their mental health. These bots can provide mental health screening tools and assessments that can help individuals determine if they are experiencing symptoms of a mental health condition. Chatbots can also provide emotional support and offer coping strategies for individuals who may be experiencing symptoms of anxiety or depression. This can help to alleviate feelings of loneliness and provide a sense of connection for those in need. Chatbots can provide educational resources and information on mental health conditions, treatments, and coping strategies. This can help individuals better understand their symptoms and find the support they need. As compared to human therapists, the chatbots may be more conveniently accessible. Chatbots can provide 24/7 access to mental health support, making it easier for individuals to seek help outside of traditional office hours or when they may not feel comfortable reaching out to a human therapist.

2.1.3 Facilitating Clinical Trials

AI also facilitates customized treatment plans, through analysing patients' data which significantly increases effectiveness and efficiency of mental health care. AI algorithms can be used to identify patient populations for clinical trials, increasing the speed and accuracy of research into new treatments for mental health conditions; this speeds up the recruitment process and reduces the time it takes to enrol participants. AI can analyse large amounts of patient data to identify potential outcomes and predict which patients are most likely to respond to a particular treatment. This can help to optimize patient selection and improve trial efficiency.

A crucial challenge for successful clinical trial is data management. AI can assist with the analysis of medical images, such as MRI scans, helping to more accurately and efficiently evaluate treatment outcomes and monitor disease progression. AI can assist with the management of large amounts of clinical trial data, helping to ensure that data is accurately captured and analysed in real time. This can help to improve the accuracy and efficiency of clinical trials. Also, AI can be used to monitor patient safety during clinical trials, detecting potential adverse events and alerting healthcare providers to take appropriate action.

2.1.4 Medication Management

AI technology in integration with sensor and other data help to manage medication schedules and dosages, improving patient outcomes and reducing the risk of adverse side effects. AI can use machine learning algorithms to analyse data from wearable devices, such as smartwatches, to monitor medication adherence in real time. This can help healthcare providers to identify when patients are not taking their medications as prescribed and intervene to address any issues. Similarly, dosage can be optimized using AI; AI algorithms can help healthcare providers to optimize medication dosing by analysing patient data, such as weight, age, and medical history, to determine the most effective dosages for each individual.

The advanced AI algorithms can identify the impact of medication on mental disorders. AI can use natural language processing to analyse patient data and detect potential drug interactions, which can help to prevent adverse drug events and improve patient safety. Moreover, AI can use predictive analytics to identify patients who may be at high risk for adverse drug reactions and alert healthcare providers to take appropriate action.

2.1.5 Limitation of AI for Mental Health Management

While AI is not a substitute for human-led mental health diagnosis, it has the potential to provide valuable support to healthcare providers. By using AI to analyse large amounts of patient data, healthcare providers can make more informed diagnoses and develop personalized treatment plans, leading to improved patient outcomes.

For the present time, it is important to note that mental health diagnosis can be complex and is best performed by qualified mental health professionals, who take into account multiple factors, including a patient's medical history, personal and family history, and symptoms. AI can assist in the diagnostic process, but it should not be relied upon as the sole source of information.

2.2 IoT

The Internet of Things (IoT) refers to the interconnected network of physical devices, vehicles, home appliances, and other items that are embedded with sensors, software, and network connectivity, enabling them to collect and exchange data.

This interconnected network allows these devices to communicate with one another and with central systems, such as cloud-based servers, allowing for the creation of smart systems and the automation of many tasks. IoT connects everyday objects to the internet and allows them to send and receive data. This opens up new possibilities for automation, monitoring, and control of a wide range of devices and systems, ranging from home appliances and personal fitness devices to industrial equipment and infrastructure. The goal of IoT is to make our lives more convenient, efficient, and sustainable by allowing us to better manage and control the things we use every day.

Due to the continuous sensing and communicating functionalities, IoT promises to revolutionize the conventional healthcare as well as psychiatry. The patients are no longer required to recall and share all the details with the therapists on their scheduled sessions, rather the information about the patient's mental health state is continuously available to the therapists on their customized dashboards and mobile applications. IoT dashboards can provide real-time data on a patient's mental health status, allowing therapists to quickly identify changes or patterns in behaviour and respond accordingly; IoT dashboards can provide valuable insights into a patient's mental health, which can be used to develop personalized treatment plans. This can help therapists to better understand a patient's needs and provide more targeted and effective treatment. Moreover, IoT dashboards can provide a platform for collaboration between therapists, allowing them to work together to develop treatment plans and monitor patient progress. Using IoT solutions targeting mental health, the therapists have even become able to categorize the risks of patients for specific mental disorders such as anxiety.

The physiological and environmental sensors as well as digital media usage today play a key role for monitoring the emotional and mental health state of the patients. Various fields such as psychology, neurology, psychophysiology, neuropsychology, and cognitive psychology all are integrated in IoT platforms to ensure timely and reliable mental health assessment and care delivery. The availability of massive amount of data captured through IoT sensors helps to realize the intersection between diverse fields of neurosciences, psychology, and physiology [6], as illustrated in Fig. 2. As a result, interaction and collaboration between experts belonging from different domains become possible and cost-effective regardless of their location and time zones. In short, IoT helps healthcare by providing real-time data, improving clinical decision-making, improving patient outcomes, better managing chronic conditions, and increasing efficiency and reducing costs.

2.2.1 Limitation of IoT for Mental Health Management

Although IoT has the potential to play a significant role in mental health management by enabling real-time monitoring and data collection. However, there are some limitations to the use of IoT for mental health management. One of the main concerns with the use of IoT for mental health management is the protection of sensitive patient data. IoT devices often collect large amounts of personal data, which

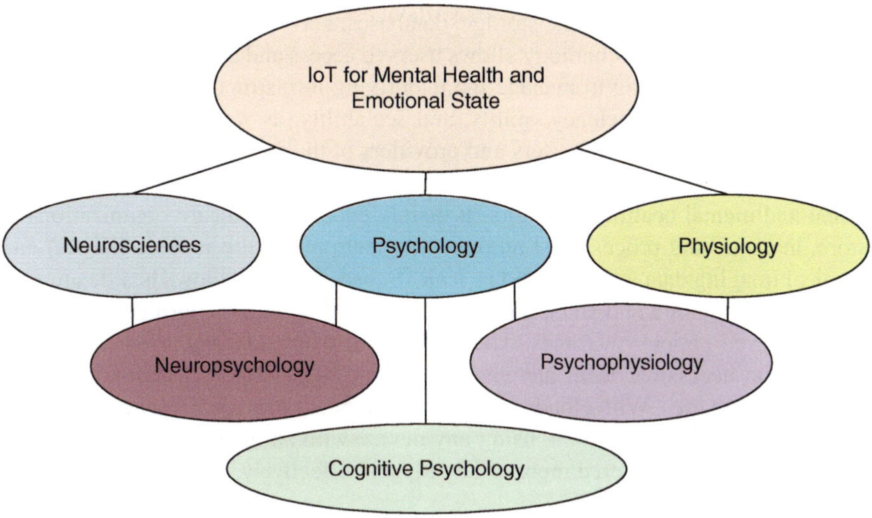

Fig. 2 Integration of IoT with psychology, neurosciences, and physiology

can be vulnerable to cyber-attacks or unauthorized access. Moreover, IoT devices can be prone to technical failures or malfunctions, which can impact their ability to accurately monitor and collect data. In addition, compatibility issues can arise when integrating different IoT devices into a single system. To be effective, IoT devices for mental health management need to be used regularly and consistently. This requires a high level of patient engagement and participation, which may be difficult to achieve for some patients.

IoT devices can be expensive, and many patients may not have the resources to purchase and maintain these devices. This can limit their availability to those who need them most. The accuracy and reliability of data collected by IoT devices can be a concern, particularly when it comes to mental health management. While these devices have the potential to provide valuable insights into a patient's mental health, the data they collect must be validated by clinical professionals to ensure its accuracy and clinical validity.

Despite the above limitations, the use of IoT for mental health management has the potential to provide valuable support to healthcare providers and improve patient outcomes. It's important to carefully consider these limitations and address any concerns before incorporating IoT devices into mental health management programs.

2.3 *Cloud Computing*

Cloud computing is a model for delivering information technology services in which resources are made available to users over the internet, rather than being provided from local servers or personal devices. The services provided by cloud computing can include servers, storage, databases, networking, software, analytics, and intelligence. This technology allows users to access and use these resources on-demand, without having to manage the underlying infrastructure themselves. This results in increased efficiency, agility, and scalability, as well as lower costs and increased flexibility for both users and providers of the services.

The technology of cloud computing brings numerous advantages to the conventional and mental healthcare sectors. It mainly enables healthcare organizations to store, manage, and process vast amounts of electronic health records (EHRs) and medical imaging data, securely and at scale. Subsequently, it allows healthcare providers to collaborate and share data securely, enabling better coordination of care and improved patient outcomes. The major goal of cloud computing is to make information accessible from anywhere any time, that reduces the constraints of physical boundaries. With cloud computing, healthcare providers can access patient information from any location, using any device with an internet connection. This enables care to be delivered more efficiently and effectively, particularly in remote or underserved areas.

Since treating mental disorders often requires lifelong information about patient's diseases, family, lifestyle, choices and preferences, cloud computing promises to aid the therapists and experts significantly. By collecting data from sensors and other devices, cloud computing ensures prolonged availability of massive information sets. The technology provides robust disaster recovery options, ensuring that critical patient data is safe and secure, even in the event of a catastrophic event. Similarly, the cost of mental healthcare delivery also reduces due to cloud computing as tens of experts may have access to the stored data and they may collaborate in no time. Therefore, by leveraging the economies of scale of cloud computing providers, healthcare organizations can reduce their IT costs, freeing up resources for other critical initiatives.

2.4 Big Data Analytics

As previously discussed, the history of healthcare industry started from generating minimal amount of data generated during sessions of patients with their practitioners. However, today, not only patients but also many sensors, wearable devices, and automated devices generate data about the patients. Furthermore, the electronic medical records and decision support systems also participate in data generation and filtering processes due to which the volume has drastically increased. As a result, advanced big data analytics techniques have been developed to examine, clean, and model the large healthcare datasets. Machine learning and statistical algorithms have frequently been used for analysing and extracting insight from large and complex datasets. These techniques help to discover useful patient's information, reach informed decisions, and improve the overall healthcare quality not only for individuals but also for communities.

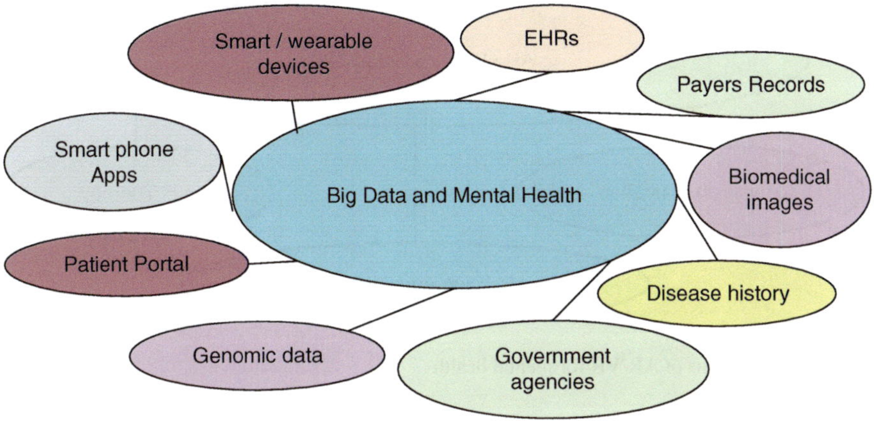

Fig. 3 Areas of mental health supported by big data techniques

Fundamentally, the goal of applying big data to the domain of healthcare is to identify patterns and trends in patient health, which allows healthcare providers to make more informed decisions about treatment and prevention strategies. Some of the major applications of big data for healthcare are illustrated in Fig. 3. Since big healthcare data is not only about patient's diseases history but also includes lifestyle and genetics information, healthcare providers can tailor treatment plans to the individual needs of each patient. Big data offers an opportunity to mental healthcare providers for developing a better understanding of a patient's mental health and make more accurate diagnoses. The patients may not be able to inform the practitioners about various important symptoms as they may consider them irrelevant. However, through the massive data collected via automated devices and sensors, it becomes possible to develop personalized treatment plans that are more effective.

Big data also identifies the problems and inefficiencies in the healthcare system which are used to optimize processes, leading to cost savings and improved outcomes.

2.5 *Augmented/Virtual Reality*

If displays, cameras, and sensors are used to overlay the real world with digital information, the application scenario is referred as Augmented Reality (AR). The creation of an entirely new vision and surrounding, the scenario is referred to as Virtual Reality (VR). AR enables bringing useful information from the digital world inside the perceptions and feelings of our own physical world. Over the recent years, we have seen promising advances in the sensor and camera technology. This advance has enabled software researchers in AR area to develop new technologies and ground-breaking applications. Though we are still in the regime of early developments of AR-based applications, over the next decade, AR devices are going to

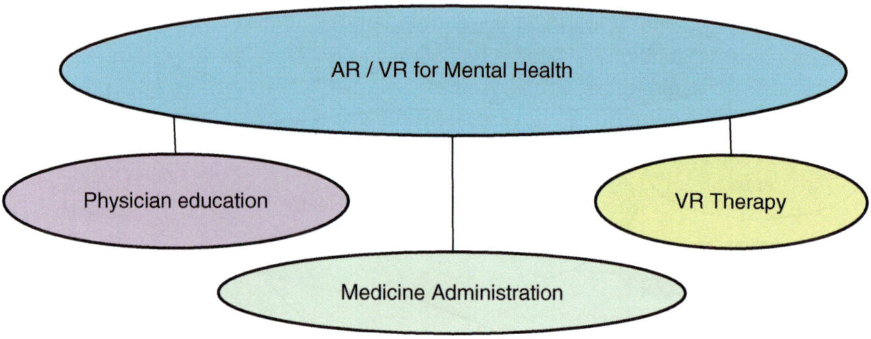

Fig. 4 Applications of AR/VR for mental health

invade every walk of life and going to impact over day-to day life in a big way. AR/VR are gradually finding different promising applications in healthcare, and doctors and nurses are interacting more and more through AR/VR applications for improving patient education and outcomes. Investment from different commercial agencies and companies over the recent years towards developing AR/VR technologies for healthcare has also pumped up the innovation in this area. Some emerging applications of AR/VR for healthcare are illustrated in Fig. 4:

2.5.1 Medicine Administration

Medicine administration has also been facilitated by novel ways introduced by AR/VR. Vein visualization is another emerging application of AR/VR. Many patients feel uncomfortable or get scared with too much pricking for drawing blood or injecting medicines/saline water. AR/VR can help project a map of the patient's veins onto their skin, making it easier for healthcare workers to find the right vein for injecting. Furthermore, since it often becomes troublesome for the family/physicians of patients suffering from mental disorders to convince them to take medications, AR/VR scenes may be set to persuade the patients.

Other most common examples of AR/VR applications in medicine and healthcare are as follows: (a) AR/VR can save lives by showing defibrillators nearby, (b) Google Glass can help new mothers with breastfeeding through interaction between counsellors and the mother herself with a projection of the reality, and (c) educating the public or kids about human physiology.

2.5.2 Physician's Education

One of the most prevalent applications of AR/VR in healthcare is education. Learning about how the body works and how they incorporate autonomy in the body functions is extremely important for the healthcare workers. AR applications can enable healthcare workers to learn and visualize with three-dimensional representation of the human bodies. On the other hand, AR/VR tools can also be used to educate patients about how to take medicines, shots, or use other simple instruments or understand surgical procedures they went through and how the after treatment will work. Another application in the same thematic area is the use of AR/VR techniques by surgeons to visualize the area on which they are to operate or improve accuracy of surgery through three-dimensional projection of the patient's anatomy.

2.5.3 Virtual Therapies

Specifically for mental health, AR/VR has been used for providing virtual therapies including "Virtual Reality Exposure Therapy (VRET)" to patients. Using these technologies, the therapies are designed in a way that patients feel completely immersed in the virtual situations. Instead of just talking and providing imaginary situations to the patients during conversations, the therapists may develop customized situations in real time using AR/VR technologies. The therapies offer full control to the therapists to put their patients under extremely customized and seemingly real, virtual scenarios; these scenarios created by the experts aid the patients to realize and modify their behaviours. Virtual therapies are more practical for the therapists and much lesser stressful for the patients [7]. VR has been found effective for providing therapies in various disorders including generic anxiety and depression, social anxiety disorder, Autism Spectrum Disorder (ASD), post-traumatic stress disorders (PTSD), schizophrenia, claustrophobia, and eating disorders.

One of the major applications of VRET is to expose the patients to their own fear. The patients are fully engaged using a 3D interactive environment to face their fear and assess the level of anxiety they may generate. For example, someone having fear of heights will be exposed by making him sit on skyscrapers using VR environment. Although various research studies have reported benefits of VRET, there are certain challenges associated with this technology at present: first, the patients may not be comfortable to be engaged in the VRET interaction due to having extreme fear; second, practical creation of the scenarios which may cause similar level of anxiety in patient as the real-world situation may not be possible; and third, the therapists may also not be very confident about the use of VRET due to their limited awareness about the technology and its possible consequences for the patients.

2.6 *Recommendation Systems*

Recommender systems, also known as recommendation systems, are a subclass of information filtering systems that seek to predict the "rating" or "preference" a user would give to an item. Recommender systems are utilized in a variety of areas and are most commonly recognized as playlist generators for video and music services, product recommenders for online stores, or content recommenders for social media platforms. In addition to generating customized contents and offering customized product advertisements, recommender systems also have applications for healthcare industry. They may offer personalized treatment recommendations, where they could analyse a patient's medical history, demographic information, and current symptoms to make personalized treatment recommendations. For example, a recommender system could recommend specific medications, therapies, or lifestyle changes based on a patient's unique needs.

One of the most crucial aspects for efficient mental healthcare delivery is identifying the best suited therapist and clinical facility. Mental healthcare is considered highly customized because mental health conditions are complex and can affect individuals in unique ways. Due to the highly diverse nature of mental disorders, recommender systems may offer significant advantage to the mental health practitioners as well as patients. Mental health conditions can manifest differently in different individuals and can be influenced by a variety of factors such as genetics, environment, and personal experiences; these conditions can be influenced by a person's unique life circumstances, such as family dynamics, work stress, and financial stability [8]. Moreover, Mental health conditions are complex and can involve multiple interacting factors such as biological, psychological, and social factors. Finally, mental healthcare treatment plans must take into account a person's personal preferences, such as their comfort level with certain types of therapy or medication. Therefore, recommender systems could assist patients in finding the best healthcare providers based on factors such as their location, specialty, and patient reviews. Furthermore, recommender systems could provide personalized health and wellness recommendations to individuals based on their lifestyle, physical activity, and dietary habits.

Also, recommender systems could match patients with clinical trials that are most suitable for their specific medical conditions and demographics. This would help to increase patient participation in clinical trials and ultimately speed up the development of new treatments.

3 Application of Healthcare 4.0 Technologies

3.1 Cost Reduction

The use of artificial intelligence, machine learning, IoT, cloud computing, etc. can significantly reduce the healthcare costs. First and foremost, the efficiency of overall healthcare delivery improves due to reducing redundancy and errors and increasing productivity. Second, the smart healthcare equipment can inform about needs of predictive maintenance, reducing the downtime as well as cost of repair. Third, telemedicine and remote patient monitoring can reduce hospital readmissions, outpatient visits, and overall costs by allowing patients to receive care from home.

Personalized medicine powered by AI tools can also help the physicians to make more accurate and timely diagnosis.

Particularly for mental health, the use of healthcare 4.0 technologies brings numerous benefits. The cost of therapy has significantly reduced due to the emerging use of mobile apps and web-based platforms for continuous monitoring and assessment. Instead of needing to visit the therapist at the physical facilities, patients could easily consult them online. The cost also reduces as the patients become able to identify their disorders at an early stage, providing more opportunity to deal with it in a cost-effective manner. Moreover, the technologies such as machine learning and big data analytics facilitate the therapists by identifying the most prevalent mental disorders in specific populations. Using this information, the practitioners may develop efficient prevention and treatment strategies in advance.

3.2 Predictive Analytics

Healthcare 4.0 technologies including big data can help mental healthcare providers anticipate and prevent potential health issues by analysing patterns and trends in patient data. IoT sensors, patient's handheld devices, and other connected medical equipment provide massive amount of data for facilitating predictive analytics. The machine algorithms can analyse vast amounts of data and identify patterns, relationships, and trends that would be difficult or impossible to detect manually. AI-powered predictive analytics tools can identify trends and predict future outcomes, allowing therapists and other care team members to take proactive measures to prevent problems or capitalize on opportunities. Moreover, since the use of social media has been increasing among all population sectors, social media analysis and opinion mining have also been emerging. The social media profiles and posts of populations may be assessed by the advanced Natural Language Processing (NLP) tools to identify any mental disorders. In short, the predictive analytics enable mental health professionals to make more informed decisions, improve operational efficiency, and stay ahead of potential health risks.

3.3 Telemedicine

Access to mental healthcare significantly enhances via telemedicine as the barriers such as distance, mobility, and scarce availability of mental healthcare professionals are reduced. Various tools and technologies facilitating telemedicine have been applied for mental healthcare, as illustrated in Fig. 5 and discussed below:

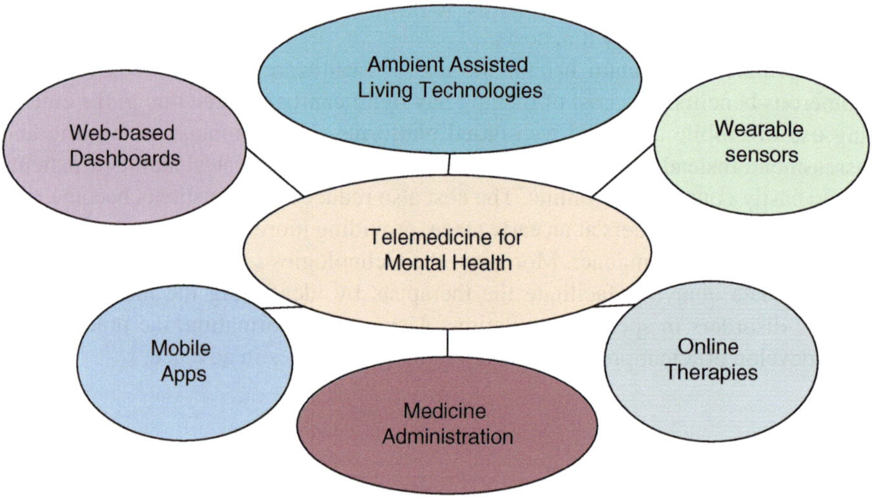

Fig. 5 Emerging healthcare 4.0 trends for mental health

3.3.1 Web-Based Dashboards and Mobile Apps for Online Therapies

Dashboards are the most common form of interfaces between man and machine for an IoT network or any other cyber-physical system. They collate, organize, analyse, and transform digital information (data) communicated in our physical world to represent them in a format that can be easily understood by everybody when read from or displayed on a mobile phone, computer, or any other user interface. The major advantages of dashboards are that they can monitor and control input/output devices in the network, can be used both for global and individual benefits, and can be operated over cloud-based data storage platforms.

There has been a recent surge in the design and development of real-time COVID-19 or pandemic-related IoT dashboards. Such dashboards have mainly been used for monitoring and managing patients, and for assisting the state authorities and healthcare professionals in situation awareness and critical decision-making. The real-time dashboard developed in [9] targeted prioritizing emergent, urgent, and semi-urgent cases requiring surgery in order to reducing risk of COVID-19 exposure for surgeons, nurses, technicians, and other health-care staff. The focus of the dashboard in [10] is to provide information on the status and location of clinical trials for avoiding any duplication and increasing chances of collaboration for vaccine development. The dashboard developed in [11] populated information about the number of patients tested, test results, availability of beds and ventilators, etc. for supporting operational decision-making like isolation procedure, etc. An interactive web-based mapping dashboard is developed in [12] for assessing changes in mobility patterns of individuals, and then reporting them over the ArcGIS dashboard. Similarly, visualization dashboards have been developed [13] to help remote consultants, tele-health operators, and emergency service providers. These dashboards provide real-time information on the number of patients requiring hospitalization, user needs, etc., which help the service providers in taking critical decisions regarding management of resources and patients. It helps authorities to keep check on whether social distancing norms are followed or not, while informing individuals about their health risk possibility owing to their mobility.

The platforms such as web-based dashboards and mobile apps have increasingly been used to provide counselling and therapy services through simple phone calls or video conferencing. The telemedicine technologies have particularly been useful for the patients who live in far off remote locations or have physical impairments. Since there is a considerable shortage of mental health professionals worldwide and also, it is not always realistic for the population to afford the high fees of clinical visits, alternative methods have been developed using healthcare 4.0 technologies. The situation of mental health is particularly worsening for the population residing at developing countries and those belonging from low socio-economic status. In fact, majority of the patients suffering from mental disorders are not even aware of their situation.

In the above scenario, the easily accessible mobile apps and web-based dashboards are being developed to assess the mental health states and manage the diseases/disorders through online service delivery. On the one hand, such services improve the accessibility to mental healthcare services, and on the other hand, they ensure accessibility while maintaining the patient's confidentiality. As previously discussed, mental health issues are yet considered taboo and people are often not comfortable to share such issues with their family. The mobile apps and other online platforms ensure that patients could avail the services of automated therapy or consultancy services at a minimum cost.

3.3.2 Medicine Administration

An important aspect of telemedicine is the possibility of regularly monitoring the patients to observe the impact of any medicine or treatment plan suggested in the past. With the help of various sensors and equipment, mental healthcare providers may track the patient's progress and response to treatment over time, which enables them to adjust a patient's treatment plan as needed. Regarding continuous monitoring, a revolutionary change is an opportunity for the physician be informed about medication administration. The novel development of digital pills ensure that the patients have taken medicine, as an alert is sent to the medical professional. Generally, Bluetooth connectivity is used to transmit an alert from the ingested tablet to patient's handheld device, which subsequently signals the remote healthcare professional; the fundamental operation of digital pill has been illustrated in Fig. 6. The digital pill technology is particularly beneficial for the patients suffering from mental diseases such as Alzheimer who tend to forget taking their medication, which could further worsen their condition.

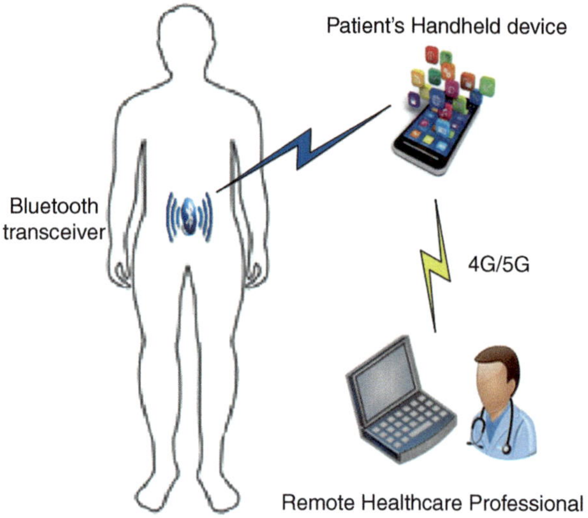

Fig. 6 Fundamental operation of digital pill

3.3.3 Wearable Sensors

Various chemical, physical, and biological sensors have been developed and sold in the wearable form to offer continuous telemedicine facilities. The most common example of wearable sensor is smart watch/Fitbit. Generally, these sensors are embedded with wearable clothing or gadgets and coordinate with the handheld devices of users via technologies such as Bluetooth/Wi-Fi. Subsequently, the information is sent over wireless links to the remote stations. Usually, the databases are managed over cloud so the remote physicians may remain informed about the users' conditions. The wearable technology has already been playing a leading role in the management of various physical and mental health conditions. It reduces the cost of care and improves the quality by real-time communication of the patient's state. Furthermore, instead of only relying on the patient as a source of information, the experts get an opportunity to have a real insight into the patient's condition through monitoring the physiological and psychological parameters of interest. For example, for various anxiety and depression use cases, the parameters such as pulse rate, SpO_2, and blood pressure are shown to be of interest.

The wearable sensors are configured according to the customized requirements of each patient. For example, the frequency of transmission of vitals or the threshold value may be set independently for each patient. The risk for patients may also be identified based on the data provided by the wearable sensors by monitoring the threshold values for each parameter. This approach facilitates the monitoring of patients for their mental health state; instead of maintaining generic appointment schedules for the patients, it becomes possible to prioritize the patients requiring immediate care which reduces the healthcare burden both on patients and providers.

3.3.4 Ambient Assisted Living Technologies

Ambient Assisted Living (AAL) is a field of research and development that focuses on using technology to improve the quality of life of elderly and disabled people, enabling them to live independently in their own homes for longer. AAL technologies aim to provide support and assistance in the home environment, by using sensors, communication systems, and other devices to monitor and respond to the needs of individuals.

The main objective of AAL is to develop intelligent systems that can detect and respond to changes in an individual's behaviour, routines, or health status, and provide them with the necessary assistance or intervention to help them maintain their independence and quality of life. This can include, for example, reminders to take medication, alerts for falls, and automatic adjustments of lighting, temperature, and other environmental factors.

AAL technologies can also provide a means of communication and connection to family members, caregivers, and healthcare professionals, improving social interaction and reducing isolation. The ultimate goal of AAL is to create a supportive, comfortable, and safe living environment that promotes independence, autonomy, and dignity for elderly and disabled people.

3.4 Personalized and Precision Medicine

4.0 technologies are providing significant novel opportunities for customizing the treatment plans. In this context, personalized and predictive medicine are two emerging domains. Personalized medicine refers to the tailoring of medical treatment to the individual patient, considering their unique characteristics such as genetic makeup, lifestyle, and environment [14]. On the other hand, precision medicine is a subset of personalized medicine, but it focuses more on using genetic and molecular information to identify the specific cause of a disease in a patient and target treatment to that specific cause. Clearly, the precision medicine is expected to be more effective as compared to standard treatment plans. All the computing technologies, specifically IoT and big data analytics play a leading role to provide an in-depth insight into the patient's lifestyle and its impact on their health. As a result, customized treatment plans and medicine may be suggested for each patient instead of the conventional generic treatment strategies.

Technologies such as machine learning and big data analytics integrate the fields of genomics to identify the genetic causes of mental disorders. The advanced computing technologies aid to identify the genetic patterns and their influence on the patient's personality since childhood. As a result, it is not only the therapist's diagnosis of patient based on their and family's history, but the facts are all stored and analysed over the patient's lifetime. Genomics facilitates creating personalized medicines for diseases such as tumours, cancers, arthritis, and Alzheimer's disease.

Both the personalized and precision medicine are particularly relevant for mental health of individuals. It is generally not possible to develop standard treatment plans for the patients requiring assistance with their mental health. Therefore, it is expected that healthcare 4.0 shall bring a revolution for psychiatry by providing a detailed insight into the health state of each patient, which shall subsequently be used for developing therapies.

3.5 Facilitating Interconnections

Healthcare 4.0 technologies are used to provide interconnection between diverse aspects of healthcare sector to create an efficient information network. The interactions between different healthcare stakeholders being facilitated by 4.0 trends are shown in Fig. 7. Firstly, the interactions between patients, caregivers, and other team members are realized using advanced hardware and software technologies to diagnose and treat the mental health conditions. This interaction between different stakeholders is vital for ensuring patient safety and mental healthcare quality. The patients and caregivers not only need to be informed about the diagnosis but their continuous engagement is crucial throughout the treatment and care process. This would enable the patients to better understand about their needs and would involve actively in the implementation of their care plan. Since mental illnesses may be chronic and complex, the engagement of patients and their caretakers becomes even more critical. In this regard, various information technology tools such as electronic medical records, patient portals, IoT data, assistive technologies, mobile apps, and video conferencing platforms all facilitate the patients and caregivers.

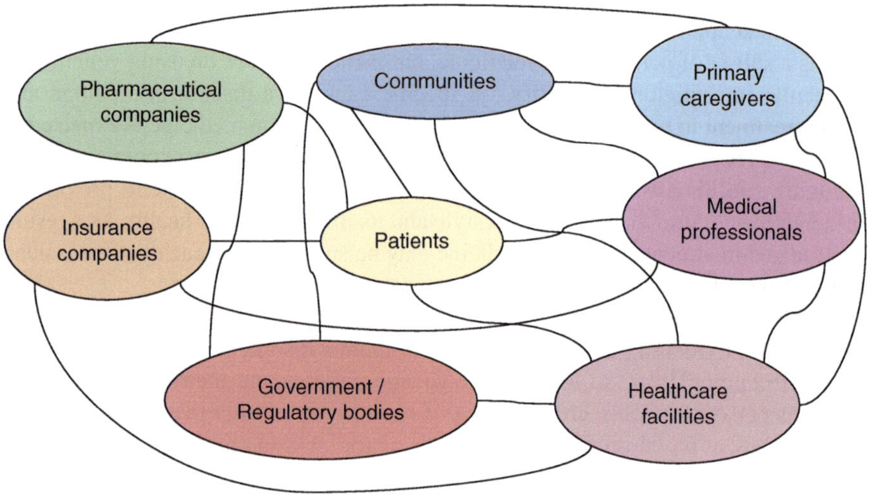

Fig. 7 Interaction between healthcare stakeholders

In addition to interaction with patients and their caregivers, the healthcare 4.0 technologies also facilitate interaction between the professional teams so they may coordinate and communicate efficiently. Particularly, when diverse team members come together to deliver therapies and other care elements, it becomes vital to use computing tools and emerging 4.0 technologies to update the status and monitor the patient's progress in the context of strategies developed by the individual team members. All team members can easily coordinate and share information using real-time dashboards. These dashboards may be integrated with the data streams being communicated via wearable and environmental sensors, patients' handheld gadgets, and any other equipment to further enhance the team's information.

Since one of the core objectives of healthcare 4.0 is to connect all the devices and equipment, it has become possible to centrally collect and maintain data generated by geographically dispersed sensors and systems. These devices facilitate additional diagnosis, prediction, and analysis with the advent of fog, edge, and cloud computing. Similarly, diverse organizations and communities may connect with other stakeholders such as small practitioner groups, pharmacies, clinics, individuals, long-term facilities, hospice care facilities, public and regional healthcare systems using advancing communication infrastructure. The collaboration between individuals and healthcare organizations would improve the quality of care. However, appropriate policies, procedures, protocols, and legislations shall be required for granting the access of data generated by each entity to others.

Due to the possibility of continuous data collection and analysis, it would become possible to study the complete mental health state of a person since their childhood. All the details about any past disease history, emotional traumas and physical accidents or incidents such as bullying shall be readily available for the therapists and other caregivers. In the present practice, where it takes multiple sessions of psychologists just to collect the details about patients' habits, their routines, lifestyle habits, social preferences, eating habits, etc., significant amount of time and cost are incurred. These details are collected to develop the treatment plans and despite spending numerous resources, it is of no guarantee that patients provide accurate details. In comparison, healthcare 4.0 technologies shall improve the situation by providing all lifestyle and health-related details in a chronological fashion, starting from the birth of patients. In future, when all the healthcare facilities worldwide will be connected, the care transition across time and space will be realized in its true sense.

In addition to the primary stakeholders of healthcare sector, patients and medical professionals, healthcare 4.0 also serves interactions between others such as pharmaceutical and insurance companies. For example, insurance companies play a significant role in determining which drugs are covered and reimbursed, as they often negotiate prices with pharmaceutical companies. If a drug is not covered or is only partially covered by insurance, it can affect its overall accessibility and affordability to patients. Using the connectivity, the pharmacy and patients may immediately know their insurance coverage. Similarly, pharmaceutical companies invest significant resources in the development of new drugs, and insurance companies often play a role in funding these research and development efforts through their payments for covered drugs. Moreover, the patients may be benefited in monetary terms through the interaction between pharmacies and insurance companies. Insurance companies and pharmaceutical companies work together to balance the cost of drugs with their effectiveness. Insurance companies often negotiate with pharmaceutical companies to reduce the cost of drugs for their clients and may encourage the use of lower-cost alternatives.

4 Future Trends

4.1 Maintaining Confidentiality

Confidentiality is a critical aspect of healthcare, and it is becoming increasingly important in the era of healthcare 4.0. In the future, smart health technology will likely include advanced security measures to protect patient information and ensure confidentiality. Data transmitted between medical devices and healthcare providers will be secured by using advanced encryption techniques to prevent unauthorized access. Encryption can be applied at the device level, network level, and data storage level. Access control policies are expected to be designed efficiently and implemented strictly. Medical devices and healthcare systems can be configured to allow access only to authorized personnel. This can be achieved through the use of passwords, biometrics, or smart cards.

Although IoT and other technologies discussed in the chapter tend to generate massive amount of data, confidentiality will require minimizing the generated data. Only the minimum amount of data necessary for a specific use case will be collected, transmitted, and stored. This strategy would reduce the potential harm that could be caused in the event of a data breach. Moreover, as hackers always remain ahead in technology, it will be crucial to ensure that even more advanced security schemes are used to maintain the patient's confidentiality. In this regard, medical devices and healthcare systems should receive regular security updates to address any newly discovered vulnerabilities. Finally, The IoMT must comply with relevant regulations, such as the Health Insurance Portability and Accountability Act (HIPAA) in the United States, which sets standards for protecting medical information [15].

4.2 Integration of Blockchains

Confidentiality and privacy appear to be the major hurdle in extending the mental healthcare services to individuals and populations. In addition to the appropriate legislation in place, the computing technology of blockchain has also been integrated with healthcare solutions to ensure immutability, traceability, transparency, security, and fault tolerance. Blockchain is based on distributed ledger, where central ledger is maintained by a trusted entity and distributed ledger is shared, replicated, and synchronized among multiple locations. Blockchain will not only ensure security, but at the same time, it will also help to maintain standardization of information across the healthcare network, which will in turn improve the accessibility of information.

As previously discussed, advancing computing and communication technologies aim at facilitating interaction between numerous healthcare stakeholders; this shall be realized by deploying secured blockchains. Since blockchain holds the inherent property of tracing the information throughout the network, only trusted entities will be allowed to update/edit the entries. The confidentiality of patients shall be guaranteed and the payment system will also become secured. Therefore, the risk of breaches will be minimized by using effective blockchain infrastructures for mental healthcare platforms. The integration of blockchain with the healthcare sector is still in infancy, and there are technical and regulatory challenges that must be overcome before its full potential can be realized.

4.3 *Enhanced Use of Big Data*

In future, the big data techniques are expected to be used to support large scale clinical trials and other research initiatives. Big data can provide detailed insight into the population disease patterns and treatment outcomes. Thus, based on the population information, big data techniques shall be used for identifying the best participants for any clinical trials; this will reduce the time and cost involved in conducting a trial. The design of clinical trials may be efficiently guided by big data analytics techniques, which shall increase the success of trials. The predictive analytics shall also be served by big data techniques for developing trials as well as treatment strategies.

The conventional electronic health records will be integrated with big data analytics algorithms to perform population health analytics. The worldwide demographics of patients shall guide the states and practitioners to develop predictive and preventive strategies for the most prevailing diseases in each population. For example, the exact mental disorders will be identified for each population, and the risks will be categorized based on parameters such as age, culture, etc. Subsequently, instead of offering generic mental healthcare strategies to the populations, specific therapy targeted at the prevalent mental disease or disorder shall be developed.

4.4 Robotics Process Automation

Robots and automated processes have already pervaded multiple quarters of the new industrial world. One more area where they are going to be prevalent is healthcare 4.0. One of the applications that is emerging and will be very common and affordable in future is the use of automated limbs, like robotic arms and legs, to replace damaged ones in individuals. Gradually, we are witnessing customized solutions for individuals who cannot move their limbs or entire body. For example, just by capturing the movement of the eye, it is possible to bring close an object or perform a particular task, like combing the hair, eating soup with a spoon, etc., through automated systems. The idea is to understand what the patient wants even though the individual cannot speak or move their limbs. As long as, it is possible to capture certain kind of gesture and map those gestures to preferred needs, the preferred action can be executed through automated processes. Another important application is the use of haptic arms in medical procedures. Smaller procedures like stitching and sutures after surgery, fitting patches, etc. can be done to utmost precision using a controlled haptic arm, sometimes even better than actual human hand. Even though, till now, actual personal care and nursing is irreplaceable, it is possible in future to have human robots or humanoids understanding our personal needs. Such humanoids can offer care, sympathy, the very needed human touch necessary for healing and overall care-and-cure of individuals.

4.5 Extended Reality

Extended Reality (ER) is a phenomenon that is going to be introduced in many possible quarters of life. It is a vision of what present reality may look like when extended to another space, verse, and time. It is a kind of a vision of the future and can be really helpful when dealing with psychological ailments. ER can assist in certain situation of clinical depression and stress in order to alleviate anxiety level. For example, a patient who is feeling traumatized in his/her current scenario that is conducive to his/her mood. Collecting extensive data on a patient, what makes the individual feel safe and complacent, it is possible to create a vision of that world. The patient in an elevated state of anxiety can actually feel safe, secure, and calm in the formulated appropriate vision of reality. ER in conjunction with AR/VR can create a vision of the alternate universe which can be used in other applications too, like gaming, metaverse, etc.

4.6 Customized Patient Experience

Customized patient experience is another application that can be unleashed through healthcare 4.0. By analysing data on both physiological and psychological parameters of a patient and applying different forms of learning and transfer learning algorithms, it will be possible to formulate customized care procedure for individual patients. A very promising example is the application of automated music therapy for treating anxiety and depression. Depending on the personal liking of the patient, list of music that helps individuals calm down, concentrate, it is possible to create a list of customized music for individual patients. If the patient is suffering from an anxiety attack, then the custom list of music can be played on the preferred choice of the individual's handheld device. This will be able to bring down the anxiety level of the patient under control. This kind of customized experience may not be able to provide ultimate solution in case of an emergency condition; but can scale down level of stress/depression and provide enough time for the actual care procedure to be implemented.

4.7 Digital Twins

Digital twins, in future, is going to offer a wonderful way of creating a digital clone of any physical entity or system. Digital twins are going to also offer emulator platform for an entire data, communication, or energy networks. With digital twins, therefore, it will be possible to monitor any system, any network in real time. Depending on the scenario, it will be possible to monitor any system, any network in real time. Depending on the scenario, it will be possible to analyse real-time signals, data, and information and then predict any impending actionable situation. It is also possible to probe the digital twin with a real signal and monitor how that will flow through a system or a network. Based on the observables, it will be possible to optimize system and network design and obtain preferable outcomes. Digital twins in healthcare 4.0 will be in the form of twin of the tele medicine platform and the monitoring dashboard with which it will be possible to monitor multiple patients/individuals cover a wide geographical area. Any patient about to suffer an impending condition can be intercepted and emergency help can arrive right on time.

4.8 Network Strategies

While so many promising applications are coming up, the possibility of cyber-discrepancies is also growing manifold. The most important feature in all applications of healthcare 4.0 is the personal data (physiological, psychological, environmental). Whether it is personalized or custom care procedure, or use of autonomous systems, robotic arms, haptic arms, it is important to use, learn, and analyse personal data gathered from individuals over a certain period of time. Sharing sensitive, personal data over the network, can be intrusive in certain cases and vulnerable to encroachment and breach of privacy. Especially, health-related data can be sensitive and very personal to a particular individual. Therefore, it is paramount to consider privacy and encryption aspects when formulating and designing network data learning and sharing strategies and protocols. Cybersecurity and data privacy are broad areas of research in itself and are beyond the scope in this short chapter.

5 Summary

The healthcare 4.0 technologies are expected to transform the healthcare delivery by providing a detailed picture of patient health. The major goal of these technologies is to enable healthcare providers to make informed and timely decisions about diagnosis and treatment strategies. At the same time, the access to mental healthcare services is expected to become more available and accessible via use of advanced computational technologies. In short, the healthcare 4.0 technologies have a potential to improve the quality and efficiency of mental healthcare delivery by providing mental healthcare providers with more accurate and actionable information about their patients.

References

1. Pavitra AR, Lawrence ID, Maheswari PU. To identify the accessibility and performance of smart healthcare systems in IoT-based environments. In: Using multimedia systems, tools, and technologies for smart healthcare services. 2023. pp. 229–245.
2. Awotunde JB, Jimoh RG, Oladipo ID, Bhoi AK. Internet of medical things for enhanced smart healthcare systems. In: Implementation of smart healthcare systems using AI, IoT, and blockchain. 2023.
3. Abbasi OH, Horowitz CD, Dauer G. Mental health stigma. In: Cases on diversity, equity, and inclusion for the health professions educator. 2023.
4. Ilangakoon TS, Weerabahu SK, Samaranayake P, Wickramarachchi R. Adoption of industry 4.0 and lean concepts in hospitals for healthcare operational performance improvement. Int J Product Perform Manag. 2022;71:2188–213.
5. Wu Z, Xuan S, Xie J, Lin C, Lu., C. How to ensure the confidentiality of electronic medical records on the cloud: a technical perspective. Comput Biol Med. 2022;147:105726.
6. Gyrard A, Boudaoud K. Interdisciplinary IoT and emotion knowledge graph-based recommendation system to boost mental health. Appl Sci. 2022;12:9712.
7. Wiebe A, Kannen K, Selaskowski B, Mehren A, Thöne A-K, Pramme L, Blumenthal N. Virtual reality in the diagnostic and therapy for mental disorders: a systematic review. Clin Psychol Rev. 2022;98:102213.
8. Rubeis G. iHealth: the ethics of artificial intelligence and big data in mental healthcare, vol. 28. Internet Interv; 2022. p. 100518.

9. Wick EC, Pierce L, Conte MC, Sosa., J. A. Operationalizing the operating room: ensuring appropriate surgical care in the era of COVID-19. Ann Surg. 2020;272:e165.
10. Thorlund K, Dron L, Park J, Hsu G, Forrest JI, Mills EJ. A real-time dashboard of clinical trials for COVID-19. Lancet Digital Health. 2020;2:e286.
11. Reeves JJ, Hollandsworth HM, Torriani FJ, Taplitz R, Abeles S, Tai-Seale M, et al. Rapid response to COVID-19: health informatics support for outbreak management in an academic health system. J Am Med Inform Assoc. 2020;27:853–9.
12. Gao S, Rao J, Kang Y, Liang Y, Kruse J. Mapping county-level mobility pattern changes in the United States in response to COVID-19. SIGSpatial Special. 2020.
13. Dixit RA, Hurst S, Adams KT, Boxley C, Lysen-Hendershot K, Bennett SS, et al. Rapid development of visualization dashboards to enhance situation awareness of COVID-19 telehealth initiatives at a multihospital healthcare system. J Am Med Inform Assoc. 2020;27:1456–61.
14. Ho D, Quake SR, McCabe ER, Chng WJ, Chow EK, Ding X, Gelb BD. Enabling technologies for personalized and precision medicine. Trends Biotechnol. 2020;38:497–518.
15. Hireche R, Mansouri H, Pathan. A-SK. Security and privacy management in internet of medical things (IoMT): a synthesis. J Cybersecurity Privacy. 2022;2:640–61.

Student's Stress Detection in Online Learning During the Outbreak

Kalpana Katiyar, Hera Fatma, and Simran Singh

Abstract The epidemic changed people's lifestyles via restrictive measures, affecting their quality of life and overall health. This study sought to examine the psychological effects of students' embrace of e-learning and their fear of the COVID-19 epidemic. The research was presented in two research applications: a quick overview of the psychological consequences of the pandemic on undergraduate students' emotional dimensions and an observational study of the impact of e-learning adoption in pandemic emergencies were switched right away to a comprehensive E-learning programme. Learning through the use of technologies for information and communication is referred to as e-learning (ICTs). The methods of instruction and learning have changed as a result of the integration of technology resources and cutting-edge educational methodologies. Earlier research has demonstrated that a variety of e-learning and web-based learning technologies, including dental emergency, are useful for educational purposes in the disciplines of health profession.

The COVID-19 epidemic has significantly impacted schooling and has emerged as a worldwide health concern. Consequently, learning techniques were offered via remote learning halfway through into the second semester year 2019/2020. (DL). We sought to assess undergraduate students' perceptions of DL in comparison to classroom learning (CL). In this paper, we aim at analyzing stress of students due to online education during the pandemic.

Keywords Online learning · SWOT · DASS-21

Supplementary Information The online version contains supplementary material available at https://doi.org/10.1007/978-981-99-6637-0_16.

K. Katiyar (✉) · H. Fatma · S. Singh
Department of Biotechnology, Dr. Ambedkar Institute of Technology for Handicapped, Kanpur, Uttar Pradesh, India
e-mail: kalpna@aith.ac.in

G. Battineni et al. (eds.), *Computational Methods in Psychiatry*,
https://doi.org/10.1007/978-981-99-6637-0_16

1 Introduction

The World Health Organization (WHO) announced a pandemic in March 2020 [1]. From an asymptomatic state to severe respiratory distress syndrome and multi-organ failure, COVID-19's clinical characteristics are diverse. Significant obstacles have to be overcome in order to stop the infection's spread and protect global health security as a result of COVID-19 [2]. Many nations enacted a variety of anti-epidemic measures due to the coronavirus's quick spread, including physical separation, face mask use, quarantine, and lockdown limitations to prevent contact with others and control transmission. Additionally, the COVID-19 outbreak had an impact on both physical and emotional health and well-being [3]. The entire population has been badly impacted by the COVID-19 epidemic. Even young people are not immune to the changes brought on by this unique circumstance [4]. Massive e-learning adoption was the safeguard implemented in academic programmes to sustain the educational demands of youngsters even in lockdown constraints. Numerous research examined how the pandemic affected young people's mental health, particularly students, in terms of social exclusion and punitive actions.

E-learning refers to learning via the internet, providing learners with a flexible and personalized platform to learn. It can be referred to be an innovative approach for an excellent provision of educational services to the learners through electronic information, aiming for continuous enhancement of their knowledge, skills, and other outcomes [5]. It offers learning-on-demand possibilities and minimizes the learning cost [6]. E-learning is the evolution of distance and remote education—a learning situation where the instructor and learner are separated by distance, time, or both. Recorded lectures by the instructors on online video streaming portals such as YouTube or on other websites are very popular among the students, especially to the ones who are learning through online education [7].

The rapid expansion of COVID-19 prompted the closure of educational institutions everywhere, leading to a shift in the teaching approach to a virtual one where students could complete their coursework at home. In addition to the prolonged confinement, the challenges posed by the switch from a face-to-face education system to a virtual one, and the mobility restriction imposed in quarantine can be stressful factors. Insufficient explanation by the teacher, and lack of materials and tools such as a computer, internet, among others. Not to mention, every student is responsible for his educational process [8]. By aiding patients in developing skills in the control and confrontation of events or circumstances viewed as stressful, early diagnosis of mental stress could help patients avoid health issues. Additionally, it significantly improves quality of life by enabling emotional responses that are aggressive toward everyday circumstances while receiving support and monitoring of professionals [9].

2 Side Effect of Online Learning

Television-based learning has been utilized in primary and secondary education to keep students' knowledge up to date while they wait to return to class. When it comes to higher education, E-learning is utilized as much as is practical in formal university courses. While previously only allowing 30% of the training programme, the Ministry of Education and Training began recognizing all outcomes of online teaching and learning by higher education institutions on March 23, 2020. High expectations and bad learning and training habits mix with the immediate switch from traditional classrooms to online learning in higher education, which can be detrimental to students' mental health [10]. Additionally, the academic setting of the COVID-19 pandemic may worsen kids' mental health. The high expectations for academic success have produced a high level of stress, which if left untreated, can be harmful to their mental health, according to earlier studies [11] found that Turkish university students experienced higher levels of depression, anxiety, and stress at levels of moderate severity or above, at 27%, 47%, and 27%, respectively. Because they have a harder time adjusting to a new situation than seniors, junior pupils react to stress more strongly than seniors [8]. Numerous studies have found that female students experience higher levels of stress, anxiety, and depression [12]. When compared to students from an urban background, university students from rural areas were found to have higher levels of stress, anxiety, and depression. Financial difficulties that can worsen depression, worry, and stress can be the cause of this [13]. We therefore use these factors to explain the sadness, anxiety, and stress experienced by Vietnamese university students participating in online learning. As far as the researchers are aware, there is currently no evidence available on the mental health of university students in Vietnam who experience an instantaneous psychological response in an e-learning environment within the context of COVID-19.

3 Methods

3.1 Sampling Procedures and Participants

Between January and February 2020, this study was conducted. Participants in the study were first, second, third, and final year of undergraduate engineering students at Dr. Ambedkar Institute of Technology for Handicapped, Kanpur. The survey was conducted through google form in which 301 students participated. On the conclusion of the semester, an online survey was administered (Supplementary Table 1).

Table 1 General information of study participants ($n = 301$)

Variable	*N* (%)	Mean preference score (SD)	*P* value
Year of study			0.001*
Class of 2017	90 (29.9%)	18.5 ± 5.7	
Class of 2018	97 (32.2%)	205 ± 6.1	
Class of 2019	114 (37.9%)	21.7 ± 5.5	
Gender			0.784**
Male	14.9%	20.4 ± 6.3	
Female	85.1%	20.3 ± 5.8	
GPA			0.393***
<3.5	121 (40.2%)	20.7 ± 5.6	
>3.51	180 (59.8%)	20.1 ± 6.0	

Although they were actively urged to complete the survey, their participation remained voluntarily. The study participants' names and other private information were kept private. The study was approved by the Faculty of Biotechnology, Dr. Ambedkar Institute of Technology for Handicapped, Kanpur. Students received information on the study and provided consent form.

3.2 *Statistical Analysis*

Cronbach's alpha was used to gauge the internal consistency reliability and questionnaire's reliability. Bivariate analyses were carried out, descriptive statistics were produced in order to determine the variables connected to the students' choice for remote learning, and logistic regression analyses were carried out. The statistical significance level was set at 0.05.

3.3 *Questionnaire*

The questionnaire was evolved to judge the student's perceptivity on the distance learning method. With the exception of questions about the best methods for distance learning (which have six options for the format of online learning) and open-ended inquiries about the difficulties and rewarding experiences of distance learning, the response options for the questionnaire items represent four Likert-type scales (0 = strongly disagree to 3 = strongly agree).

There were 22 statements total, divided into 4 parts: A broad description of the student's gender, academic year, and GPA; B their preferences; C their effectiveness; and D their level of learning satisfaction as shown in Table 1 and Fig. 1.

Statements	Likely score				
	Strongly Disagree	Disagree	Agree	Strongly Agree	Domain Mean Preference ± SD
A. Preference Domain					**1.89 ± 0.58**
1.Clarification sessions is more suitable in distant learning	1.33%	23.59%	53.49%	21.59%	
2. Assessment is more suitable delivered in distant learning	1.66%	28.24%	55.48%	14.62%	
B. Effectiveness Domain					**1.84 ± 0.56**
3. I don't experience any problem during distant learning	11.63%	54.15%	28.24%	5.98%	
4. I don't experience any stress during distant learning	5.98%	29.24%	45.18%	19.60%	
5. I have more time to prepare learning materials before group discussion with distant learning	2.66%	9.63%	57.48%	30.23%	
6. I have more time to review all the learning materials after class with distant learning	2.33%	10.63%	59.14%	27.90%	
C. Learning Satisfaction Domain					**1.53 ± 0.59**
7. Distant learning gives similar learning satisfaction than classroom learning	10.30%	51.49%	33.89%	4.32%	
8. Distant learning can be implemented in the next semester	4.65%	30.56%	52.49%	12.30%	
9. Distant learning gives motivation for self-directed learning and eager to prepare learning materials before group discussion	5.65%	32.56%	47.51%	14.28%	
10. Communication with lecturers and fellow students is easier with distant learning	6.31%	53.49%	30.23%	9.97%	
11. I like distant learning than classroom learning	10.30%	45.51%	34.22%	9.97%	
12. I study more efficiently with distant learning	6.64%	41.20%	39.53%	12.63%	

Fig. 1 Percentage of student agreement with online learning

4 Impact of "e-Learning Crack-Up" Perception on Psychological Distress Among College Students During COVID-19 Pandemic: A Mediating Role of "Fear of Academic Year Loss"

The COVID-19 virus, often referred to as SARS-CoV-2 or COVID-19, was initially discovered in Wuhan, China, in late December 2019 [14], and it afterwards spread to more than 200 other nations. On March 11, 2020, the World Health Organization (WHO) swiftly declared the situation to be a global pandemic. 11,125,245 confirmed cases across the globe as of July 5, 2020, with 203,836 new cases and a total of 528,204 fatalities reported. Public health, particularly mental health, is now at risk because COVID-19 has been labeled a global pandemic. The national governments compelled millions of citizens, including researchers, academics, businesspeople, and students, to isolate themselves or implement a full or partial lockdown worldwide in order to keep safe [15]. The classroom has had limited physical access as a result of the prolonged lockout. A total of 1.5 billion pupils who are enrolled in schools and universities have been affected by closures of institutions due to the COVID-19 pandemic. Children and young people are most affected when educational institutions close [9]. In this historic period, online courses are in high demand as a substitute to institution closure. However, a prior study revealed that students' anxiety is related to their lack of interest in the classroom [4]. An online meta-analysis found that e-Learning is (on average) comparable to conventional training and that it is better than nothing. Additionally, a study by, which included 7143 college students as participants, discovered that 25% of students were experiencing acute anxiety as a result of the e-Learning crack-up. According to another study, almost 83% of students are in the worst possible position, and 26% of students are unable to obtain mental health support. Due to the poor view of the e-Learning system, this condition gives a situational requirement to evaluate psychological discomfort among college students. However, there hasn't been any extensive research done on psychological anguish as a result of college students' unfavorable perceptions of e-Learning during this epidemic. Therefore, the primary goal of this study is to evaluate how psychological suffering among college students during in the COVID-19 pandemic is affected by the perception of "e-Learning crack-up."

5 Online Education Evaluation of College Students Through SWOT Analysis During COVID-19

The COVID-19 outbreak has interfered with university teaching and learning as usual, which presents serious difficulties for college education. Online (distance) learning has replaced the conventional face-to-face learning style, which has a variety of effects on students' academic achievement. It is crucial to look into and advance online learning in the framework of COVID-19 since higher education is essential for the advancement of society and technology. In order to evaluate online education, the SWOT analysis was used to develop 16 different internal and external assessment elements as well as 4 different improvement plans. The questionnaire survey provides the fundamental information for the subjective weight method (AHP), and the findings of the questionnaire survey are used to calculate the weight value of the SWOT components. For its successful implementation, the best possible methods are chosen using the fuzzy MARCOS technique. In the post-pandemic period, several coping mechanisms are proposed to enhance online education, which is crucial for higher learning and the advancement of a civilized and sustainable society [16].

5.1 SWOT Analysis

SWOT analysis can be used to evaluate the effectiveness of online education for college students during the COVID-19 pandemic. Here is an example of how SWOT analysis can be applied:

- Strengths: These are the internal factors that contribute to the success of online education for college students during the pandemic. Some of the strengths associated with online education during the pandemic could include increased flexibility in scheduling, reduced commuting time and expenses, access to online resources, and the ability to participate in classes from anywhere.
- Weaknesses: These are the internal factors that hinder the effectiveness of online education for college students during the pandemic. Some of the weaknesses associated with online education during the pandemic could include a lack of face-to-face interaction, difficulty in staying motivated, limited access to hands-on training, and a lack of opportunities for networking and socializing.
- Opportunities: These are the external factors that can be leveraged to improve the effectiveness of online education for college students during the pandemic. Some of the opportunities associated with online education during the pandemic could include the development of new digital tools and technologies, the availability of online resources, and the potential for greater collaboration and partnerships between institutions and organizations.
- Threats: These are the external factors that pose a challenge to the effectiveness of online education for college students during the pandemic. Some of the threats associated with online education during the pandemic could include the potential for technological challenges and glitches, limited access to high-speed internet and digital devices, and the potential for distractions and disruptions in a home learning environment.

By conducting a SWOT analysis of online education for college students during the pandemic, educational institutions can identify the strengths, weaknesses, opportunities, and threats associated with online learning. This information can be used to develop more effective strategies to support students, improve the quality of online education, and address the challenges and limitations associated with remote learning.

An effective strategic analytical method for determining an organization's strengths and weaknesses as well as prospective opportunities and threats is the SWOT analysis. The SWOT analysis technique cannot, however, assess the relative significance of the various aspects objectively or scientifically, nor can it statistically examine the components. Based on its dimensions and components, such as strength-opportunity (SO), weakness-opportunity (WO), a SWOT matrix can also incorporate different methods [16].

5.2 *The Marcos Method*

A ground-breaking MCDM technique created by Stevi'c et al. [17]. Measurement Alternatives and Ranking According to Compromise Solution (MARCOS) assigns utility scores to both alternatives after evaluating a number of selection criteria based on ideal and non-perfect solutions using the just-proposed MARCOS method. The MARCOS technique is built on specifying how alternatives and reference values relate to one another (ideal and anti-ideal alternatives). The value functions of alternatives are established based on the stated relationships, and compromise rankings with respect to ideal and anti-ideal solutions are created. Utility functions are used to define decision preferences [17] which has been merged with the AHP technique in the references, is more flexible than other approaches since it can examine expert preferences without taking scale into account. Despite the wide range of standard and alternative, it is nevertheless stable. They illustrated the benefits of the MARCOS methodology in comparison to conventional multi-criteria techniques: Comparison of the Multi-Attributive Border Approximation area (MABAC).

5.3 *The AHP Method*

As part of a more comprehensive assessment study, American operations research experts in the 1970s supported AHP as a well-liked MCDM technique [18]. Planning for the environment and natural resources may be done very well using it. This strategy requires far less quantitative data while being useful and simple to use. The SWOT model must be put into a hierarchical structure utilizing the AHP technique in order to measure its usefulness. The AHP technique is therefore entirely suitable for our inquiry [18].

6 Electronic Devices for Stress Detection in Academic Contexts During Confinement Because of the COVID-19 Pandemic

Stress is viewed as a physiological response in which many defensive systems interact when confronted with a scenario or an impending threat that prompts the body to fight or flee [19]. By aiding patients in developing skills in the control and confrontation of circumstances or events viewed as stressful, early recognition of psychological stress can avert health issues. Additionally, it contributes significantly to improving quality of life by enabling emotional responses that are forceful against everyday circumstances under the guidance and supervision of trained experts [20].

The COVID-19 pandemic has had a significant impact on the academic community, with many individuals experiencing high levels of stress and anxiety due to the changes in their daily routines and increased academic pressures. Electronic devices can be useful for stress detection and management in academic contexts during confinement. Here are some possible options:

- Wearable devices: There are a number of wearable devices on the market that can track biometric data such as heart rate, breathing rate, and skin conductance. These can be useful for detecting and monitoring stress levels over time.
- Mobile apps: There are several mobile apps that can be used to track stress levels and provide tools for stress management. Examples include Headspace, Calm, and Pacifica.
- Smartwatches: Smartwatches can be used to track physical activity, heart rate, and sleep patterns. These can be useful for detecting patterns of activity and rest that can contribute to stress.
- Biofeedback devices: Biofeedback devices such as the HeartMath emWave can provide real-time feedback on heart rate variability, which is a measure of stress levels. This can be useful for developing relaxation techniques and managing stress.
- Virtual reality: Virtual reality technology can be used to create immersive environments that can promote relaxation and reduce stress. There are a number of virtual reality apps and devices available that can be used for this purpose.

Overall, electronic devices can be useful for stress detection and management in academic contexts during confinement. However, it's important to remember that these devices are not a substitute for professional medical advice and treatment. If you are experiencing significant stress or anxiety, it's important to seek help from a qualified healthcare provider.

6.1 Liner Discriminant Analysis (LDA)

Linear discriminant analysis (LDA) is a statistical method used for classification of data into two or more classes. It is a supervised learning method, which means that it requires labeled data to learn the class boundaries. LDA aims to find a linear combination of features that best separates the different classes in the data. The goal is to project the data onto a lower-dimensional space while preserving the class separation as much as possible. This is achieved by finding the directions in the data that maximize the between-class variance while minimizing the within-class variance. The resulting linear discriminants can then be used to classify new observations based on their feature values.

LDA has several advantages over other classification methods, such as its ability to handle high-dimensional data and its ability to perform well even when the assumptions of normality and equal covariance matrices are not met. However, LDA assumes that the data is normally distributed and that the covariance matrices of the classes are equal, which may not always be the case in practice. LDA has many practical applications in various fields, such as image recognition, face recognition, and medical diagnosis [12].

6.2 SVM

Support Vector Machine (SVM) is a popular machine learning algorithm used for classification and regression analysis. SVMs work by finding a hyperplane in a high-dimensional space that can best separate data into different classes. The hyperplane is chosen such that it maximizes the margin, which is the distance between the hyperplane and the nearest points from each class. In the case of a binary classification problem, the SVM tries to find a hyperplane that separates the two classes with the largest margin possible. If the data is not linearly separable, SVM uses a kernel function to transform the data into a higher dimensional space where it can be linearly separable. Commonly used kernel functions include linear, polynomial, and radial basis function (RBF) kernels.

In addition to classification, SVM can also be used for regression analysis by finding a hyperplane that fits the data as closely as possible while still satisfying a certain tolerance level. This is called support vector regression [19]. SVM has several advantages, including the ability to handle high-dimensional data, the ability to handle non-linearly separable data through kernel functions, and the ability to find the optimal hyperplane that maximizes the margin. However, SVM can be computationally expensive, especially for large datasets, and it can be sensitive to the choice of kernel function and parameters. SVM has many practical applications in various fields, such as image classification, bioinformatics, and finance.

6.3 SISCO Inventory

SISCO stands for the "Stock Inventory Sales and Control System." It is a computerized system used for managing inventory and sales in retail businesses. The system is designed to automate the inventory tracking and management process, including purchasing, receiving, pricing, and selling of products.

SISCO inventory system typically includes several features such as:

- Inventory management: It helps to track the inventory levels, monitor product movement, set reorder levels, and generate reports for managing inventory.
- Sales management: It helps to track the sales made, generate invoices, manage customers, and monitor sales performance.
- Purchase management: It helps to track the purchase orders, manage suppliers, receive goods, and monitor the procurement process.
- Pricing and discounts: It helps to set prices for products and apply discounts based on various criteria, such as quantity or customer type.
- Reports and analytics: It provides various reports and analytics on inventory levels, sales trends, profit margins, and other key performance indicators.

SISCO inventory system can help businesses to streamline their inventory and sales management processes, reduce manual errors, and improve overall efficiency. The system can also provide real-time visibility into inventory levels and sales performance, which can help businesses to make data-driven decisions and improve profitability.

6.4 Electronic Nose

An electronic nose, also known as an e-nose, is a device that is designed to detect and identify odors or volatile compounds. It is inspired by the human sense of smell and uses a combination of sensors, signal processing algorithms, and machine learning techniques to analyze and classify odors. An e-nose typically consists of a sensor array that is composed of various chemical sensors, such as metal oxide sensors, conducting polymers, and quartz crystal microbalances. Each sensor in the array is sensitive to different types of volatile compounds, and when exposed to an odor, it generates an electrical signal that is proportional to the concentration of the compound.

The electrical signals generated by the sensor array are then processed using signal processing algorithms, such as principal component analysis (PCA) or artificial neural networks (ANN), to extract features and classify the odor. Machine learning techniques are often used to train the e-nose to recognize specific odors or to distinguish between different odors. E-noses have many practical applications, such as in the food and beverage industry for quality control, in the medical industry for disease diagnosis, and in environmental monitoring for detecting pollutants.

They can also be used for detecting explosives and other dangerous substances, as well as for detecting spoilage in food and other perishable items. E-noses have several advantages over traditional chemical analysis methods, including their ability to quickly detect and identify multiple volatile compounds simultaneously, their low cost and portability, and their ability to perform non-invasive and real-time analysis. However, e-noses also have some limitations, such as their limited sensitivity and selectivity compared to traditional analytical methods.

7 Result

The study included 301 dental undergraduates first-, second-, and third-year students from Universitas Indonesia's School of Dentistry. 84.3% of respondents responded. Eighty-five percent of the subjects were women, which is representative of the majority of our graduate dentistry students (Table 1). The questionnaire's Cronbach alpha was 0.880. Each domain's Cronbach's alpha coefficient was over 0.8, which was regarded as excellent.

The overall mean preference score, which ranged from 2 to 36, was 20.3 5.9. The majority of students (75.1%) believed that classroom learning interactions are essential for group discussions. The academic year had an impact on how students felt about distant learning. When compared to their seniors, first-year students choose distant learning more (p 0.001). Students' preferred learning techniques were not significantly correlated with their genders or grade point average (GPA). When it came to group discussions and explanation sessions, the majority of students (87.4%) favored synchronized learning sessions. Also, 58.8% of students expressed their worry about the results of the online tests because of possible student dishonesty.

Although there were still technological limitations when using distant learning, students thought that they had more learning time. Just 34.2% of students reported no issues with distant learning. The bulk of the issues with distant learning were classified as external reasons, such as an inconsistent internet connection and an additional financial load for internet quota, according to data from open inquiries about the obstacles. Additional issues stemming from internal causes were time management, difficulty focusing when using a computer for extended periods of time, and student preparation for the new learning approach (Fig. 1). These difficulties might be a factor in the stress that 35.2% of students experience during distant learning.

8 Conclusion

The study provided proof that, despite certain difficulties, undergraduate dentistry students could adjust to the new teaching techniques of remote learning and that, on average, distant learning was more effective than classroom instruction. Even if it is unwelcome, the abrupt shutdown of universities throughout the globe due to the COVID-19 epidemic offers a huge window of opportunity for cultural change in the educational system. Dental educators must include blended learning into the curriculum in order to develop the best elements of in-person and online learning in order to enhance the learning environment as more "tech-savvy" generations enroll in higher education [5].

References

1. Amir LR, Tanti I, Maharani DA, Wimardhani YS, Julia V, Sulijaya B, Puspitawati R. Mir-2020. pdf. BMC Med Educ. 2020;20(392):1–6.
2. Quinn B, Field J, Gorter R, Akota I, Manzanares MC, Paganelli C, Davies J, Dixon J, Gabor G, Amaral Mendes R, Hahn P, Vital S, O'Brien J, Murphy D, Tubert-Jeannin S. COVID-19: the immediate response of European Academic Dental Institutions and future implications for dental education. Eur J Dent Educ. 2020;24(4):811–4. https://doi.org/10.1111/eje.12542.
3. Donkin R, Askew E, Stevenson H. Video feedback and e-learning enhances laboratory skills and engagement in medical laboratory science students. BMC Med Educ. 2019;19(1):1–12. https://doi.org/10.1186/s12909-019-1745-1.
4. Saiz- Manzanares MC, Escobar-Llamazares M-C, Gonzalez AA. Effectiveness of blended learning in nursing education. Int J Environ Res Public Health. 2020;17:1–15.
5. Saxena C, Baber H, Kumar P. Examining the moderating effect of perceived benefits of maintaining social distance on E-learning quality during COVID-19 pandemic. J Educ Technol Syst. 2021;49(4):532–54. https://doi.org/10.1177/0047239520977798.
6. Katiyar K, Kumari P, Srivastava A. Interpretation of biosignals and application in healthcare. In Information and communication technology (ICT) frameworks in telehealth. Springer; 2022. pp. 209–229.
7. Srivastava A, Seth A, Katiyar K. Microrobots and nanorobots in the refinement of modern healthcare practices. In: Robotic technologies in biomedical and healthcare engineering. Boca Raton: CRC Press; 2021. p. 13–37.
8. Katiyar K. AI-based predictive analytics for patients' psychological disorder. In: Predictive analytics of psychological disorders in healthcare: data analytics on psychological disorders. Springer; 2022. pp. 37–53.
9. Zubair M, Yoon C. Multilevel mental stress detection using ultra-short pulse rate variability series. Biomed Signal Process Control. 2020;57:101736. https://doi.org/10.1016/j.bspc.2019.101736.
10. Lan HTQ, Long NT, Van Hanh N. Validation of depression, anxiety and stress scales (Dass-21): immediate psychological responses of students in the e-learning environment. Int J Higher Educ. 2020;9(5):125–33. https://doi.org/10.5430/ijhe.v9n5p125.
11. Katiyar S, Katiyar K. Recent trends towards cognitive science: from robots to humanoids. In: Cognitive computing for human-robot interaction. Elsevier; 2021. pp. 19–49.
12. Rutkowska A, Liska D, Cieślik B, Wrzeciono A, Brod'áni J, Barcalová M, Gurín D, Rutkowski S. Stress levels and mental well-being among Slovak students during e-learning in the covid-19 pandemic. Healthcare (Basel). 2021;9(10):1–10. https://doi.org/10.3390/healthcare9101356.
13. Alqahtani AY, Rajkhan AA. E-learning critical success factors during the covid-19 pandemic: a comprehensive analysis of e-learning managerial perspectives. Educ Sci. 2020;10(9):1–16. https://doi.org/10.3390/educsci10090216.
14. Hasan N, Bao Y. Impact of "e-Learning crack-up" perception on psychological distress among college students during COVID-19 pandemic: a mediating role of "fear of academic year loss". Child Youth Serv Rev. 2020;118(August):105355. https://doi.org/10.1016/j.childyouth.2020.105355.

15. Chandra Y. Online education during COVID-19: perception of academic stress and emotional intelligence coping strategies among college students. Asian Educ Dev Stud. 2021;10(2):229–38. https://doi.org/10.1108/AEDS-05-2020-0097.
16. Wang H, Wu J, Muhedaner M, Maihemuti S. College students online education evaluation through SWOT analysis during COVID-19. IEEE Access. 2022;10(June):88371–85. https://doi.org/10.1109/ACCESS.2022.3198082.
17. Stević Ž, Brković N. A novel integrated FUCOM-MARCOS model for evaluation of human resources in a transport company. Logistics. 2020;4(1):4. https://doi.org/10.3390/logistics4010004.
18. Wu J, Wang H, Yao L, Kang Z, Zhang Q. Comprehensive evaluation of voltage stability based on EW-AHP and fuzzy-TOPSIS. Heliyon. 2019;5(10):e02410. https://doi.org/10.1016/j.heliyon.2019.e02410.
19. Durán-Acevedo CM, Carrillo-Gómez JK, Albarracín-Rojas CA. Electronic devices for stress detection in academic contexts during confinement because of the covid-19 pandemic. Electronics (Switzerland). 2021;10(3):1–23. https://doi.org/10.3390/electronics10030301.
20. Pourmohammadi S, Maleki A. Stress detection using ECG and EMG signals: a comprehensive study. Comput Methods Prog Biomed. 2020;193:105482. https://doi.org/10.1016/j.cmpb.2020.105482.

GPSR Compliance

The European Union's (EU) General Product Safety Regulation (GPSR) is a set of rules that requires consumer products to be safe and our obligations to ensure this.

If you have any concerns about our products, you can contact us on ProductSafety@springernature.com

In case Publisher is established outside the EU, the EU authorized representative is:

Springer Nature Customer Service Center GmbH
Europaplatz 3
69115 Heidelberg, Germany

Batch number: 10726060

Printed by Printforce, the Netherlands